Preservation Rhinoplasty

Editor

SAM P. MOST

FACIAL PLASTIC SURGERY CLINICS OF NORTH AMERICA

www.facialplastic.theclinics.com

Consulting Editor
J. REGAN THOMAS

February 2021 • Volume 29 • Number 1

ELSEVIER

1600 John F. Kennedy Boulevard • Suite 1800 • Philadelphia, Pennsylvania, 19103-2899

http://www.theclinics.com

FACIAL PLASTIC SURGERY CLINICS OF NORTH AMERICA Volume 29, Number 1
February 2021 ISSN 1064-7406, ISBN-13: 978-0-323-75726-3

Editor: Stacy Eastman
Developmental Editor: Julia McKenzie

Facial Plastic Surgery Clinics of North America (ISSN 1064-7406) is published quarterly by Elsevier Inc., 360 Park Avenue South, New York, NY 10010-1710. Months of issue are February, May, August, and November. Business and Editorial Offices: 1600 John F. Kennedy Blvd., Suite 1800, Philadelphia, PA 19103-2899. Periodicals postage paid at New York, NY, and additional mailing offices. Subscription prices are $412.00 per year (US individuals), $895.00 per year (US institutions), $459.00 per year (Canadian individuals), $944.00 per year (Canadian institutions), $546.00 per year (foreign individuals), $944.00 per year (foreign institutions), $100.00 per year (US students), $100.00 per year (Canadian students), and $255.00 per year (foreign students). Foreign air speed delivery is included in all *Clinics* subscription prices. All prices are subject to change without notice. POSTMASTER: Send address changes to *Facial Plastic Surgery Clinics*, Elsevier Health Sciences Division, Subscription Customer Service, 3251 Riverport Lane, Maryland Heights, MO 63043. **Customer service: 1-800-654-2452 (US and Canada); 1-314-447-8871 (outside US and Canada); Fax: 314-447-8029; E-mail: journalscustomerservice-usa@elsevier.com (for print support); journalsonlinesupport-usa@elsevier.com (for online support).**

Reprints. For copies of 100 or more of articles in this publication, please contact the Commercial Reprints Department, Elsevier Inc., 360 Park Avenue South, New York, NY 10010-1710. Tel.: 212-633-3874; Fax: 212-633-3820; E-mail: reprints@elsevier.com.

Facial Plastic Surgery Clinics of North America is covered in *MEDLINE/PubMed* (*Index Medicus*).

Contributors

CONSULTING EDITOR

J. REGAN THOMAS, MD
Professor, Facial Plastic and Reconstructive Surgery, Department of Otolaryngology–Head and Neck Surgery, Northwestern University School of Medicine, Chicago, Illinois, USA

EDITOR

SAM P. MOST, MD
Chief, Division of Facial Plastic and Reconstructive Surgery, Director, Fellowship in Facial Plastic and Reconstructive Surgery, Professor, Departments of Otolaryngology–Head and Neck Surgery and Surgery (Plastic), Stanford University School of Medicine, Stanford, California, USA

AUTHORS

MOHAMED ABDELWAHAB, MD, MS
Research Fellow, Department of Otolaryngology–Head and Neck Surgery, Division of Facial Plastic and Reconstructive Surgery, Stanford University School of Medicine, Stanford, California, USA; Assistant Lecturer, Department of Otolaryngology–Head and Neck Surgery, Division of Facial Plastic and Reconstructive Surgery, Mansoura University, Faculty of Medicine, Dakahlia Governorate, Egypt

ALI MURAT AKKUŞ, MD
Specialist, Plastic, Reconstructive and Aesthetic Surgery

EUGENE B KERN, MD, MS
Professor of Rhinology and Facial Plastic Surgery, Department of Otorhinolaryngology–Head and Neck Surgery, Mayo Clinic, Emeritus, Mayo Clinic Alix School of Medicine, George M. and Edna B. Endicott Professor of Medicine, Mayo Foundation for Medical Education and Research, Rochester, Minnesota, USA; Professor of Otolaryngology University at Buffalo-State University of New York, Director, Gromo Foundation for Medical Education and Research, Buffalo, New York, USA

BARIŞ ÇAKIR, MD
Specialist, Plastic, Reconstructive and Aesthetic Surgery

WILSON DEWES, MD
Otolaryngology and Head and Neck Surgery Specialist, Facial Plastic Surgeon, Facial Plastic Surgery Clinica Dewes, Lajeado, Brazil

CHARLES EAST, MD, FRCS
Consultant Surgeon and Associate Clinical Professor, University College London, Rhinoplasty London, London, United Kingdom

MARIO FERRAZ, MD, IBCFPRS
International Board Certified, Facial Plastic and Reconstructive Surgery IBCFPRS, Otolaryngology and Head and Neck Surgery Specialist, Campinas, Brazil

OREN FRIEDMAN, MD
Director of Facial Plastic Surgery, Associate Professor, Otorhinolaryngology, University of Pennsylvania School of Medicine, Philadelphia, Pennsylvania, USA

JENNIFER C. FULLER, MD
Assistant Professor, Department of Otolaryngology–Head and Neck Surgery, Division of Facial Plastic and Reconstructive Surgery, Loma Linda University, Loma Linda, California, USA

ABDÜLKADIR GÖKSEL, MD
Facial Plastic Surgeon, ENT Facial Plastic Surgery, Rino Istanbul, Istanbul, Turkey

BÜLENT GENÇ, MD
Specialist, Plastic, Reconstructive and Aesthetic Surgery

PETER A. HILGER, MD
Professor, Department of Otolaryngology–Head and Neck Surgery, Division of Facial and Plastic and Reconstructive Surgery, University of Minnesota, Edina, Minnesota, USA

EUGENE B. KERN, MD, MS
Emeritus Professor, Department of Otorhinolaryngology–Head and Neck Surgery, Mayo Clinic, Rochester, Minnesota, USA; Clinical Professor, Department of Otolaryngology, University at Buffalo, State University of New York, Buffalo, New York, USA

AARON M. KOSINS, MD
Clinical Assistant Professor, Plastic Surgery, UC Irvine School of Medicine, Newport Beach, California, USA

MILOS KOVACEVIC, MD
Private Practice, Hamburg, Germany

HEATHER A. LEVITES, MD
Resident, Division of Plastic, Maxillofacial and Oral Surgery, Duke University, Durham, North Carolina, USA

JEFFREY R. MARCUS, MD
Professor and Chief, Division of Plastic, Maxillofacial and Oral Surgery, Duke University, Durham, North Carolina, USA

JOSE JUAN MONTES-BRACCHINI, MD
Private Practice, Cirugia Facial Polanco, Ejercito Nacional, Mexico City, Mexico

SAM P. MOST, MD
Chief, Division of Facial Plastic and Reconstructive Surgery, Director, Fellowship in Facial Plastic and Reconstructive Surgery, Professor, Departments of Otolaryngology–Head and Neck Surgery and Surgery (Plastic), Stanford University School of Medicine, Stanford, California, USA

JOSÉ CARLOS NEVES, MD, EBCFPRS
Board Certified in Facial Plastic and Reconstructive Surgery EBCFPRS, Otolaryngology and Head and Neck Surgery Specialist, MyFace, Clinics and Academy, Lisbon & Coimbra, Portugal

PRIYESH N. PATEL, MD
Assistant Professor, Division of Facial Plastic and Reconstructive Surgery, Department of Otolaryngology–Head and Neck Surgery, Vanderbilt University Medical Center, Nashville, Tennessee, USA

DIEGO ARANCIBIA TAGLE, MD, FEBORL
Fellow of the European Academy of Facial Plastic Surgery, Otolaryngology and Head and Neck Surgery Specialist, Hospital Son Espases, Palma de Mallorca, Spain

ANALISE B. THOMAS, MD
Resident, Division of Plastic, Maxillofacial and Oral Surgery, Duke University, Durham, North Carolina, USA

DEAN M. TORIUMI, MD
Clinical Professor, Department of Otolaryngology–Head and Neck Surgery, Rush University Medical School, Chicago, Illinois, USA

FAUSTO LOPEZ ULLOA, MD
Director of Facial Plastic Surgery, ENT Department, Angeles Lomas Hospital, Mexico City, Mexico

Contents

Foreword: Preservation Rhinoplasty: Revitalization of an Age-Old Technique xi

J. Regan Thomas

Preface: Preservation Rhinoplasty: Revitalization of an Age-Old Technique xiii

Sam P. Most

History of Dorsal Preservation Surgery: Seeking Our Historical Godfather(s) for the "Push Down" and "Let Down" Operations 1

Eugene B. Kern

There are 2 approaches for lowering the osseocartilaginous nasal dorsum. The most frequently used method includes resection of the osseocartilaginous nasal dorsum. The second method is based on preservation of the osseocartilaginous nasal dorsum. The concept of dorsal preservation surgery is to preserve, not resect, the nasal bones and upper lateral cartilage. Reduction rhinoplasty with preservation of the nasal dorsum is not only possible, but results in a natural appearing postoperative dorsal esthetic line. Thus, the rhetorical question: Why reconstruct the nasal dorsum when you can simply preserve it?

Conventional Resection Versus Preservation of the Nasal Dorsum and Ligaments: An Anatomic Perspective and Review of the Literature 15

Mohamed Abdelwahab and Priyesh N. Patel

Preservation rhinoplasty may refer to preserving several anatomic components including: the nasal bones, upper lateral cartilages, the keystone area and/or ligaments of the nose. Preserving the osseocartilaginous framework or "dorsal preservation" minimizes or completely avoids violation of the dorsal aesthetic lines' architecture. Conventional hump reduction in open rhinoplasty disrupts these lines; however, it also provides versatility to reshape the entire dorsum. Surgical success with either technique requires a thorough understanding of the underlying nasal anatomy.

Dorsal Preservation Rhinoplasty: Method and Outcomes of the Modified Subdorsal Strip Method 29

Priyesh N. Patel, Mohamed Abdelwahab, and Sam P. Most

There has been particular recent interest in dorsal preservation rhinoplasty techniques because of claims of superior functional and aesthetic results relative to conventional hump reductions. The septum in dorsal preservation rhinoplasty is managed in a variety of ways with differences largely based on the location of septal excision (subdorsal resection, midseptal resection, and inferior septal resection). The technical considerations of a modified subdorsal strip method using a structural preservation technique are described. This technique maintains a subdorsal and caudal strut of cartilage. Patient-reported measures demonstrate significantly improved functional and aesthetic outcomes postoperatively with this procedure.

Key Points in Subperichondrial-Subperiosteal Dissection 39

Bülent Genç, Ali Murat Akkuş, and Barõş Çakõr

"Subperichondrial-subperiosteal dissection technique (SSDT) decreases soft tissue injury to a minimum by protecting soft tissues from dissection and retraction traumas. The fact remains that dissecting the perichondrium of the nasal tip cartilages is not effortless. Cartilages may be harmed if dissection is not initiated at the right location. The aforementioned surgeons have routinely used the SSDT between the years 2008 and 2019 in more than 4000 rhinoplasties. The number of the surgeons making use of the SSDT will increase with the understanding of the key points in dissection, their ordering, and use of correct instrumentation."

Tip Ligament Preservation and Suspension: Why and How? 47

Jeffrey R. Marcus, Analise B. Thomas, and Heather A. Levites

This issue of Clinics explores the concept of "preservation" rhinoplasty. At present, this topic is gaining considerable attention. As proponents of preservation suggest, a great number of problems we encounter in rhinoplasty are problems that were not present before the surgery; therefore, they can often be attributable to the deconstruction and reconstruction that took place. Preservation rhinoplasty should be viewed generally as a mindset to limit deconstructive steps in rhinoplasty when possible, understanding that these steps and those to later reconstruct provide the potential to create new problems that did not previously exist.

Preservation Rhinoplasty (Let-Down Technique) for Endonasal Dorsal Reduction 59

Jose Juan Montes-Bracchini

Preservation rhinoplasty has been a trending topic in the rhinoplasty literature. There is no single technique that can correct all structures; therefore, patient analysis is paramount. This article focuses on the anatomy of the keystone area and the dynamics of the dorsum explained through the biotensegrity concept. Differences between push-down and let-down techniques are addressed from a nasal valve physiology point of view. The let-down technique maintains the tensegrity of the nasal pyramid. Preservation should be preferred, in most cases, over resection, as well as reposition over manipulation.

Preservation Rhinoplasty: The Endonasal Cottle Push-Down/Let-Down Approach 67

Oren Friedman, Fausto Lopez Ulloa, and Eugene B. Kern

Preservation rhinoplasty is a new term for an old technique. The authors have used the endonasal push-down and let-down techniques that are attributed to Dr Maurice Cottle throughout their careers on select patients with excellent success. The endonasal Cottle technique allows the authors to manage the nasal dorsum in a conservative fashion, reducing the need for routine restructuring of the middle third and nasal dorsum. The details of their approach are presented in this publication.

Piezoelectric Osteotomies in Dorsal Preservation Rhinoplasty 77

Abdülkadir Göksel, Priyesh N. Patel, and Sam P. Most

Dorsal preservation rhinoplasty requires precise management of the osseocartilaginous vault. Ultrasonic piezo instruments offer several advantages compared with traditional tools such as hand saws, rasps, and osteotomes. As always, an understanding of the dynamics of manipulation of the vault, anatomy, and proper technique are paramount and are reviewed herein.

A Segmental Approach in Dorsal Preservation Rhinoplasty: The Tetris Concept 85

José Carlos Neves, Diego Arancibia Tagle, Wilson Dewes, and Mario Ferraz

Video content accompanies this article at http://www.facialplastic.theclinics.com.

Rhinoplasty has become a detail-dependent surgery. With precise techniques better results have been achieved. We are continually searching for the ideal technique to offer predictable, accurate, and desired long-term results. Conservative rhinoplasty techniques have been described for more than 100 years as an alternative to dorsal resective surgeries and have reemerged as the new fashion among rhinoplasty surgeons. This article presents our philosophy when approaching the nasal dorsum regarding its segments and their specific anatomic aspects and surgical demands. We describe our intermediate septal strip approach, the intermediate split and the Tetris concept, and discuss their advantages and limitations.

Incorporating Dorsal Preservation Rhinoplasty into Your Practice 101

Aaron M. Kosins

For rhinoplasty surgeons, surgery of the dorsum has never been so dynamic or as easily learned. Reproducible techniques offer excellent results that can be difficult to achieve in certain patients using component reduction. An expanding repertoire of dorsal preservation (DP) techniques is evolving. Each DP operation builds on the others. To understand DP requires a new appreciation of the cartilaginous septum, the perpendicular plate of ethmoid, nasal osteotomies, and anatomy of the nose where surgeons do not operate with traditional component reduction. The result is more beautiful noses where the normal anatomy is preserved.

Combined Functional and Preservation Rhinoplasty 113

Priyesh N. Patel, Mohamed Abdelwahab, and Sam P. Most

Dorsal preservation rhinoplasty has aesthetic advantages over conventional hump takedown rhinoplasty. In dorsal preservation surgery, the nasal vault is treated en bloc. The internal nasal valve angle is not disrupted and there is no need for midvault reconstruction. Two techniques for management of the bony vault exist in dorsal preservation surgery: the let-down and the push-down techniques. There are a variety of techniques used for management of the septum in dorsal preservation. Available patient-reported outcomes of suggest positive results in nasal breathing. More robust data are needed to clarify the functional results of dorsal preservation and compare breathing outcomes.

Preservation Rhinoplasty and the Crooked Nose 123

Charles East

Crooked or deviated noses pose a specific challenge as many of the elements in a deviated nose are not symmetric and therefore not ideal for preservation techniques. Deviated noses are often where a hybridization between preservation and structural rhinoplasty is required. Careful preoperative evaluation of the soft tissue and bony anatomy of the patient is very important and congenital or post-traumatic asymmetry may involve more than the nasal pyramid. Full exposure of the nasal pyramid allows for visualization and appropriate osteotomy or rhinosculpture.

Modified Skoog Method for Hump Reduction **131**

Jennifer C. Fuller and Peter A. Hilger

Dorsal hump reduction is a key component of rhinoplasty. Spreader grafts are the most frequently used technique; however, dorsal irregularities may result. The modified Skoog method involves removal of the osseocartilaginous dorsal hump, its modification, further reduction of the nasal dorsum, replacement of the modified dorsal segment, and suspension of the upper lateral cartilages. The dorsal segment acts as an onlay spreader graft, preserves the middle vault, closes the open roof deformity, and creates a smooth dorsal contour from radix to anterior septal angle. The modified Skoog method produces optimal functional and aesthetic outcomes in appropriately selected patients.

Dorsal Preservation Rhinoplasty: Measures to Prevent Suboptimal Outcomes **141**

Dean M. Toriumi and Milos Kovacevic

Preservation rhinoplasty is making a resurgence as a reliable method of performing primary rhinoplasty. Dorsal preservation is an important part of the approach to preserve favorable nasal contours when performing rhinoplasty. Keys to success require proper patient selection and careful execution. There are potential sequelae, such saddle nose deformity, recurrence of the dorsal convexity, cerebrospinal fluid leak, and radix step-off. This article discusses methods and adjustments in technique to help minimize these potential problems when performing dorsal preservation.

FACIAL PLASTIC SURGERY CLINICS OF NORTH AMERICA

FORTHCOMING ISSUES

May 2021
Oculoplastic Surgery
Guy Massry and John Bryan Holds, *Editors*

August 2021
Facial Paralysis
Travis Tollefson and Jon-Paul Pepper, *Editors*

November 2021
Facial Plastic Surgery Procedures in the Non-Caucasian Population
Yong Ju Jang, *Editor*

RECENT ISSUES

November 2020
Day-to-Day Challenges in Facial Plastic Surgery
William H. Truswell, *Editor*

August 2020
Facelift Surgical Techniques
Andrew A. Jacono, *Editor*

May 2020
Techniques for Hair Restoration
Lisa E. Ishii and Linda N. Lee, *Editors*

Foreword

Preservation Rhinoplasty: Revitalization of an Age-Old Technique

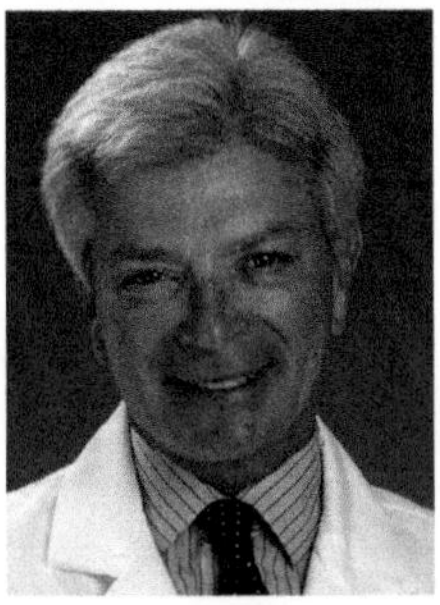

J. Regan Thomas, MD
Consulting Editor

Rhinoplasty historically has been, and perhaps continues to be, the primary procedure associated with Facial Plastic Surgery. Indeed, in many facial plastic surgeon's practices, rhinoplasty is the primary procedure provided and performed. Various techniques, approaches, and surgical philosophies have been utilized and periodically popularized by rhinoplasty surgeons throughout its history. It is understandably a potentially confusing environment at this time to the novice rhinoplasty surgeon, residents and fellows in training, and perhaps many experienced rhinoplasty surgeons. New descriptive procedural terms and titles are now utilized, presented, and published. These include techniques and approaches entitled Push Down, Let Down, Preservation, Precision, as well as others, and are being supported and promoted by surgical colleagues. Discussion of techniques described by now historical names, such as Cottle and Skoog, has been updated and popularized by some surgeons. Others continue to support and maintain resection and reduction techniques, and interestingly, all groups are understandably reinforced with excellent postoperative results. New technology is also discussed frequently and highly recommended by some such as piezoelectric instrumentation.

Dr Most has assembled an outstanding group of experienced authors to discuss and describe their views on these rhinoplasty techniques. There have been perhaps differing preferred and popularized approaches based on geographic location through the years. Now with much more interaction of rhinoplasty colleagues in the international community, an insightful and active discussion of these approaches and techniques is enjoyed and ostensibly of benefit to the specialty at large. The international makeup of this issue's contributing authors is an excellent example of these benefits.

Rhinoplasty, though a frequent and popular surgical procedure, can be a very challenging operation. Understanding and evaluating various approaches and the expertise of others can prove to be very valuable. Rhinoplasty and its techniques have continued to evolve and change and perhaps to recycle in some aspects. This issue of *Facial Plastic Surgery Clinics of North America*, which Dr Most has organized, and with the experience and expertise of the contributing authors, provides valuable insights to our specialty readership. The outstanding group of contributors who have been assembled and their coordinated contributions through this issue add an important and practical reference for our specialty.

J. Regan Thomas, MD
Facial Plastic and Reconstructive Surgery
Department of Otolaryngology–
Head and Neck Surgery
Northwestern University
School of Medicine
60 East Delaware Place
Chicago, IL 60611, USA

E-mail address:
jreganthomas@gmail.com

Facial Plast Surg Clin N Am 29 (2021) xi
https://doi.org/10.1016/j.fsc.2020.09.012
1064-7406/21/© 2020 Published by Elsevier Inc.

Preface

Preservation Rhinoplasty: Revitalization of an Age-Old Technique

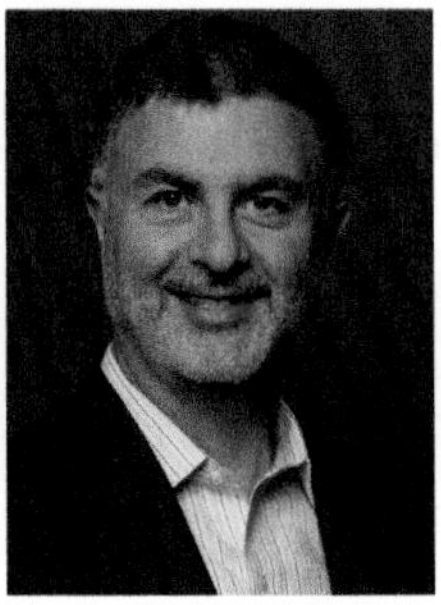

Sam P. Most, MD
Editor

I was first introduced to the concept of dorsal reduction with simultaneous osseocartilaginous vault preservation at the Portland Rhinoplasty Course in the early 2000s. Only a few years out of fellowship, I was stunned by my friends and colleagues Drs Fausto-Lopez Ullua's and Jose-Juan Montes' talks in which they described the "Let-Down" and "Push-Down" rhinoplasty. I had never heard of such methods previously, and I was highly skeptical. Year after year, I heard my friends from Mexico City speak of these methods. Never an early adopter, I chose to continue to practice the methods of external structural rhinoplasty and dorsal resection that I learned from my fellowship mentors, Drs Craig Murakami and Wayne Larrabee, and continued to learn from luminaries such as Drs Dean Toriumi, Rod Rohrich, and Steve Perkins, to name a few.

It turns out the idea that one could preserve rather than resect the nasal dorsum has been around since the late nineteenth century, as so nicely described in Dr Eugene Kern's enclosed article, "History of Dorsal Preservation Surgery: Seeking Our Historical Godfather(s) for the 'Push Down' and 'Let Down'." And while only a few surgeons in the United States have continued to practice this method, Dr Kern included, the technique has been very much alive and well outside of the United States. In particular, surgeons in Brazil, France, Portugal, and Mexico have continued to teach this method.

In the past 5 years, the adoption of ultrasonic piezotomes in rhinoplasty, as championed by Dr Olivier Gerbault in Paris, as well as the revelation that one could combine osseocartilaginous preservation with open structural techniques was demonstrated, opening the door for many more surgeons to try the method. Seminal primary publications on the matter by Daniel, Cakir, Palhazi, Saban, Goksel, and others further elaborated the anatomy and rationale for osseocartilaginous as well as ligamentous preservation. And, of course, the "Preservation Rhinoplasty" textbook and accompanying meetings have allowed many more to learn these techniques.

Herein, we have not tried to duplicate the steps of those before us, but rather to highlight and review important concepts and, it is hoped, introduce these to an even wider audience. These concepts include osseocartilaginous vault approaches, septal approaches, and preservation of ligamentous/cartilaginous structures of the nasal tip. Many of the authors included are those who have published extensively in this area. In this small issue, we could not include all, but many are referenced, and I encourage the reader to see this as a starting point, an introduction, and to seek further knowledge through attending meetings on this topic, attending cadaver dissections, and observing cases prior to trying this on your own.

Furthermore, as is true of much of our work in Facial Plastic Surgery, the levels of evidence of our literature lag behind those of our colleagues in

Facial Plast Surg Clin N Am 29 (2021) xiii–xiv
https://doi.org/10.1016/j.fsc.2020.09.011
1064-7406/21/© 2020 Published by Elsevier Inc.

medicine. In most cases, what you read is expert opinion only, telegraphed via case series. While expert opinion is of course valuable, in the age of evidence-based medicine, it does not allow us to definitively compare methods or outcomes. Studies using quantifiable determinants of outcome, such as validated outcome instruments, rhinomanometry, CT scans, or other methods, will help us answer some of the questions regarding the superiority of nonpreservation or preservation techniques. I hope that younger surgeons reading this will see this as a call to action to do such studies.

Finally, I would like to thank all the contributors who have worked hard to make this issue come together. And a special thank you to Fausto and Jose-Juan, who introduced the "Let-Down" and "Push-Down" methods to me nearly 2 decades ago.

Sam P. Most, MD
Division of Facial Plastic and Reconstructive Surgery
Stanford University School of Medicine
801 Welch Road
Stanford, CA 94304, USA

E-mail address:
smost@stanford.edu

History of Dorsal Preservation Surgery

Seeking Our Historical Godfather(s) for the "Push Down" and "Let Down" Operations

Eugene B. Kern, MD, MS[a,b,c,d,*,1]

KEYWORDS

• Dorsal preservation surgery • "Push down" operation • "Let down" operation • Renaissance
• Preservation rhinoplasty revolution

KEY POINTS

- Dorsal preservation surgery preserves the osseocartilaginous nasal dorsum, allowing reduction rhinoplasty without nasal dorsal (roof) resection; in the Joseph rhinoplasty, the osseocartilaginous nasal dorsum is regularly resected.
- Dorsal preservation surgery first appeared in the American literature over 100 years ago, described by Goodale ("push down" 1899) and Lothrop ("let down" 1914).
- The French contributed to dorsal preservation surgery with Sebileau and Dufourmentel ("let down" 1926) and Maurel ("push down" 1940).
- Fomon (1939) observed that previous surgeons, including Goodale, Lothrop, Eitner, and Dufourmentel were able to "correct the deformity without attacking the hump itself."
- In 2018, Saban, Daniel, Polselli, Trapasso, and Palhazi published a reassessment of the push down technique (320 cases), heralding a reemergence or renaissance (rebirth) of dorsal preservation surgery.

WHY BOTHER READING HISTORY?

History is a living breathing access laboratory, an expedition into the human experience, delivering knowledge; affording evidence of the thoughts, contributions, and achievements of our predecessors; and providing perspective and insight as to our origins and the consequent contemporaneous state.

Today in corrective rhinoplasty, there are primarily 2 distinctive and disparate approaches for lowering the osseocartilaginous nasal dorsum ("hump"). The most frequently used method, described by Jacques Joseph (**Fig. 1**) in 1898 and 1904, includes resection of the osseocartilaginous nasal dorsum.[1] The second method is based on preservation of the osseocartilaginous nasal dorsum and was illuminated, advocated, and

[a] Department of Otorhinolaryngology–Head and Neck Surgery, Mayo Clinic, 200 First Street Southwest, Rochester, MN 55905, USA; [b] Department of Otolaryngology, University at Buffalo-State University of New York, Buffalo, NY, USA; [c] Emeritus, Mayo Clinic Alix School of Medicine, Rochester, MN, USA; [d] Gromo Foundation for Medical Education and Research, Buffalo, NY, USA

[1] Portions of this paper were presented at the Preservation Rhinoplasty meeting in Nice, France, February 2 to 4, 2019.

* Department of Otorhinolaryngology–Head and Neck Surgery, Mayo Clinic, 200 First Street Southwest, Rochester, NY 55905.
E-mail address: ekern@mayo.edu

Facial Plast Surg Clin N Am 29 (2021) 1–14
https://doi.org/10.1016/j.fsc.2020.08.003

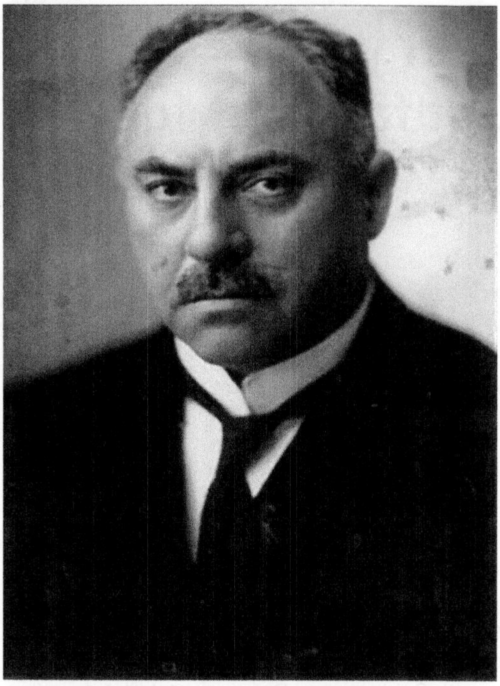

Fig. 1. Dr Jacques Joseph (1865–1934).

taught by Maurice Cottle in 1954 (**Fig. 2**). Cottle labeled the procedure a "push down" operation.[2] His surgical conception was elimination of the dorsal hump, not by resection but rather by downward displacement of the intact osseocartilaginous nasal pyramid with retention (preservation) of the anatomic and physiologic integrity of the nasal roof (vault, or osseocartilaginous nasal dorsum).

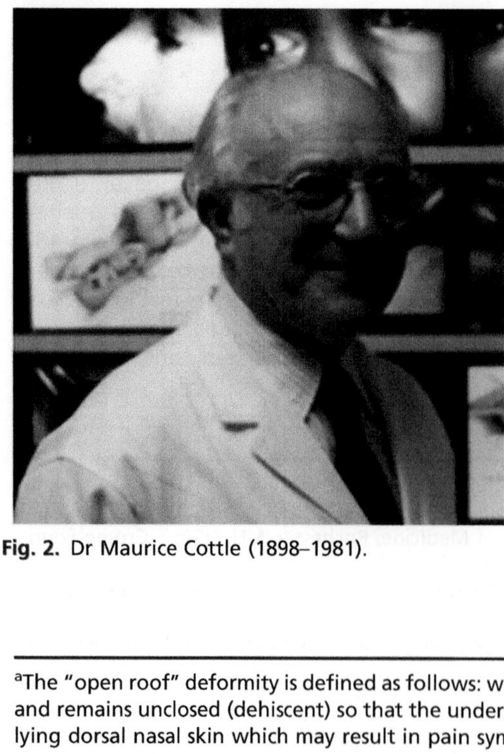

Fig. 2. Dr Maurice Cottle (1898–1981).

WHAT IS DORSAL PRESERVATION SURGERY?

Dorsal preservation surgery preserves both the nasal bones and the upper lateral cartilage, thereby maintaining an intact osseocartilaginous nasal dorsum. Photographs of cadaver dissections in the masterwork text *Rhinoplasty: An Anatomic and Clinical Atlas*, by Rollin Daniel and Peter Palhazi,[3] captures this anatomy beautifully (**Fig. 3**).

WHY DORSAL PRESERVATION SURGERY?

At a 2016 rhinoplasty meeting in Versailles, France, Daniel (**Fig. 4**) suggested that surgeons reconsider the push down operation, alluding to the undesirable consequences of hump resection as practiced in the Joseph rhinoplasty. The Joseph rhinoplasty embraces the "en bloc" removal (resection) of a portion of the nasal bones, along with portions of the upper lateral cartilage and nasal septum, which can result in the following postoperative consequences:

1. Dorsal esthetic irregularities (the "operated look").
2. Neurogenic pain syndromes secondary to an "open roof" deformity.[a]
3. Breathing dysfunction secondary to a narrowed nasal airway, especially in the critical internal nasal valve area.

With dorsal preservation surgery, a term coined by Daniel, it is possible to preserve the osseocartilaginous nasal dorsum, including the "K-area." The K-area refers to the keystone, or bedrock region of the nose, where the distal end of the nasal bones and the cephalic end of the upper lateral cartilage joins the underlying perpendicular plate of the ethmoid and the quadrangular (septal) cartilage.

The result is a more natural postoperative dorsal esthetic line that does not require the obligatory midvault reconstruction with spreader grafts or spreader flaps.[4–6]

TWO METHODS OF DORSAL PRESERVATION SURGERY: THE PUSH DOWN AND LET DOWN

In 2018, Saban and colleagues[7] (**Fig. 5**) published "Dorsal Preservation: The Push Down Technique

[a]The "open roof" deformity is defined as follows: when the nasal dorsum (osseocartilaginous roof) is removed, and remains unclosed (dehiscent) so that the underlying nasal mucosa contacts the under surface of the overlying dorsal nasal skin which may result in pain symptoms.

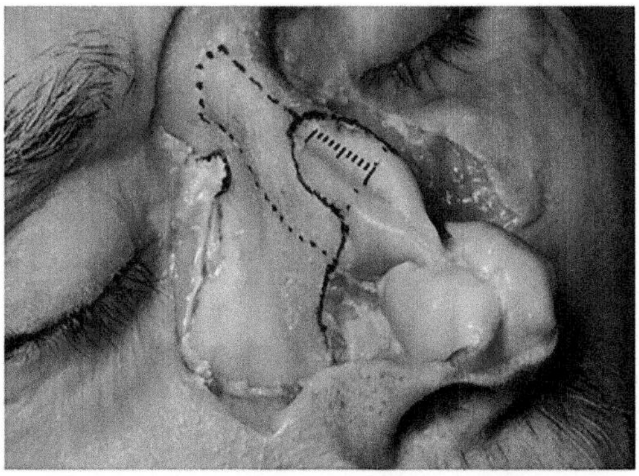

Fig. 3. Photograph of the external nose from Daniel and Palhazi. (*From* Daniel RK and Palhazi P. Rhinoplasty: An Anatomical and Clinical Atlas. Springer, Cham (Switzerland) 2018; 345 p.)

Reassessed," the senior author and surgeon reviewed 740 septo-rhinoplasties performed, over 5 years, in which 320 clinical cases of dorsal preservation surgery occurred. There were 286 females to 34 males. The mean follow-up was 2 years and 5 months (range, 6 months to 5.5 years) amid a revision rate of 3.4% (11/320). Using the endonasal approach, a strip of septal cartilage is removed from the subdorsal region. This step is followed by complete lateral and transverse osteotomies at the radix, thereby achieving a dorsal reduction by either a push down operation or a let down operation. The push down operation consists of downward impaction of the fully mobilized osseocartilaginous nasal dorsum into the pyriform aperture and is used in patients with humps of less than 4 mm (**Fig. 6**). The "let down" entails resection of a "maxillary wedge" from the ascending (frontal) process of the maxilla, along with some septal resection and is implemented in patients requiring more than 4 mm of dorsal reduction (**Fig. 7**). Saban and colleagues[7] clearly presented the difference between these operations:

1. *"Push down"*
   a. Septal phase: strip cartilage excision; after Saban and associates,[7] a high subdorsal resection (excision) of septal cartilage; after Cottle,[2] a low septal resection (excision) of septal cartilage; Cottle's "inferior strip" removal of septal cartilage.
   b. Bone phase: lateral and transverse osteotomies, then the bony and cartilaginous dorsum is depressed downward ("pushed down") into the pyriform aperture.
2. *"Let down"*
   a. Septal phase: strip cartilage excision; after Saban and colleagues,[7] a high subdorsal resection (excision) of septal cartilage; after Cottle,[2] a low septal resection (excision) of septal cartilage; Cottle's "inferior strip" removal of septal cartilage.
   b. Bone phase: resection of a portion maxillary wedge of the ascending (frontal) process of the maxilla followed by transverse osteotomies; next the bony and cartilaginous dorsum is depressed downward (let down) onto the ascending (frontal) process of the maxilla.

SEEKING THE GODFATHER(S) OF DORSAL PRESERVATION SURGERY

A godfather is additionally defined as a pioneer, a person who is influential in a specific movement or

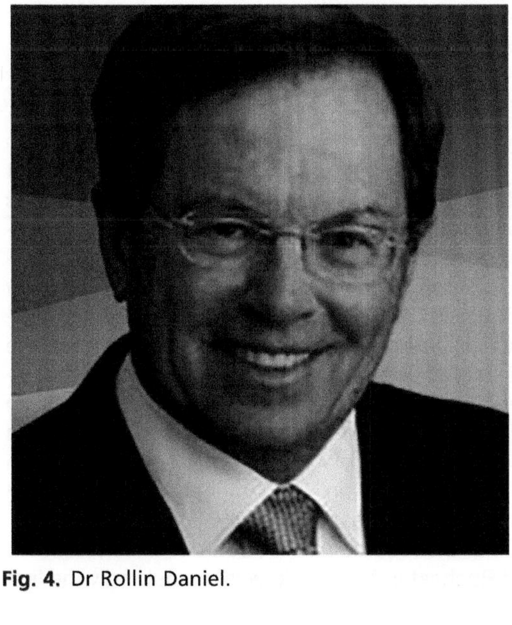

Fig. 4. Dr Rollin Daniel.

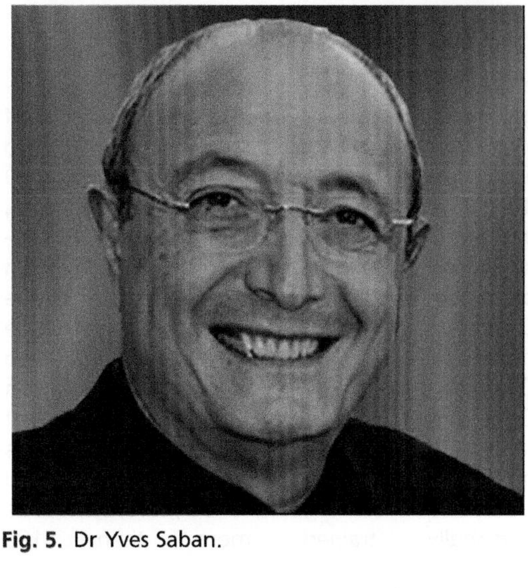

Fig. 5. Dr Yves Saban.

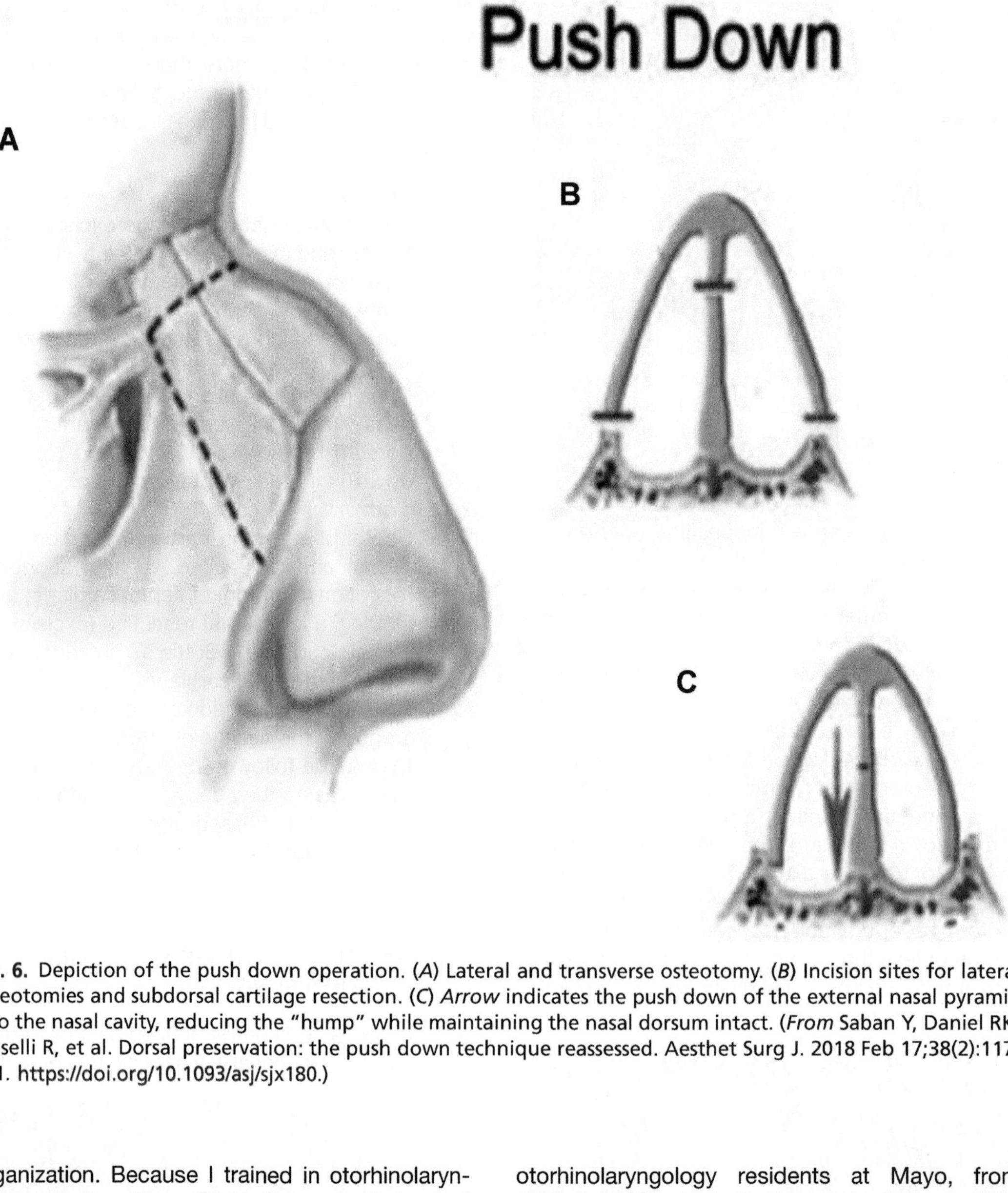

Fig. 6. Depiction of the push down operation. (*A*) Lateral and transverse osteotomy. (*B*) Incision sites for lateral osteotomies and subdorsal cartilage resection. (*C*) *Arrow* indicates the push down of the external nasal pyramid into the nasal cavity, reducing the "hump" while maintaining the nasal dorsum intact. (*From* Saban Y, Daniel RK, Polselli R, et al. Dorsal preservation: the push down technique reassessed. Aesthet Surg J. 2018 Feb 17;38(2):117-131. https://doi.org/10.1093/asj/sjx180.)

organization. Because I trained in otorhinolaryngology at the Mayo Clinic Graduate School of Medicine in Rochester, Minnesota, from 1964 to 1968, my teachers included Clifford Lake, MD (**Fig. 8**) of Mayo Clinic in Rochester, Minnesota, and Pat Barelli, MD (**Fig. 9**) of Kansas City, Missouri, and both surgeons taught the push down operation; each were professors at the "Cottle Courses" and proficient practitioners of the Cottle push down. My friend and colleague at Mayo Clinic is the accomplished and skillful surgeon George W. Facer, MD (**Fig. 10**). We both first attended and later taught at the Cottle Courses and cochaired the Mayo Clinic Rhinologic Surgical Courses on alternate years for 30 years; each of us personally trained more than 120 otorhinolaryngology residents at Mayo, from 1970 to 2003, in both the push down and let down operations. Until quite recently, it was believed, by this author (E.B.K.), that dorsal preservation surgery embodied in the push down operation was first presented to the profession by Cottle in 1954.[2] This misapprehension was corrected and clarified while preparing a talk on the history of dorsal preservation surgery for the Preservation Rhinoplasty meeting in Nice, France, in February 2019. Astonishingly, dorsal preservation surgery is an old idea, published more than 100 years ago in the American literature and more than 90 years ago in the French literature.

For the record, in 1887, John Orlando Roe, MD, of Rochester, New York, was undoubtedly the first

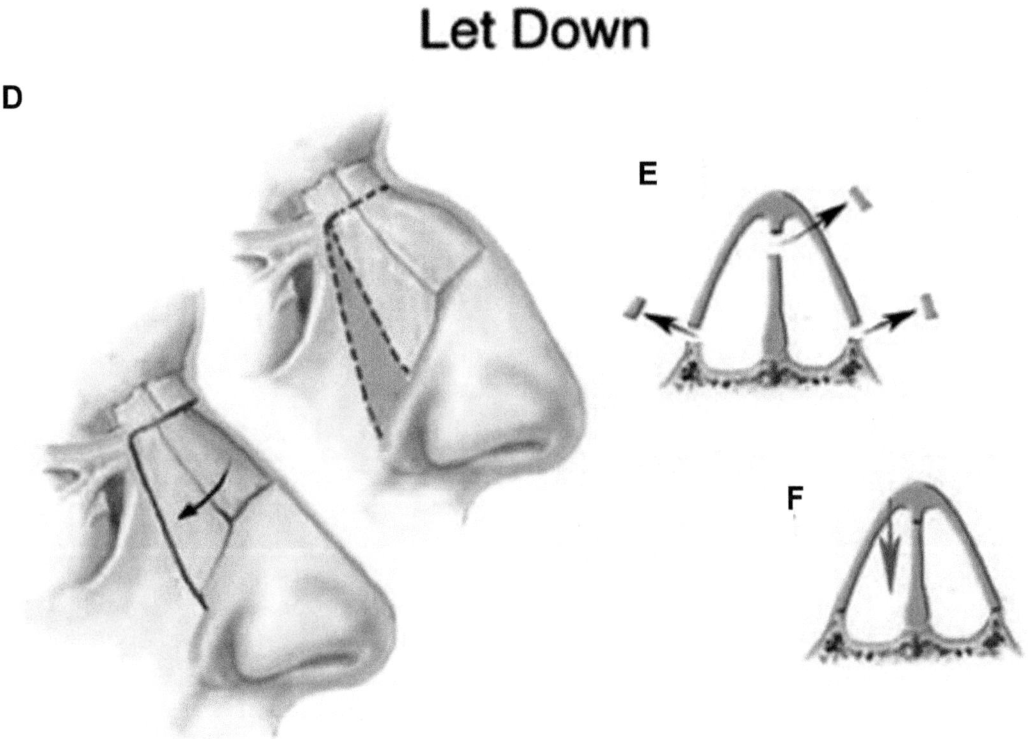

Fig. 7. Depiction of the let down operation. (*D*) Bony wedge-shaped resection of a portion of the frontal (ascending) process of the maxilla and the site of the transverse osteotomy (*dotted line*). (*E*) *Arrow* indicates the subdorsal septal cartilage excision and bony wedge resection from the frontal (ascending) process of the maxilla. (*F*) *Arrow* indicates the let down and lowering of the external nasal pyramid onto the frontal (ascending) process of the maxilla, reducing the "hump" while keeping the nasal dorsum intact. (*From* Saban Y, Daniel RK, Polselli R, et al. Dorsal preservation: the push down technique reassessed. Aesthet Surg J. 2018 Feb 17;38(2):117-131. https://doi.org/10.1093/asj/sjx180.)

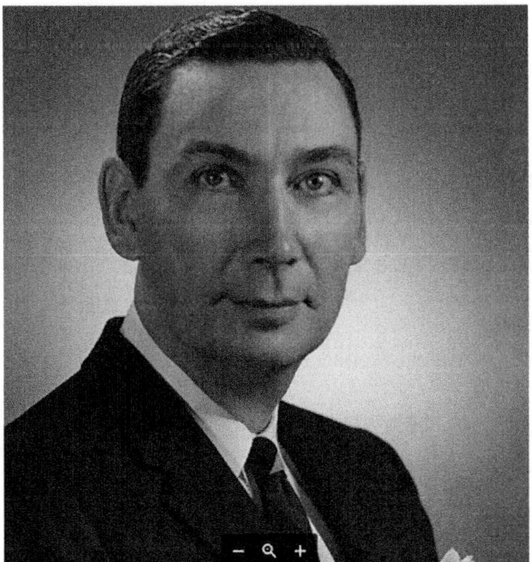

Fig. 8. Dr Clifford Lake (1913–1989).

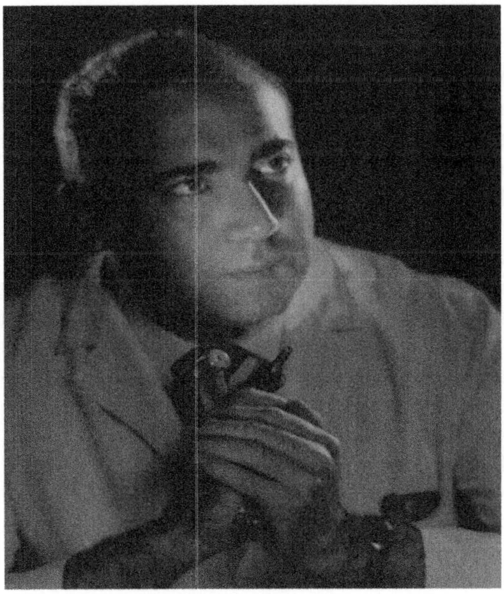

Fig. 9. Dr Pat Barelli (1919–2011).

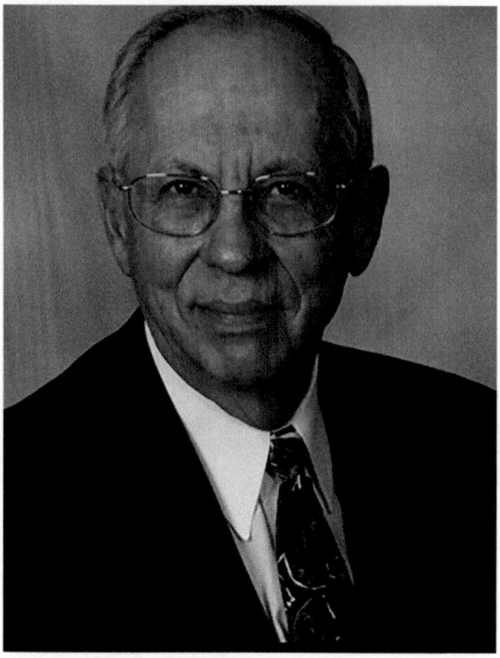

Fig. 10. Dr George Facer (1937-2020).

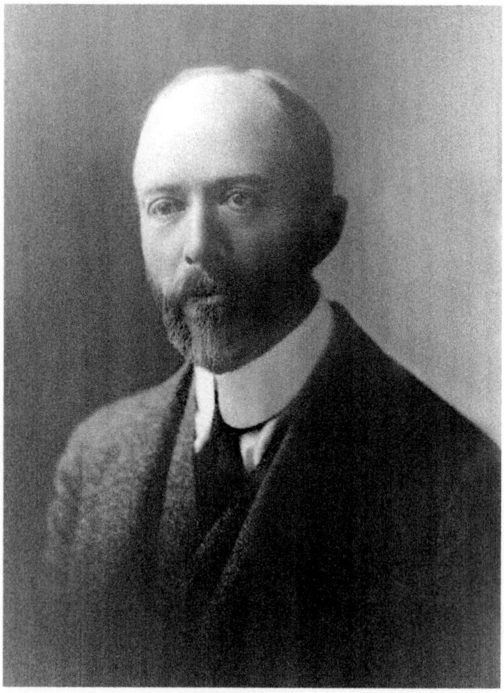

Fig. 11. Dr J.L. Goodale (1868–1957).

to publish a cosmetic surgical procedure of the nasal tip.[8] In 1891, he reported a cosmetic correction of an angular deformity of the nasal dorsum using bone scissors for the reduction of a dorsal deformity without septal surgery or osteotomies in 3 patients.[9]

In the mission to accurately discover the godfathers of dorsal preservation surgery, the journey stretched back in time and place to nineteenth-century Boston, Massachusetts.

J.L. GOODALE

The contributions of Roe[8,9] aside, the first "push down" operation and the first article on dorsal preservation appeared in the Boston Medical and Surgical Journal 1899 authored by J.L. Goodale, MD (**Fig. 11**). At that time, neither dorsal preservation surgery nor the "push down" operation was part of the lexicon. Goodale, an assistant physician for diseases of the throat in the Massachusetts General Hospital and in the Boston Children's Hospital, described a case of dorsal preservation surgery on June 21, 1898, on a 13-year-old girl, incorporating photographs. The description of the operation was read on October 12, 1898, at the Middlesex South District Medical Society and published in 1899 (**Figs. 12** and **13**).[10] Goodale's operation was conceptually a "push down". The septal phase used 2 scissor cuts: first a curved scissors convex side uppermost and then a lower cut with a straight scissor. Both cuts were transmucosal as septal flaps were not raised.

> *A small saw was introduced teeth uppermost into the left nasal passage and the articulation of the nasal and maxillary bones sawn through from below upwards. A similar saw cut was made on the corresponding articulation on the right side. The nasal bones were thus left articulating with the frontal bone and with each other. A few comparatively gentle taps upon the nasal bones sufficed to break the frontal articulation and depress them, still firmly united with each other, until they came*

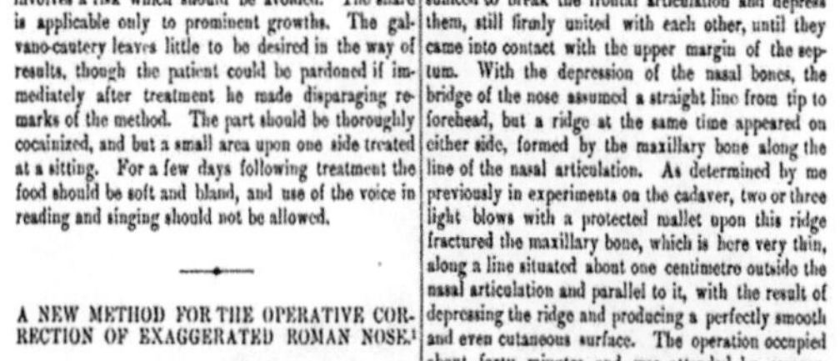

112 *BOSTON MEDICAL AND SURGICAL JOURNAL.* [FEBRUARY 2, 1899.

involves a risk which should be avoided. The snare is applicable only to prominent growths. The galvano-cautery leaves little to be desired in the way of results, though the patient could be pardoned if immediately after treatment he made disparaging remarks of the method. The part should be thoroughly cocainized, and but a small area upon one side treated at a sitting. For a few days following treatment the food should be soft and bland, and use of the voice in reading and singing should not be allowed.

A NEW METHOD FOR THE OPERATIVE CORRECTION OF EXAGGERATED ROMAN NOSE.[1]

BY J. L. GOODALE, M.D.,

Assistant Physician for Diseases of the Throat in the Massachusetts General Hospital and in the Boston Children's Hospital.

sufficed to break the frontal articulation and depress them, still firmly united with each other, until they came into contact with the upper margin of the septum. With the depression of the nasal bones, the bridge of the nose assumed a straight line from tip to forehead, but a ridge at the same time appeared on either side, formed by the maxillary bone along the line of the nasal articulation. As determined by me previously in experiments on the cadaver, two or three light blows with a protected mallet upon this ridge fractured the maxillary bone, which is here very thin, along a line situated about one centimetre outside the nasal articulation and parallel to it, with the result of depressing the ridge and producing a perfectly smooth and even cutaneous surface. The operation occupied about forty minutes and was attended by comparatively slight hemorrhage. An external splint was applied to hold the nasal bones and the fragments of

Fig. 12. First paper of dorsal preservation, Goodale 1899. (*From* Goodale JL. A New Method for the Operative Correction of Exaggerated Roman nose. Boston Med Surg J. 140:112, 1899.)

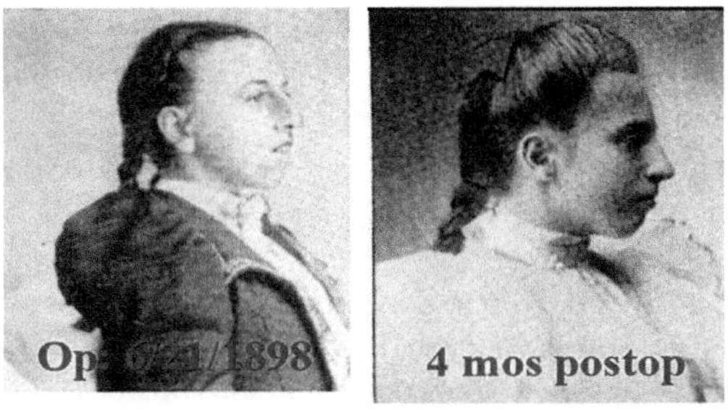

Fig. 13. First patient, dorsal preservation "push down" operation, Goodale 1899. (*From* Goodale JL. A New Method for the Operative Correction of Exaggerated Roman nose. Boston Med Surg J. 140:112, 1899.)

into contact with the upper margin of the septum. With the depression of the nasal bones, the bridge of the nose assumed a straight line from tip to forehead, but a ridge at the same time appeared on either side, formed by the maxillary bone along the lines of the nasal articulation. As determined by me previously in experiments on the cadaver, two or three light blows with a protected mallet upon this ridge fractured the maxillary bone, which is here very thin, along a line situated about 1 cm outside the nasal articulation and parallel to it, with the result of depressing the ridge and producing a perfectly smooth and even cutaneous surface. The operation occupied about 40 minutes and was attended by comparatively slight hemorrhage.[10]

In 1901, Goodale reported on 22 additional cases (including photographs) of dorsal preservation surgery; again, the language used was unlike current narrative vocabulary, but the surgery was clearly the "push down" technique.[11]

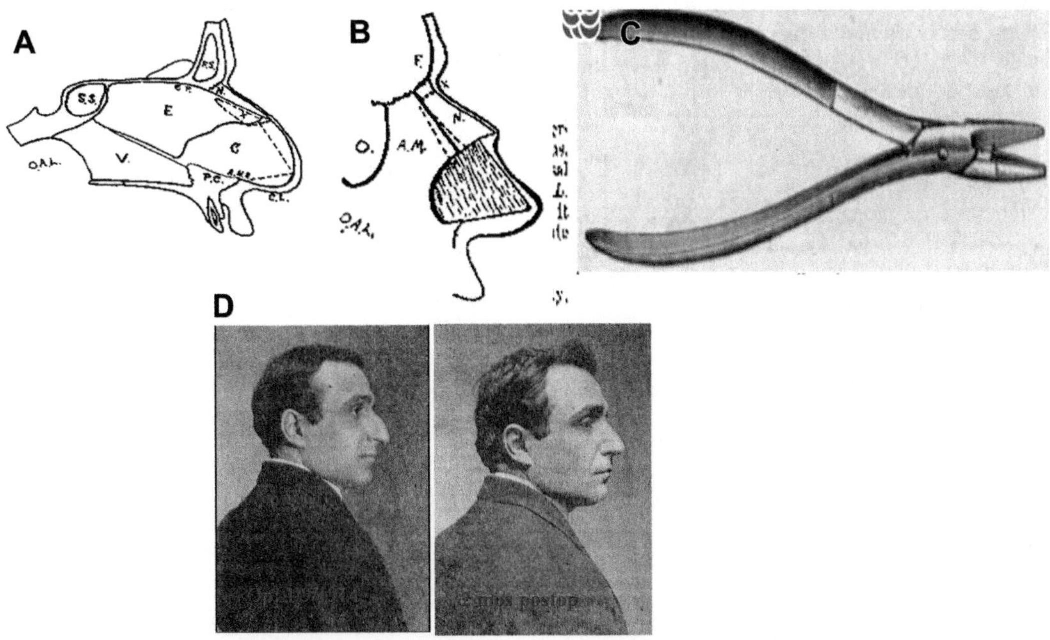

Fig. 14. (*A*) Drawing from Lothrop. This is the septal portion of the let down operation. Note the dorsum (nasal bone) remains intact. E indicates perpendicular plate of the ethmoid; V, vomer; SS, sphenoidal sinus; CP, region of cribriform plate; FS, frontal sinus; N, nasal bone; PC, premaxillary crest; ANS, anterior nasal spine; CL, columella; C, septal cartilage (the broken lines showing where it is cut to form the new borders); X, section of the perpendicular plate of the ethmoid just beneath nasal bones which must be removed. (*B*) Drawing from Lothrop. F indicates frontal bone; O, orbit; N, nasal bone; AM, ascending process of the maxilla; X, site of the transverse osteotomy (the broken lines depicting the v-shaped wedge resection from a portion of the nasal bone (N) and a portion of the frontal process of the maxilla (FM). This is the bony portion of the let down operation; note the dorsum (nasal bone is maintained intact. (*C*) Bone punch from Lothrop. A new bone punch designed to remove a V-shaped section of bone from a portion of the nasal bone and a portion of the frontal (ascending) process of the maxilla. The bone punch facilitates removal of bony portions of the let down operation, which includes bone punch removal of a portion of the bony perpendicular plate of the ethmoid and bone punch removal of a portion of the nasal bone and of the frontal (ascending) process of the maxilla. (*D*) Lothrop's first patient, 1914. (*From* Lothrop OA. An operation for correcting the aquiline nasal deformity; the use of new instrument; report of a case. Boston Med Surg J. 1914; 170:835-837.)

O.A. LOTHROP

The first "let down" was performed in 1914 by Oliver A. Lothrop, MD, as he described 1 case of dorsal preservation surgery that appeared in the same *Boston Medical Surgical Journal*.[12] Lothrop was an assistant otologist at Massachusetts General Hospital and clinical assistant at Massachusetts Charitable Eye and Ear Infirmary. He clearly described dorsal preservation surgery and illustrated both a septal cartilage phase and bone phase to the surgery (**Fig. 14**A, B). Lothrop also introduced a new bone punch instrument to remove a V-shaped section of bone (**Fig. 14**C).

Preoperative and postoperative photographs of Lothrop's patient are clearly pictured (**Fig. 14**D).[12]

Technic.

An incision is made on one side of the columella down to the free edge of the septal cartilage. The muco-perichondrium is now elevated for a short distance on either side. If the septal cartilage has grown too long in this direction, so that the nose is too long and hangs over the upper lip, a suitable amount of the denuded cartilage is now removed.

The muco-perichondrium is then elevated on both sides of the septum close under the nose bridge up to and under the nasal bones. The free border of the cartilage forming the bridge is now shaved down to the line desired for the reconstructed bridge. A piece of the perpendicular plate of the ethmoid close under the nasal bones is now removed, relieving all support at that point. The step in the operation consists in making an incision within the nostril along the free border of the nasal bone and ascending process of the superior maxilla. This incision cuts the mucous membrane and underlying tissues adherent to the free border of the bones and brings the operator beneath the periosteum covering the external surface of the nasal bone and ascending process. The periosteum elevator now raises all the periosteum over the nasal

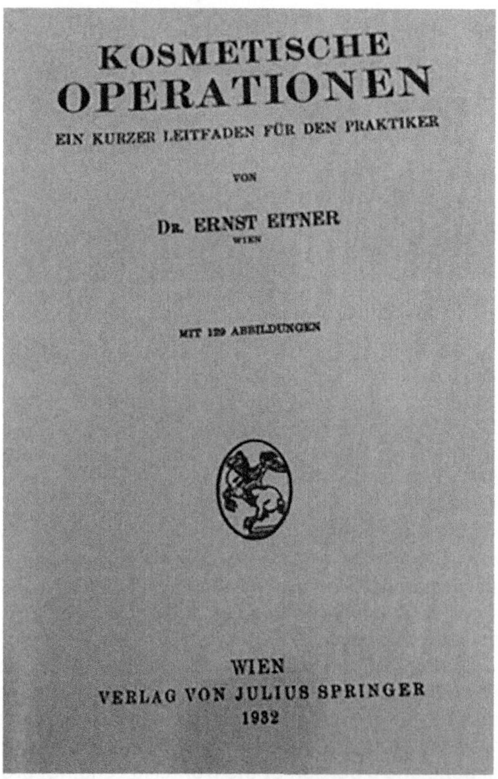
KOSMETISCHE OPERATIONEN

EIN KURZER LEITFADEN FÜR DEN PRAKTIKER

VON

DR. ERNST EITNER

WIEN

MIT 129 ABBILDUNGEN

WIEN

VERLAG VON JULIUS SPRINGER

1932

Fig. 15. Title page of Eitner's book. Translated from German: "Cosmetic Operations: A Short Guide for the Practitioner." (*From* Eitner E. Kosmetische Operationen: Ein Kurzer Leitfaden fur den Praktiker. Wein: J. Springer 1932.)

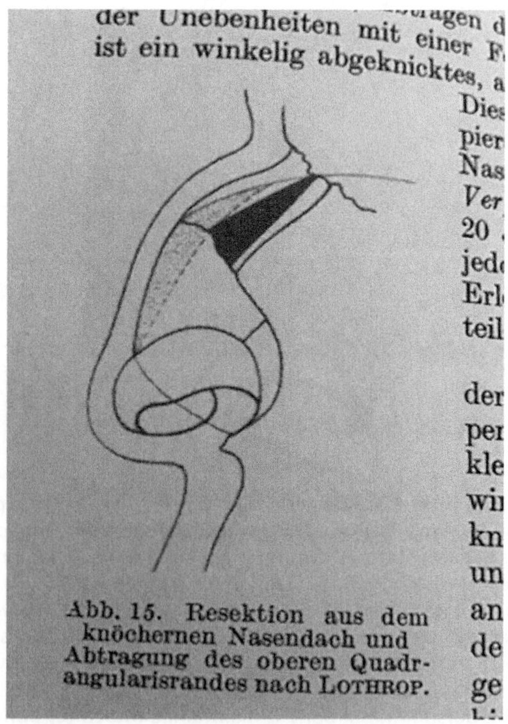

Fig. 16. Eitner's citation of Lothrop's "let down." Translated from German: "Resection from the bony roof (dorsum) of the nose and reduction of the quadrangular cartilage (septum) after Lothrop. (*From* Eitner E. Kosmetische Operationen: Ein Kurzer Leitfaden fur den Praktiker. Wein: J. Springer 1932.)

bone and ascending process of that side. The above technique is now repeated on the other side. A triangular or V-shaped piece of bone is next removed subperiosteally from either side of the nose. This section includes a little of the nasal bone and some of the ascending process and has its acute angle near the fronto-nasal suture. In order to remove this section cleanly, symmetrically and quickly, a new bone punch was devised for this operation. It is heavy forceps just small enough to enter the vestibule, having a male blade and a female blade. The female blade has a triangular aperture, one-quarter of an inch at the base and seven-eighths of an inch on each of the other sides. The male blade fits into this area so that with one closure of the forceps the desired section can be removed. After the lateral V-shaped sections have been removed the nasal bones are fractured near the fronto-nasal suture with a narrow straight chisel. Protecting the soft tisues[b] over the nasal bones, the latter can now be easily depressed with a blow from the mallet flush with the newly shaped, free border of the septal cartilage. If the nose is of the proper length the operation is finished. No packing or splinting is required. Light gauze pressure may be used over the nose for a few hours if desired to prevent hematoma.[12]

Surprisingly, although both Goodale and Lothrop likely lived in the Boston area and were attached to Massachusetts General Hospital, Lothrop neither mentioned nor referenced the work of his predecessor, Goodale, in the bibliography of his 1914 paper.[12]

P. SEBILEAU AND L. DURFOURMENTEL

Pierre Sebileau and his father-in-law Leon Durfourmentel published their work, Correction Chirurgicale Des Difformites Congenitales et Acquises De La Pyramide Nasale in 1926 (Surgical Correction of Congenital and Acquired Deformities of the Nasal Pyramid).[13] These surgeons, University of Paris, France faculty members, illustrated the details of the let down procedure, according to the French surgeon Raymond Gola and colleagues.[14] Sebileau and Durfourmentel resected a portion of the ascending (frontal) process of the maxilla and removed an "inferior strip" of septal cartilage to reduce the dorsal profile line while preserving the K-area and maintaining the osseocartilaginous dorsum intact.

OTHER CONTRIBUTORS

In the 1932 book entitled *Kosmetische Operationen: Ein Kurzer Leitfaden fur den Praktiker* (*Cosmetic Operations: A Short Guide for the Practitioner*) (**Fig. 15**),[15] Eitner illustrated and

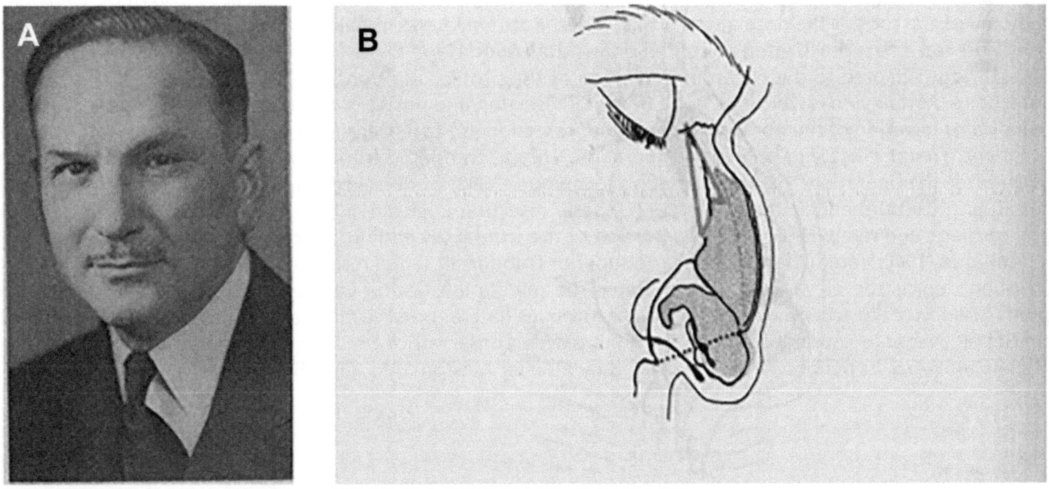

Fig. 17. (*A*) Dr Sam Fomon (1889–1971). (*B*) Fomon's citation of Lothrop's "let down". The legend reads, "Lothrop's method for the elimination of nasal hump. Wedge-shaped sections excised from the nasal bones and septum. Dorsal hump forced back into space thus created, to produce a normal profile." (*From* Fomon S. The Surgery of Injury and Plastic Repair: The Williams & Wilkins Company, Baltimore 1939.)

[b]Note the typographical correction of tisues is tissues.

acknowledged the dorsal preservation operation in rhinoplasty by citing the 1914 let down work of Lothrop (**Fig. 16**).[15]

Sam Fomon contributed a monumental opus: *The Surgery of Injury and Plastic Repair* in 1939.[16] Quoting directly from page 688 (**Fig. 17**A, B) of Fomon's book, which compellingly and convincingly reads:

Some surgeons find the technique of Goodale (84) (1899), Lothrop (184) (1914), Eitner (56) (1924)[c] *Dufourmentel (50,51), and Moskovicz, correct the deformity without*

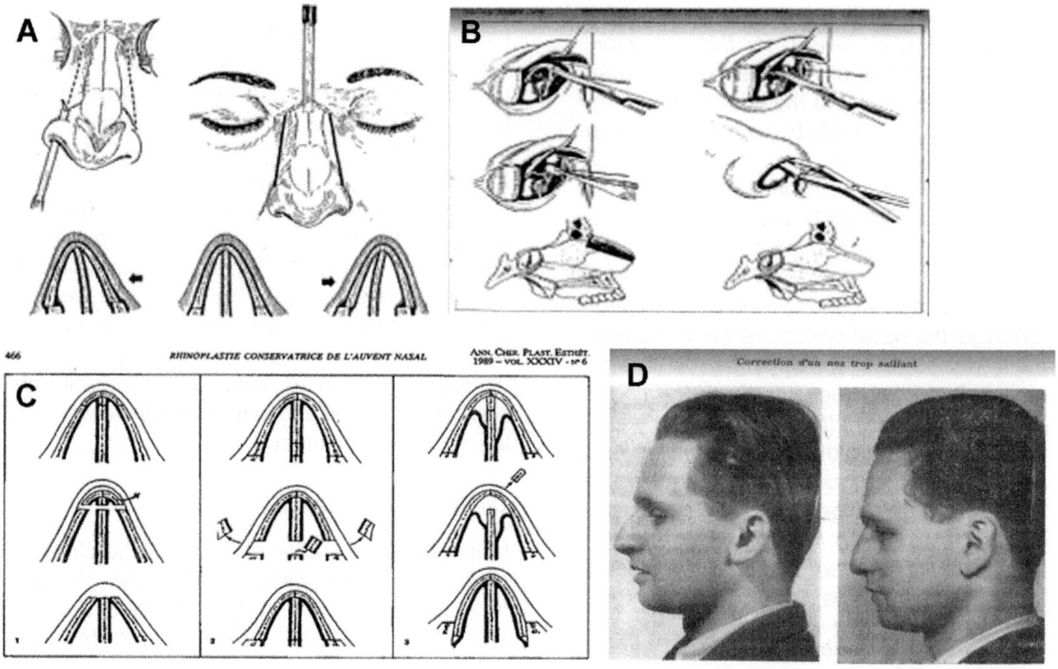

Fig. 18. Maurel's "push down," 1940. (*A*) *Top left*, low lateral osteotomy along broken lines. *Top right*, transverse osteotomy of the root of the nose along broken lines. *Bottom*, lateral mobilization of the nasal canopy (dorsum or roof). (*B*) *Top left*, septal section under the bony ridge. *Middle and lower left*, resection of a septal band under the nasal ridge adapted to the necessary reduction of the profile. *Top right*, resection of the nasal spine of the frontal bone. *Middle and lower right*, zone of septal resection and posterior displacement of the nasal ridge. *Arrow* indicates lowering of the bony dorsum without resection. (*C*) *Left*, translated from French: "A photograph of the patient from the left side before the operation." *Right*, translated from French: "Same patient, left profile 15 days after the operation." (*D*) *Left*, Joseph's technique (1898) of dorsal resection with an open roof. *Middle*, Sebileau and Dufourmentel's technique (1927): basal resection ("let down"), removal of an "inferior strip" of septal cartilage and removal (*arrows*) of a portion of the frontal (ascending) process of the maxilla. *Right*, Maurel's technique (1940): lateral basal section and superior (subdorsal) septal resection ("push down"). Note: the top illustration depicts the elevation of septal flaps. The middle illustration depicts (*arrow*) removal of subdorsal septum. The lower illustration depicts lateral osteotomies (lateral basal section) and "push down." (*Reproduced from* Gola R, Nerini A, Laurent-Fyon C, et al. Rhinoplastie Conservatrice De L'Auvent Nasal. Ann Chir Plast Esthet 1989;34(6):465-475. Copyright © 1989 published by Elsevier Masson SAS. All rights reserved.)

[c]Note: The date 1924 of Eitner's book is incorrectly quoted above by Fomon, actually it is 1932, as noted in the list of Fomon's references (No. 56) and from the title page of Eitner's book (see **Fig. 15**). Unfortunately, Fomon did not reference Moskovicz's paper(s) in his voluminous (342 citations) bibliography; using PubMed, I have been unable to unearth any nasal surgical references by the author Moskovicz. Eitner's 1932 book[15] and Fomon's 1939 book,[16] both clearly referenced Lothrop's work with illustrations and the contributions of Goodale and Durfourmentel were noted by Fomon, but unfortunately all these offerings were totally disregarded or ignored by a subsequent generation of surgeons; somewhat embarrassingly, this author (E.B.K.) is included among those legions.

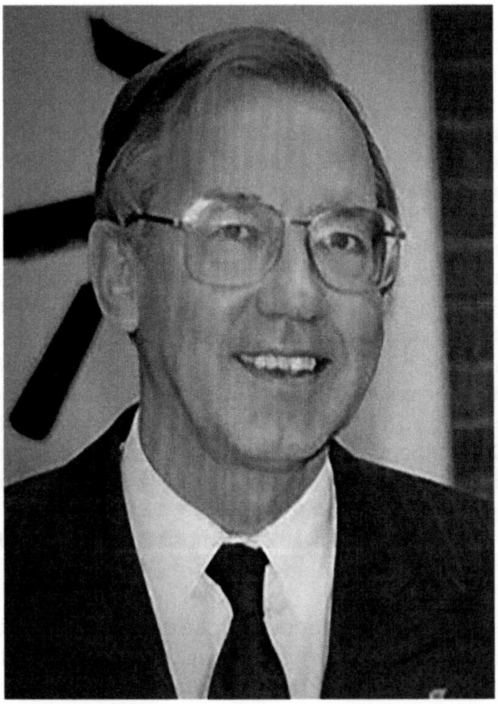

Fig. 19. Dr Egbert Huizing.

> *attacking the hump itself. They excise a wedge-shaped section from the septum and also a wedge of bone from each side of the nose (see **Figs. 3** and **11**). The space created by the removal of these substrata permits of the depression of the hump to the normal profile level.*

In 1989, Gola[14] cited the work of fellow French surgeon Maurel, illustrating Maurel's practice, which was clearly a "push down" rendition of dorsal preservation surgery. The technique included a bone phase with a low lateral osteotomy followed by a transverse osteotomy mobilizing the nasal dorsum ("canopy," according to Maurel). The cartilage phase included a subdorsal septal resection under the bony bridge with resection of the nasal spine of the frontal bone allowing the displacement of the osseocartilaginous nasal dorsum into the nose thereby "improving" the profile line (**Fig. 18**A–D).[17] The let down of Sebileau and Durfourmentel published in 1927 and the "push down" of Maurel published in 1940, both works in the French language, were obviously well before Cottle's 1954 push down[2] or Huizing's 1975 "let down".[18] Cottle (see **Fig. 2**) and Huizing (**Fig. 19**) were apparently unacquainted with the French contributions nor did they cite the work of Goodale,[10,11] Lothrop,[12] Eitner,[13] or Fomon.[16] In fact, there are numerous other surgeons who contributed to the literature carrying on the work of Cottle and Huizing but did not reference any of the early godfathers of dorsal preservation surgery. Although dorsal preservation surgery, popularized by Cottle in the 1960s and 1970s under the rubric "push down" operation, was abandoned by many, if not most, plastic and facial plastic surgeons because they principally preferred the Joseph canon of dorsal resection rhinoplasty. Dorsal preservation surgery was, however, still practiced at diverse sites in Europe and the Americas. Some scattering of papers and books added to the dorsal preservation literature, including the contributions of Gola (France),[14,19] Huizing (the Netherlands),[18] Willemot and colleagues (Belgium),[20] Wayoff and Perrin (France),[21] Hinderer (United States),[22] Sulsenti (Italy),[23] Drumheller (United States),[24] Barelli (United States),[25] Pirsig and Konigs (Germany),[26] Pinto (Brazil),[27] Kienstra and colleagues (United States),[28] and Lopez Ulloa (Mexico).[29]

ANOTHER RECENT CONTRIBUTION

After the 2018 influential contribution of dorsal preservation surgery written by Saban and colleagues[7] the latest article by Santos and

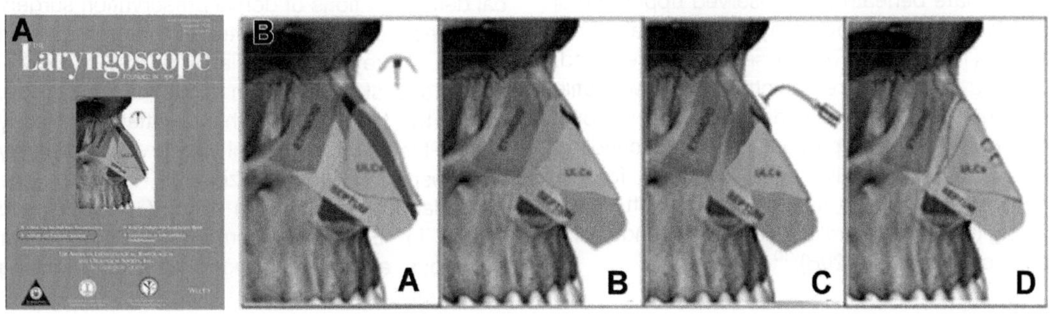

Fig. 20. (*A*) Front cover of journal, *Laryngoscope*. (*B*) Spare roof technique in reduction rhinoplasty: Prospective study of the first one hundred patients. (*From* Santos M, Rego AR, Coutinho M, Almeida e Sousa C, and Ferreira MG. Spare Roof Technique in Reduction Rhinoplasty: Prospective Study of the First One Hundred Patients. Laryngoscope, 129:2702-2706, 2019.)

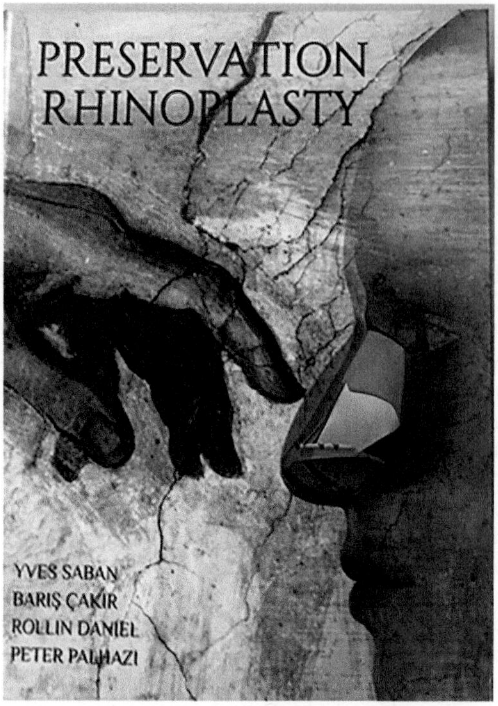

Fig. 21. Preservation rhinoplasty by Saban, Çakir, Daniel, and Palhazi book cover. (*From* Ferreira MG, Monteiro D, Reis C, Almeida e Sousa C. Spare Roof Technique: A Middle Third New Technique. Facial Plast Surg. 2016 Feb;32(1):111-6.)

colleagues[30] graced the cover of the December 2019 issue of *Laryngoscope* in their rendition of dorsal preservation surgery (**Fig. 20**A).[30] This work by Santos and colleagues[30] is a summary and continuation, with additional cases, of the spare roof technique concept developed by Ferreira and colleagues in 2016.[31] Santos and colleagues[30] advocate the subdorsal cartilage removal similar to Maurel[14] and Saban and colleagues[7] describing an initial "longitudinal cut" of 1 mm of septal cartilage from the anterior inferior corner of the septum back to the ethmoid perpendicular plate beneath the preserved upper lateral cartilage. This is followed by the removal of the excess (1–5 mm) of dorsal septum as required, adjusting for the desired height of the new profile line. Next, is the delicate diamond burr removal of the bony cap and a portion of frontal (ascending) process of the maxilla, again adjusting for the desired height of the new profile line, afterward fixating the upper lateral cartilage to the underlying septal cartilage (**Fig. 20**B).[30]

SUMMARY

After investigating the literature, it is clear that dorsal preservation surgery was practiced more than 100 years ago, and the pioneers, or godfathers, in the United States include Goodale, with his paper in 1899[10] with an actual description of the "push down", followed by Lothrop's 1914[12] authentic account of what we would currently term the "let down". Although these early surgeons did not engage the terms "push down" or "let down", the idea of preserving the dorsum was unmistakably and distinctly described in these primary works by these American godfathers Goodale and Lothrop. In Europe, it seems that the French surgeons Sebileau, Durfourmentel, and Maurel deserve the mantel of godfathers of dorsal preservation surgery on the continent. According to Gola and coworkers,[14] Sebileau and Durfourmentel in 1926[13] clearly practiced the "let down" operation, whereas Maurel performed the "push-down" operation (see **Fig. 18**A–D).[14]

It was Fomon in 1939[16] who impressively and insightfully observed that previous surgeons, including Goodale, Lothrop, Eitner, and Dufourmentel were able to "correct the deformity without attacking the hump itself." Fomon understood that these results could be achieved by excising a wedge of tissue from both the septum and from the bony pyramid to produce: "The space created by the removal of these substrata permits of the depression of the hump to the normal profile level."[16]

The realization is inescapable, that it is possible to lower the dorsal profile line *without* en bloc removal of any portion of the nasal bones or upper lateral cartilage; consequently, hump reduction without hump resection is possible. Therefore, dorsal preservation surgery is achievable and indeed preferable in many primary rhinoplasty cases. The existence of a number of unpublished surgeons who practice dorsal preservation surgery using either the "push down" or the "let down" technique is well-known in rhinology and rhinoplasty circles. In fact, recent, 2019, intensive courses with lectures, dissections, and live surgical demonstrations of dorsal preservation surgery have been formally presented to the profession in France, Turkey, and Russia by a host of experienced and skilled veteran surgeons. In Europe, during the latter part of the twentieth and early twenty-first century dorsal preservation surgery was espoused by Huizing in Utrecht, the Netherlands; Rettinger in Ulm, Germany; and Wurm in Erlangen, Germany, through their numerous annual teaching programs, reaching hundreds of students from various countries, for more than 2 decades. In France, Gola,[14,19] was the written advocate for dorsal preservation surgery and these precepts were recently resurrected, as it were, through the leadership and writing of the French surgeon Saban[7,32] and by the prominent American surgeon Daniel.[3,7,32–34] The well-known goal of dorsal preservation surgery is designed to evade the unfavorable esthetic and functional (breathing) consequences of the Joseph dorsal en bloc resection rhinoplasty, with its obligatory middle third reconstruction with spreader grafts or spreader flaps. The ideas of dorsal preservation rhinoplasty, preserving the bony and cartilaginous dorsum, avoiding midvault and keystone (K-area) disruption, is gaining absorbed attention while germinating a comprehensive newer concept embracing the entirety of rhinoplasty. The new term, coined by Daniel, is preservation rhinoplasty. The principles of preservation rhinoplasty are extending past just dorsal preservation alone and are enumerated in the 2018 seminal text *Preservation Rhinoplasty* edited by Saban, Çakir, Daniel, and Palhazi (**Fig. 21**).[32]

These contemporary preservation rhinoplasty ideas, plausibly heralding a new rhinoplasty epoch, as suggested and summarized by Daniel[33] and Kosins with Daniel[34] which include:

1. Subperichondrial-subperiosteal dissection plane
2. Negligible resections, if any
3. Replacing extensive resections with preservation and or repositioning of soft and skeletal tissues, including safeguarding the dorsal soft tissue envelop, ligaments and saving the osseocartilaginous dorsum
4. Preserving as much of the lobular cartilages as possible, choosing suturing over excision
5. Using advanced suturing techniques for tissue stabilization

Kosins and Daniel closed with the following sentence: "Some patients will benefit from total preservation (rhinoplasty) where nothing is removed/disrupted and underlying structures are reshaped."[34]

As fundamental as it is to keep an open airway for breathing, it is also imperative to keep an open mind, sustaining your scientific skepticism still seeking evidence and objectivity while avoiding the hardening of surgical practices into rock solid biases. In my opinion, in the energetic pursuit of excellence, it is prudent to accede the challenge of striving for modifications, enhancements, and improvements by maintaining your inquisitive questioning mind. Reflect on becoming part of the great renaissance, rebirth, of dorsal preservation surgery; contemplate making these preservation principles, maintaining an intact osseocartilaginous nasal dorsal roof, an integral part of your modern rhinoplasty thinking while processing and assessing the latest philosophies embodied in the cutting-edge preservation rhinoplasty revolution. Generally, in the end, I think the best operation is the one you do not do; the second-best operation is the one you do the least on. Specifically, considering preservation rhinoplasty, according to Daniel, "the best operation is the one you resect the least and preserve the most" (Daniel RK. Personal communication).

ACKNOWLEDGMENTS

The author must acknowledge librarians Joyce R. Mc Fadden and Julie A. Swenson of the Mayo Medical Library, Rochester, Minnesota, who orchestrated the collection of original papers and books—some in French, others in German—from the Mayo collection and by inter-library loan; a most grateful thank you to you both. I am most fortunate to count Michael A. Hohberger as a friend who is both cheerful and a very smart, effective Mayo Clinic editor, with appreciation.

DISCLOSURE

This work was partially funded by an educational grant from Gromo Foundation for Medical Education and Research. The author has no conflicts of interest to declare.

REFERENCES

1. Cottle MH. Nasal roof repair and hump removal. AMA Arch Otolaryngol 1954;60(4):408–14.
2. Joseph J. The classic reprint: nasal reductions. Plast Reconstr Surg 1971;47(1):79–83.
3. Daniel RK, Palhazi P. Rhinoplasty: an anatomical and clinical atlas. Cham (Switzerland): Springer; 2018. p. 345.
4. Sheen JH. Spreader graft: a method of reconstructing the roof of the middle nasal vault following rhinoplasty. Plast Reconstr Surg 1984;73(2):230–9.
5. Kovacevic M, Wurm J. Spreader flaps for middle vault contour and stabilization. Facial Plast Surg Clin North Am 2015;23(1):1–9.
6. Wurm J, Kovacevic M. A new classification of spreader flap techniques. Facial Plast Surg 2013; 29(6):506–14.
7. Saban Y, Daniel RK, Polselli R, et al. Dorsal preservation: the push down technique reassessed. Aesthet Surg J 2018;38(2):117–31.
8. Roe JO. The deformity termed pug-nose and its correction by a simple operation. Med Rec 1887.
9. Roe JO. The correction of angular deformities of the nose by a subcutaneous operation. Med Rec 1891.
10. Goodale JL. A new method for the operative correction of exaggerated Roman nose. Boston Med Surg J 1899;140:112.

11. Goodale JL. The correction of old lateral displacements of the nasal bones. Boston Med Surg J 1901;145:547.
12. Lothrop OA. An operation for correcting the aquiline nasal deformity; the use of new instrument; report of a case. Boston Med Surg J 1914;170:835–7.
13. Sebileau P, Dufourmentel L. (Surgical correction of congenital an acquired deformities of the nasal pyramid). Paris: Arnette; 1926. p. 104–5 [in French].
14. Gola R, Nerini A, Laurent-Fyon C, et al. Rhinoplastie Conservatrice De L'Auvent Nasal. [(Conservative rhinoplasty of the nasal canopy)]. Ann Chir Plast Esthet 1989;34(6):465–75 [in French].
15. Eitner E. (Cosmetic operations: a short guide for the oractitioner). Wein: J. Springer; 1932 [in German].
16. Fomon S. The surgery of injury and plastic repair. Baltimore (MD): The Williams & Wilkins Company; 1939.
17. Maurel G. Chirurgie maxilla-faciale. Paris: Le François; 1940. p. 1127–33 [in French].
18. Huizing EH. Push-down of the external nasal pyramid by resection of wedges. Rhinology 1975;13(4): 185–90.
19. Gola R. Functional and esthetic rhinoplasty [Review]. Aesthetic Plast Surg 2003;27(5):390–6.
20. Willemot J, Vrebos J, Pollet J, et al. Plastic surgery and otorhinolaryngology. Acta Otorhinolaryngol Belg 1967;21(5):463–732 [in French].
21. Wayoff M, Perrin C. Global mobilization of the nasal pyramid according to Cottle's technic: its possibilities in functional nose surgery. Acta Otorhinolaryngol Belg 1968;22(6):675–80 [in French].
22. Hinderer KH. Fundamentals of anatomy and surgery of the nose. Ann Arbor (MI): Aesculapius Publishing Co; 1971. p. 193.
23. Sulsenti G. Chirugia Funzionale ed Estetica del Naso, Ghedini. Milan (Italy): 1972. 2nd edition. 1994 [in Italian].
24. Drumheller GW. The push down operation and septal surgery. In: Daniel RK, editor. Aesthetic plastic surgery: rhinoplasty. Boston: Little Brown; 1973. p. 739–66. Chapter 30.
25. Barelli PA. Long term evaluation of the push down procedures. Rhinology 1975;13(1):25–32.
26. Pirsig W, Königs D. Wedge resection in rhinosurgery: a review of the literature and long-term results in a hundred cases [Review]. Rhinology 1988;26(2): 77–88.
27. Pinto RM. On the let-down procedure in septorhinoplasty. Rhinology 1997;35(4):178–80.
28. Kienstra MA, Sherris DA, Kern EB. The Cottle vs Joseph rhinoplasty. In: Larrabee WF, Thomas RT, editors. Facial plastic surgery clinics of North America. Philadelphia: W.B. Saunders; 1999. p. 279–94.
29. Ulloa FL. Let down technique. Available at: http://www.rhinoplastyarchive.com/articles/let-down-technique. Accessed September 24, 2019.
30. Santos M, Rego AR, Coutinho M, et al. Spare roof technique in reduction rhinoplasty: prospective study of the first one hundred patients. Laryngoscope 2019;129:2702–6.
31. Ferreira MG, Monteiro D, Reis C, et al. Spare roof technique: a middle third new technique. Facial Plast Surg 2016;32(1):111–6.
32. Saban Y, Çakir B, Daniel R, et al. Preservation rhinoplasty. Istanbul (Turkey): Septum Publishing; 2018. p. 435.
33. Daniel RK. The preservation rhinoplasty: a new rhinoplasty revolution. Aesthet Surg J 2018;38(2): 228–9.
34. Kosins AM, Daniel RK. Decision making in preservation rhinoplasty: a 100 case series with one-year follow-up. Aesthet Surg J 2020;40(1):34–48.

Conventional Resection Versus Preservation of the Nasal Dorsum and Ligaments

An Anatomic Perspective and Review of the Literature

Mohamed Abdelwahab, MD, MS[a,*], Priyesh N. Patel, MD[b]

KEYWORDS

• Preservation rhinoplasty • Hump resection • Nasal dorsum • Internal nasal valve • Keystone area • Ligaments of the nose • Upper lateral cartilage • Dorsal aesthetic lines

KEY POINTS

- Preservation and conventional rhinoplasty techniques require a thorough understanding of the surface and soft tissue nasal anatomy, and its integration with the underlying osseocartilaginous framework.
- Preservation of the keystone area (divided into a dorsal and lateral components) contributes to the continuity of the dorsal aesthetic lines.
- For more in-depth description, the reader is referred to the primary literature referenced herein.

INTRODUCTION

A hallmark of rhinoplasty is the maintenance of anatomic and structural components of the nose, while still allowing for changes in the external contour. Although preservation rhinoplasty has been advocated and performed by expert surgeons around the world,[1–5] open structural approaches with Joseph or conventional hump reduction techniques have predominated rhinoplasty teaching and practice.[6] Recently, there has been increased interest in the preservation rhinoplasty concept, particularly as the anatomic knowledge of the nasal skeleton and soft tissue envelope (STE) has been explained further by anatomists and experts such as Palhazi, Daniel, and Saban.[2,7–10] Preservation rhinoplasty may refer to several elements including (1) elevation of the STE in a subperichondrial–subperiosteal plane, (2) preservation of alar cartilages while minimizing excision. and (3) maintaining the bony/cartilaginous dorsum without violation of the osseocartilaginous interface.[2,3] The latter of these, or dorsal preservation rhinoplasty (DPR), can be performed with or without the other. Although conventional hump resection (CHR) or the traditional method described by Joseph disrupt the dorsal aesthetic lines (DALs), these methods provide versatility to reshape the entire dorsal architecture. Surgical success with either DPR or CHR techniques requires a thorough understanding of external and underlying nasal anatomy, particularly the dorsal hump.[11] In this article, essential elements of nasal anatomy as they pertain to DPR and CHR are discussed.

[a] Department of Otolaryngology–Head & Neck Surgery, Mansoura University, Faculty of Medicine, Gomhoreya Street, Mansoura 35516, Egypt; [b] Division of Facial Plastic and Reconstructive Surgery, Department of Otolaryngology–Head and Neck Surgery, Vanderbilt University Medical Center, Nashville, TN, USA
* Corresponding author.
E-mail addresses: m.wahab.plasty@gmail.com; m.wahab@mans.edu.eg

Facial Plast Surg Clin N Am 29 (2021) 15–28
https://doi.org/10.1016/j.fsc.2020.08.005

SURFACE AND SOFT TISSUE ANATOMY

An initial assessment of the nose involves an analysis of its relationship with other facial landmarks on different views (**Fig. 1**). On the frontal view, the ratio of the length of the nose to the middle third of the face is 0.9:1.0. The width of the nasal root to the alar width is 0.5:1.0. The ratio of nasal projection on profile view to nasal length is 0.4:1.0, and the tip length is nearly 45% of the projection.[12,13] When a line is drawn from the deepest aspect of the nasal root at the nasion, to the appropriately projected nasal tip, the dorsum should lie at or just posterior and parallel to this line.

The nasal pyramid can be subdivided topographically into surgical thirds (**Figs. 2** and **3**). The upper third is composed of a pair of nasal bones and the middle third is formed by the paired upper lateral cartilages (ULCs) that are responsible for forming the midvault and the internal nasal valves (INV). The nasal keystone area refers to the underlying junction between the upper and middle thirds of the nose[14,15]; thus, a dorsal hump has contribution from both bone and cartilage (see **Fig. 3**). The lower third of the nose consists of the tip, soft tissue triangles, alar lobule, and columella, all of which are related to the shape and orientation of the lower lateral cartilages (LLCs).

Anatomic description of the STE mirrors layers of the face: dermis, superficial areolar (fatty) layer, superficial muscular aponeurotic system (SMAS) layer, deep areolar layer, and perichondrium/periosteum. Dissection in rhinoplasty can be performed in a subcutaneous, sub-SMAS, or subperichondral plane.[2,7,16] In DPR, subperichondral dissection has been advocated. In open structural approaches or CHR techniques, a similar dissection can also be performed although many surgeons ultimately dissect in the sub-SMAS plane. It remains unclear if dissection in the sub-SMAS plane is aesthetically or functionally inferior to a subperichondrial plane of dissection, although there is theoretically less disruption of ligamentous nasal structures that are discussed elsewhere in this article and potentially less soft tissue edema.

The STE varies in thickness among ethnicities and along the length of the dorsum (see **Fig. 2**),[17] with an average of 1.25 mm at the radix and thinnest at the rhinion at 0.6 mm.[18] There is greater mobility of the STE over the upper two-thirds than the lower third of the nose because of less adherence of the SMAS to the perichondrium,[16] and more abundance in sebaceous and sweat glands in the lower third.[19] In DPR, the thickness of the STE at the radix allows for the camouflage of any underlying stop-off after a transverse osteotomy (see **Fig. 2**). Because the STE is thinnest at the rhinion, irregularities can appear with the CHR, whereas the DPR has the benefit of minimal disruption to the dorsum at this site. In addition, in CHR techniques, as discussed elsewhere in this article, leaving the rhinion slightly more pronounced needs to be considered to compensate for differential skin thickness.

DORSAL AESTHETIC LINES

On the frontal view, 2 concave divergent reflection lines are seen extending from the orbital rim to the tip where they become slightly divergent again (see **Fig. 1**C).[20] These reflections are formed as a result of the contours of the underlying nasal osseocartilaginous structures. Conventionally,

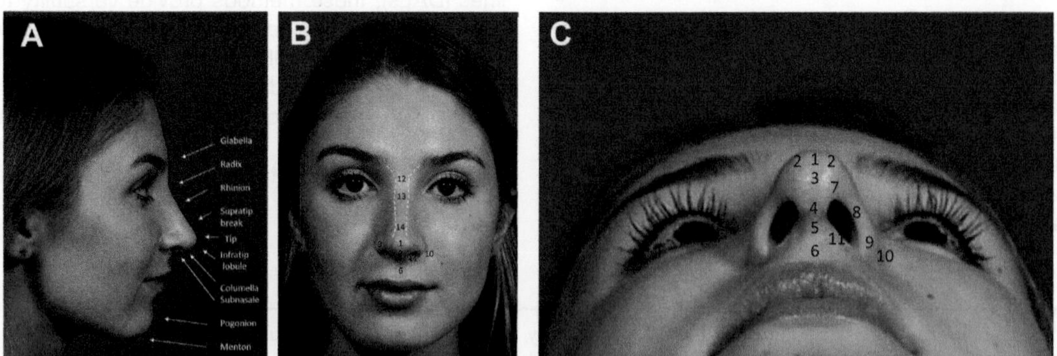

Fig. 1. Surface landmarks in a patient's profile view (*A*), basal view (*B*), and frontal view (*C*). Relevant landmarks of the external nose include (1) nasal tip, (2) tip defining points, (3) infratip lobule, (4) columella, (5) base of the columella, (6) philtrum, (7) soft tissue triangle, (8) alar margin, (9) alar lobule, (10) alar crease, (11) nasal sill, (12) radix, (13) keystone area (rhinion), and (14) supratip break.

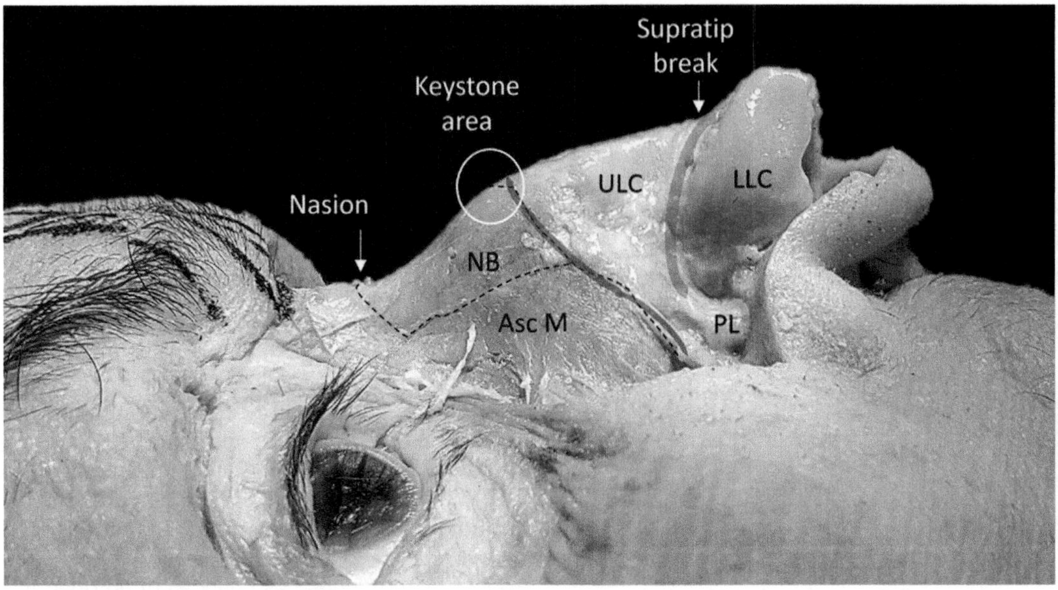

Fig. 2. Lateral view of the osseocartilaginous side wall (cadaveric). This shows contributors to a dorsal hump. Asc-M, ascending maxillary process; LLC, lower lateral cartilage; NB, nasal bones; PL, pyriform ligament; ULC, upper lateral cartilage. *Blue*, scroll ligament complex; *red*, pyriform attachment ligament.

these lines were thought to be narrowest at the keystone area. However, it has been proposed that these lines are instead fusiform, being narrowest at the radix, wider at the keystone, and again narrow at the supratip.[21] This widening at the keystone area corresponds with the caudal flare of the nasal bones and is relatively higher in males. The anatomic contributions to the DALs include the curvature at the junction between the dorsal and lateral aspects of the nasal bones in addition to the architecture of the underlying ULCs (**Fig. 4**). In CHR, DALs are violated, requiring meticulous care restoring their continuity and symmetry; however, it provides the surgeon with freedom to reshape these lines when asymmetric or broken as in severe or S-shaped deviations. In DPR, these lines are preserved providing a natural dorsal architecture, provided they are desirable.

NASAL BONES

The nasal bones' cephalic attachment to the frontal bones corresponds topographically with the radix or nasal root, forming the upper limit of the nasal height. The radix angle is obtuse with variations in values and position with gender; in males it tends to lie at the level of the superior tarsal crease and is less obtuse, whereas in females it is at the level of the upper lashes. The nasal bones on a profile view demonstrate 4 main points (**Fig. 5**):[22]

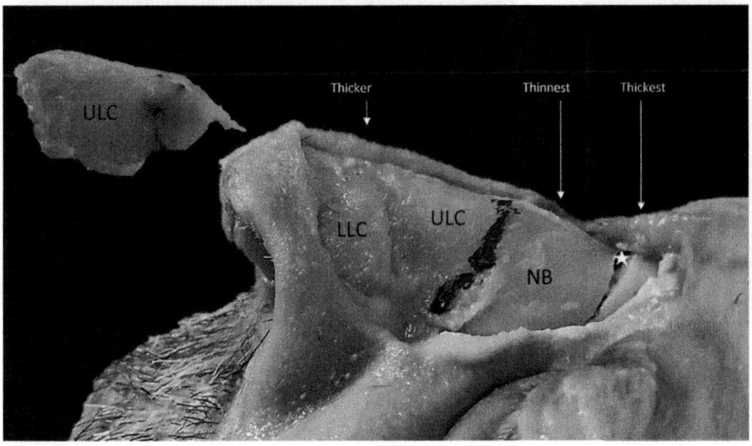

Fig. 3. Surgical thirds of the nose. An upper (NB, nasal bones) middle (ULC) and lower (LLC) third, each covered by skin of variable thickness along the nasal dorsum. Blue transparency outlines the ULC extension underneath the nasal bones and alar cartilages. *Transverse osteotomy for dorsal preservation, with intact osseocartilaginous complex.

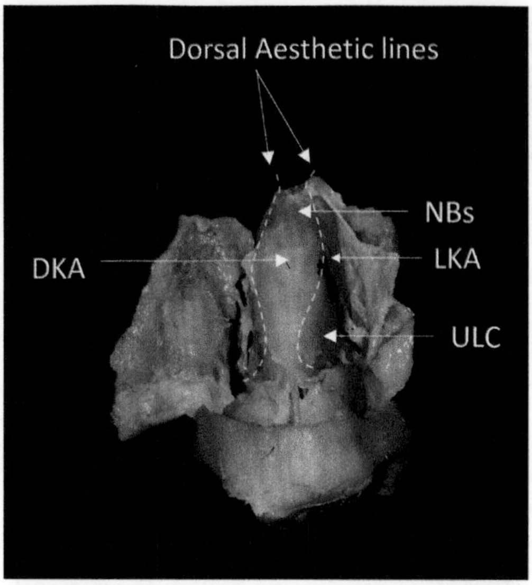

Fig. 4. DALs. Their anatomic contribution includes the ULC, nasal bones (NB), and dorsal and lateral keystone area (DKA/LKA).

1. The nasion: midpoint of the nasofrontal suture line.
2. The sellion: deepest depression of the nasal bones and is used in pretreatment plans.
3. The kyphion: most prominent point of the bony dorsum.
4. The rhinion: most caudal point of the nasal bones and marks the midpoint of the osseocartilaginous vault.

These points have led to dividing the bony dorsum into 2 configurations:

1. S-shaped nasal bones have a curve which begins at the sellion, with an apex at the kyphion, and plateaus at the rhinion (see **Fig. 5**).
2. V-shaped nasal bones have a nearly straight configuration from the sellion through the rhinion and thus one locus of angulation at the sellion (**Fig. 6**).

In DPR, as the nasal vault is pushed inferiorly, the kyphion is not resected, and therefore patients with S-shaped nasal bones may be at higher risk of a residual hump. In CHR, the kyphion is removed, thereby minimizing this risk. In nonpreservation hump removal, dorsal reduction can be performed in either a component or composite (en bloc) resection. The original description by Joseph was a composite resection,[6] yet with evolution toward more conservative techniques, component resection has gained popularity. Although the latter procedure is time consuming, it allows more gradual reduction and thereby precise control over the bony dorsum reduced. Importantly, it allows for preservation of structures when possible and decreases chances of an open roof deformity with every dorsal reduction. With the thinning of the bone at the rhinion, and extension of ULCs under the nasal bones, when the bony cap is removed, it is possible to preserve the underlying cartilage if dorsal reduction is done gradually in a component rather than in a composite fashion.

Nasal bones attach to the ascending maxillary processes that hosts the attachment of the medial canthal ligament.[23] Lateral osteotomies in (push-down or CHR) or lateral wedge resection (in let-down procedures) should be placed such that the medial canthal ligament is preserved (**Fig. 7**). In DPR, a transverse osteotomy across the dorsum connects the 2 lateral osteotomies. The level of the transverse osteotomy determines the starting cephalic point for the hump reduction. In CHR, the starting point of the nose is determined

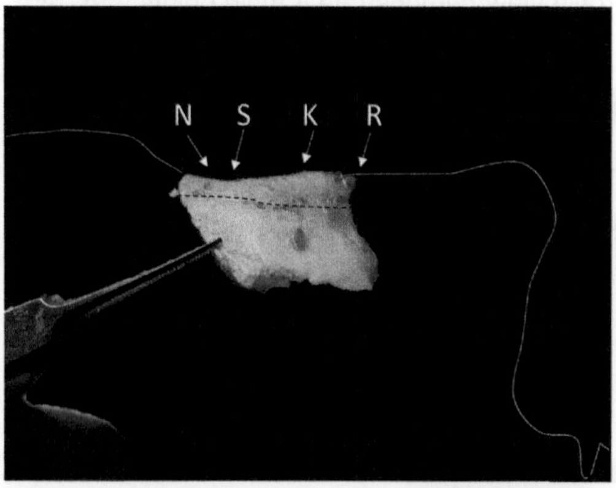

Fig. 5. Example of S-shape bony hump. This type has 4 main dorsal landmarks: the nasion (N), syllion (S), kyphion (K) (prominent), and rhinion (R). *Dotted line*, nasomaxillary suture line.

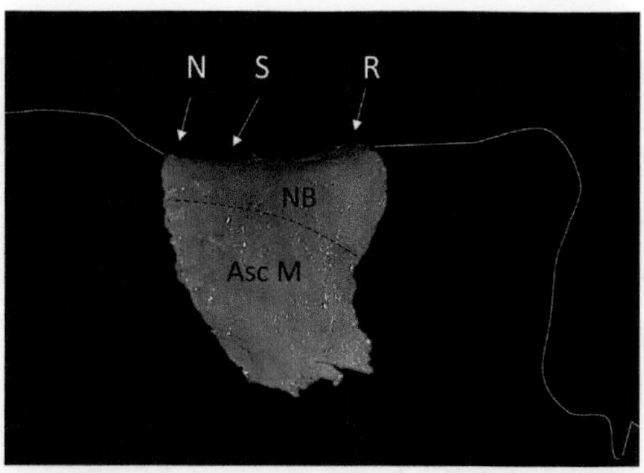

Fig. 6. Example of V-shaped bony hump. This type lacks kyphion prominence. Asc M, ascending process of the maxilla; N, nasion; NB, nasal bones; R, rhinion; S, syllion.

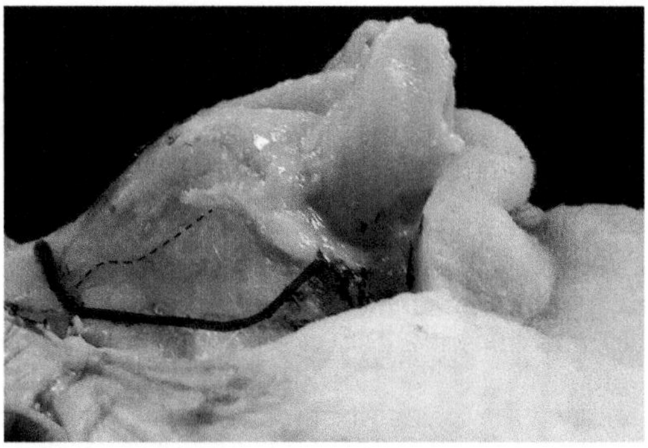

Fig. 7. Osteotomy planning in DPR. Right high-low-high lateral osteotomy is combined with a transverse osteotomy preserving the medial canthal ligament (MCL) cephalically (*red*) and the Webster triangle caudally (*blue*).

directly by where the reduction terminates. In subjects with convexity at the nasofrontal junction (shallow radix), the use of a curved radix rasp can help to reduce the nasal bone at this site, determining the start point of hump reduction.

THE KEYSTONE AREA (DORSAL KEYSTONE AREA AND LATERAL KEYSTONE AREA)

There are 2 surfaces of the nasal bones: dorsal and lateral. Thinner bone exists at the junction between these surfaces bilaterally, that hosts the convex curvature of the ULCs (**Fig. 8**). This junction, along with the ULCs, contributes to the DALs and is considered a portion of the lateral keystone area (LKA; see **Fig. 8**).[9] The attachment of the ULC to both the undersurface of the nasal bone and the cartilaginous septum at the midline is known as the dorsal keystone area (DKA; **Figs. 9** and **10**).[24,25] This complex also involves the fusion between the periosteum of the nasal bones and the perichondrium of the ULC (**Figs. 11** and **12**). The overlap between the ULCs and nasal bones is variable in length (average 9 mm; **Fig. 13**).[14,26] This overlap extends both under the dorsal surface of the nasal bones, thereby contributing to the DKA, and under the lateral aspect of the nasal bones. This lateral overlap makes up the LKA. **Fig. 10** shows a coronal section at the level of the keystone area, showing the overlap of the bony and cartilaginous components of both the DKA and LKA (see **Figs. 8** and **10**). Laterally, the transition of the cartilaginous component from the DKA to the LKA has been reported to be either continuous, rounded stepped, sharp-edged stepped, or a minimal joint.[9]

In DPR, the DKA and LKA are preserved, whereas they are resected in composite CHR. In component resection, the bony cap is incrementally rasped, allowing for preservation of the cartilaginous components of the keystone area where possible. At the midline, the cartilaginous component of the DKA, including the septal cartilage and ULCs, is seen extending under the nasal bones (see **Fig. 9**), with a cartilage to bone ratio of 1.6:1 in the specimens we dissected. The overlap between ULC and the maxillary side wall fades laterally.[1,8]

UPPER LATERAL CARTILAGE AND THE INTERNAL NASAL VALVE

The middle third of the nose is formed anatomically by the paired ULCs that fuse with the septum

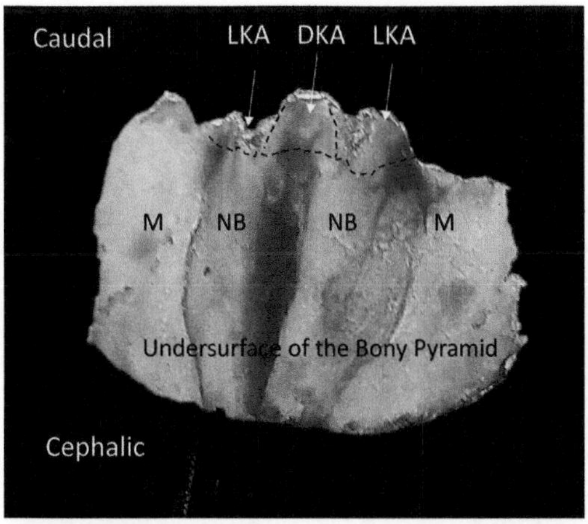

Fig. 8. Undersurface of the nasal pyramid. Under surface demonstrates dorsal and lateral surfaces of the nasal bones (NB) that correspond with the DKA and LKA. Thinner bone exists between them to host the ULC curvatures. M, maxilla.

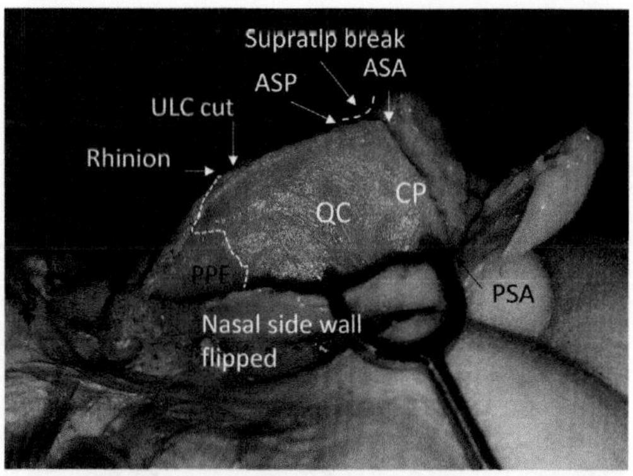

Fig. 9. Sagittal view of the DKA. The osseocartilaginous structure of the DKA in a sagittal view shows the quadrangular cartilage (QC) extension under the nasal bones (NB). ASA, anterior septal angle; ASP, anterior septal prominence; CP, caudal point; PPE, perpendicular plate of ethmoid; PSA, posterior septal angle.

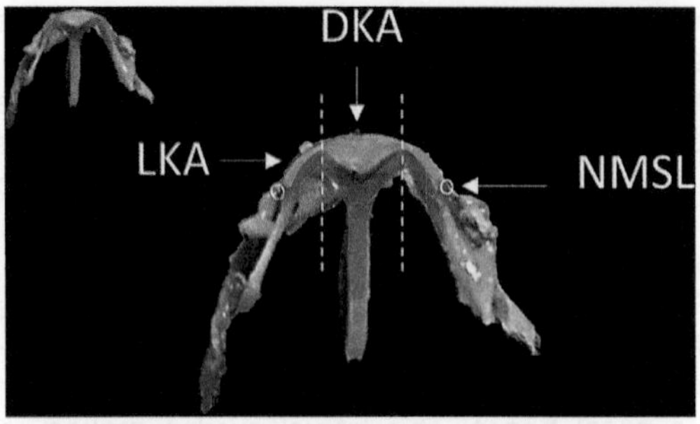

Fig. 10. Coronal cross-section at the keystone area. *Yellow* shows bony component of the DKA. *Green,* bony component of the LKA. *Light blue,* cartilaginous component of the DKA (medial wings of the ULC + septal cartilage). Darker blue: cartilaginous component of the LKA. *White circles,* nasomaxillary suture line (NMSL).

at the midline and superiorly to nasal bones. Dorsally, The ULCs are closely related to the septal quadrangular cartilage (QC), where 3 regions of this relationship can be identified:

a. Cephalically, there is an anatomic fusion between the QC and ULC.[27] On cross-section, the shape of this fusion evolves from a cephalic Y-shaped fusion, to a T shape, and then a caudal inverted V (**Fig. 14**).
b. More caudally, the medial edge of the ULC are seen separate from the septal cartilage. However, the transverse fibers of the perichondrium hold the ULC and QC complex together. This relationship, known as the paraseptal cleft, can be appreciated upon dissection of the inner nasal lining (**Fig. 15**).[28] Upon dissection of multiple cadaveric specimens, we have found this cleft to measure between 3 and 15 mm.
c. The W point (or caudal separation), where the ULCs have a free distal medial border. At this point, the ULCs edges end before the anterior septal angle (ASA) (see **Fig. 15**A).

DPR preserves the dorsal configuration of the ULC and its attachments. Therefore, it theoretically maintains the INV angle,[29] bounded by the septum medially and cephalic edge of the ULC laterally.[29,30] In the push-down technique, the lateral nasal wall is pushed medially, which is transmitted to the ULCs. This results in objective narrowing of the INV, as we have demonstrated in a cadaveric study.[29] In the let-down technique, the nasal wall and subsequently ULCs are not medialized, preserving the INV dimensions.[29]

In component CHR resection, the cartilaginous structure of the keystone area can be preserved, providing autospreader flaps to reconstruct the midvault.[31–33] This helps to reestablish a functional valve and an aesthetically pleasing dorsal contour.[34–36] We have demonstrated that the CHR with osteotomies to close an open roof defect and autospreader flaps preserves the INV dimensions.[29] Autospreader flaps also minimize development of an inverted V deformity, particularly when resecting a high dorsum. In composite CHR, this may not be feasible, requiring additional grafting material for spreader grafts. Regardless, some form of midvault reconstruction is necessary in CHR.

The ULCs has 3 lateral attachments (**Fig. 16**):

a. A superolateral attachment to the lateral undersurface of the nasal bones forming the LKA.

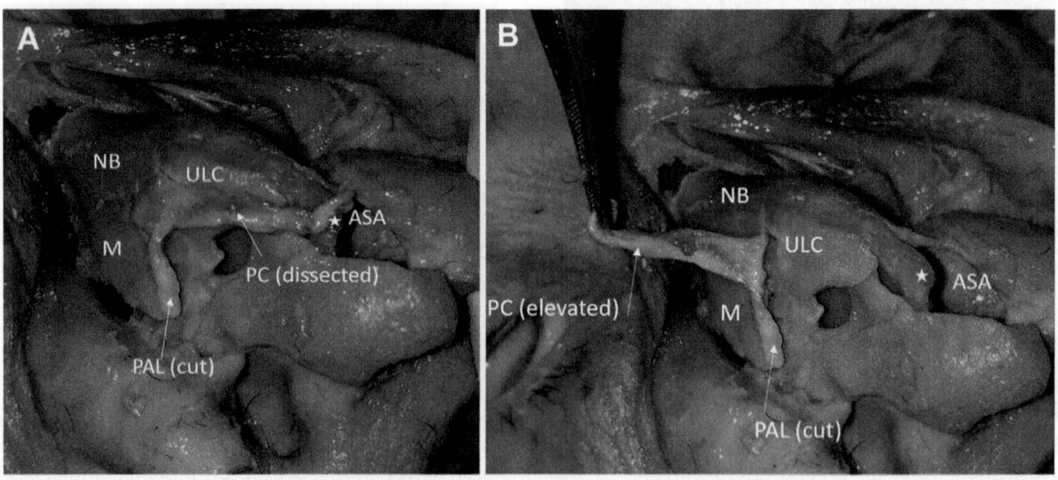

Fig. 11. Perichondrium structure at the keystone area. Dissection of perichondrium (PC) over the ULC demonstrates its continuity under nasal bones (NB). ASA, anterior septal angle; M, maxillary bone; PAL, pyriform attachment ligament. The star represents the ASA.

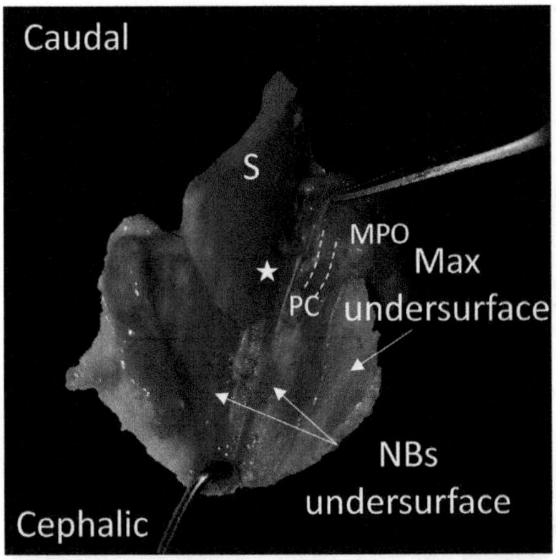

Fig. 12. Mucoperiosteum structure at the keystone area. Mucoperiosteum (MPO) of the bony dorsum is being stripped from the undersurface, showing the adherent fusion with the perichondrium (PC). Asterisk is at the undersurface of the keystone area. Max, maxillary bone; NB, nasal bones; NBs, nasal bones; S, septum.

This forms the junction between the dorsum and the lateral side wall, corresponding with the midpoint of the nasal portion of the DAL. Preserving this attachment is a key aspect of DPR.

b. A lateral attachment to the maxillary ascending process undersurface reinforced by the pyriform attachment ligament. Its release gives flexibility to allow flexion of the convex configuration of the dorsum (see **Fig. 11**).
c. An inferolateral edge ends in a region called the external lateral triangle.[25] This region contains small sesamoid cartilages that may act as pillows for support.[37] The fusion of the inner and outer periosteum from the ascending process of the maxilla forms the pyriform ligament which attaches to the ULCs laterally (**Fig. 17**).[38]

The relation between the caudal edge of the ULC and the lateral crura of the LLCs is referred to as the scroll area, and could be either apposition, alar overlap, or alar underlap.[14,39] This consists of a fibrous attachment known as the scroll ligament complex (longitudinal and vertical).[8,40]

NASAL SEPTUM

The nasal septum is a midline composite structure composed of QC anteriorly and a bony portion posteriorly. The bony septum is formed of 4 bones: the vomer, the perpendicular plate of the ethmoid bone, the maxillary bone, and the palatine bones.[24] The latter 2 bones form the septal crest.

The QC is of hyaline type and is greatly variable. It is responsible for supporting the nasal dorsum from its junction at the DKA to the depression cephalic to the tip (the supratip break; see **Fig. 9**). The QC is securely attached to the ethmoid and vomer posteriorly and maxillary crest and anterior nasal spine inferiorly.[24,41] The interlacing fibers of both the periosteum and perichondrium at these sites results in an adherent junction that can be difficult to dissect.[42] Anatomic landmarks include the following (see **Fig. 9**).

a. The caudal point: most caudal projection of the septum
b. The ASA at the junction between the dorsal and caudal septum. The domes project anterior and caudal to the ASA.[43]

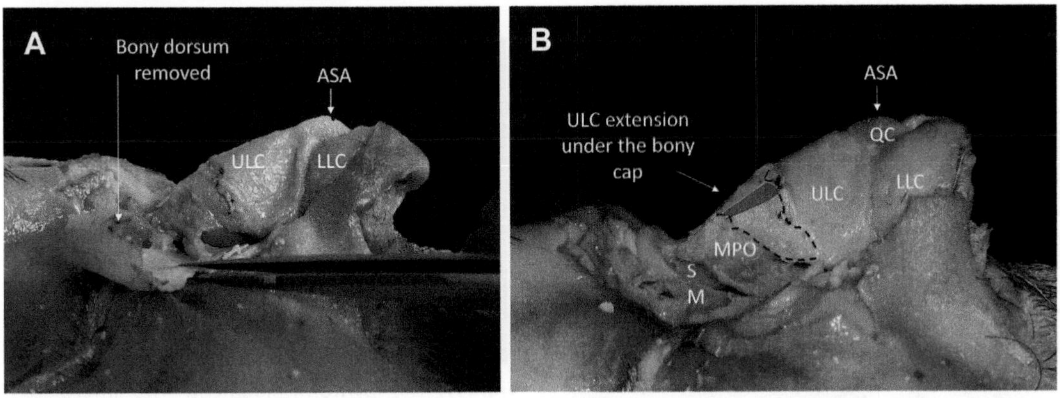

Fig. 13. Cartilaginous component of the keystone area. After bony cap removal in (*A*), ULC extends underneath covered by perichondrium and continues cephalically to fuse with mucoperiosteum (MPO) in (*B*). *Blue transparency* is the cartilaginous component of the DKA, and *red* is the cartilaginous component of the LKA. ASA, anterior septal angle; QC, quadrangular cartilage; SM, septal mucosa.

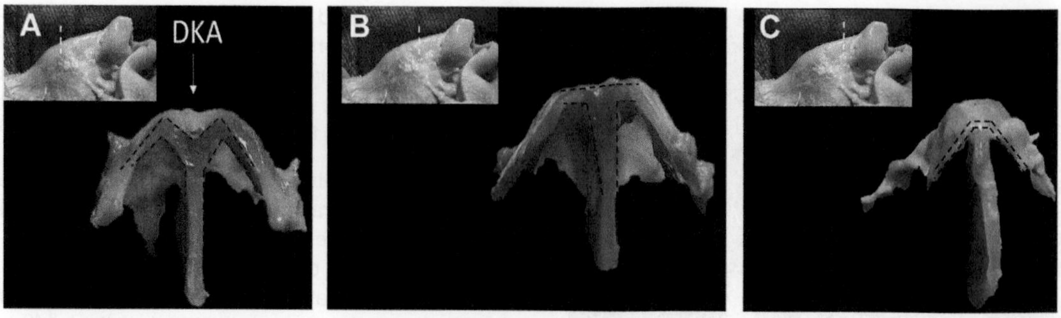

Fig. 14. Configuration of the ULC–septum attachment (*A–C*). Subsequent coronal cross-sections of the cartilaginous complex at 3 different levels showing the change in configuration of the ULC–septal attachment.

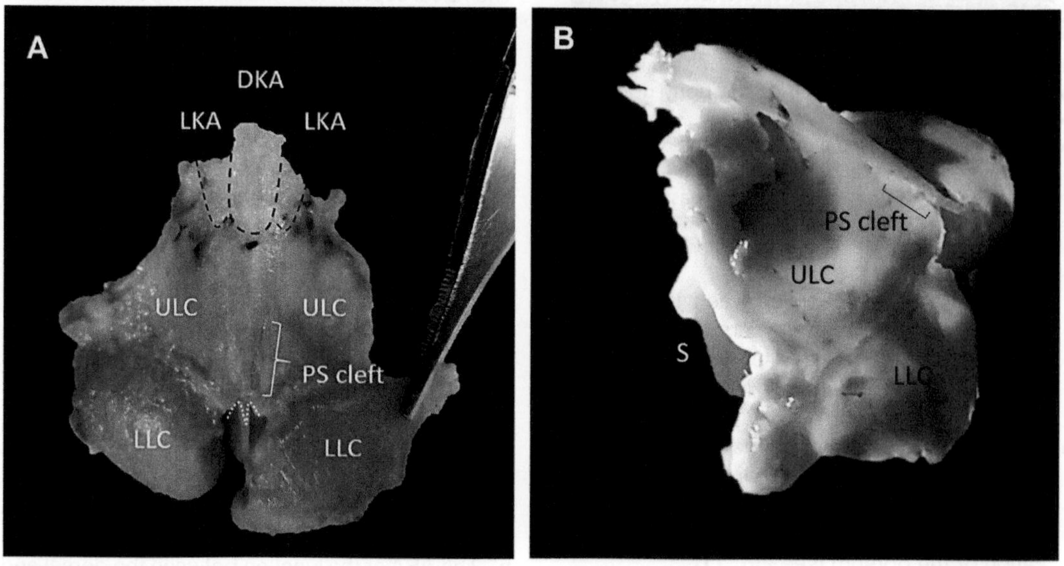

Fig. 15. The cartilaginous framework structure. (*A*) Different components. PS-cleft, paraseptal cleft. *Dotted line*, W-point. (*B*) Transillumination of the PS-cleft.

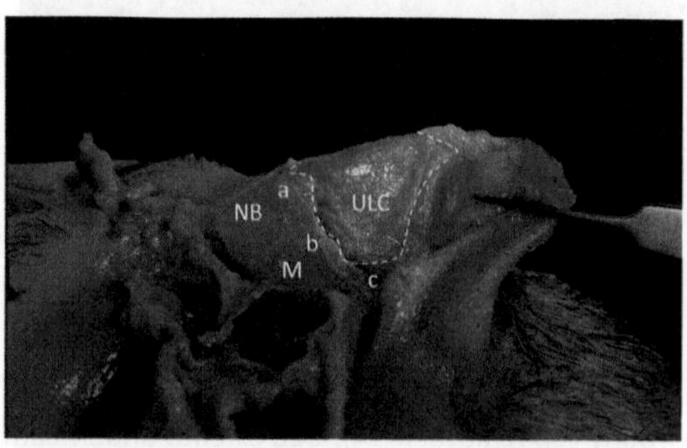

Fig. 16. ULC attachments. The ULC attaches laterally to the (a) nasal bones (NB), (b) the ascending maxillary process (M), and (c) external lateral triangle.

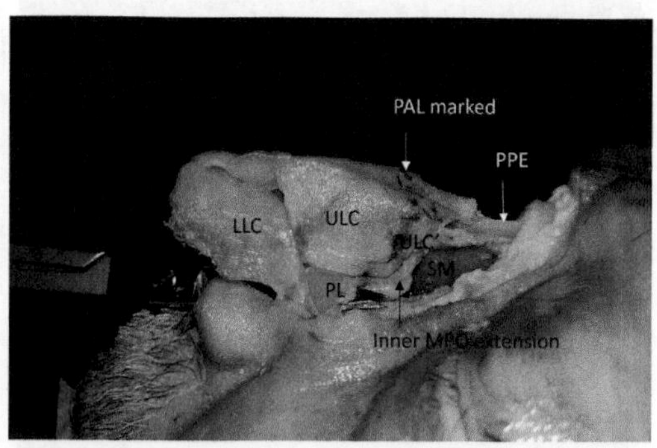

Fig. 17. The pyriform ligament. The inferolateral attachment of the ULC is the pyriform ligament (PL, *blue*). PAL, pyriform attachment ligament; PPE, perpendicular plate of the ethmoid; MPO, mucoperiosteum.

c. The anterior septal prominence, which is the most prominent point on the dorsal cartilaginous septum. This can vary in location from the DKA to the ASA.
d. The posterior septal angle, which is the inferior angle of the caudal septum in contact with the anterior nasal spine.[10]

The expansion of the cartilaginous septum is responsible for elevating the nasal bridge and thereby contributes to dorsal hump development.[44] As previously described, the cartilaginous septum extends under the nasal bones (see **Fig. 9**). This extension in specimens that we have dissected was an average of 59% the length of the nasal hump. This extension is one of the properties that supports the feasibility of DPR, in which removal of a cartilaginous strip with minimal or even without subdorsal septal bone removal allows for dorsal hump descent. Different variations of cartilage resection have been described in DPR with success.[1,4,11,45]

An important consideration in CHR is the need to reduce the dorsal hump before resecting the septum for deviations or grafting needs to preserve a sufficient width of dorsal septal cartilage. In DPR, the septum is resected in part for dorsal descent first, however further resection can be performed for deviations or grafting needs after the hump has been lowered. Unlike in CHR, the amount of septum that can be resected could be less in DPR to preserve the stability of the septum.

Another consideration is the correction of external deviations in the presence of high septal deviations. In this setting, the attachment of the septum to the undersurface of the bony cap may be toward or away from the external dorsal deviation. In DPR, this does not have to be considered because the high septal deviation is not exposed and the entire nasal vault is treated en bloc. Correction of a deviation in DPR is done via asymmetric wedge resections along the lateral nasofacial junction. In CHR, a high septal deviation that is exposed after a hump takedown may limit the correction of the external deviation (**Fig. 18**). In a favorable high deviation (see **Fig. 18**B), the septum is deviated in the same direction of the desired nasal bone movement (opposite to the preoperative dorsal deviation) and, therefore, the nasal bone can be effectively mobilized medially toward the deviated septum. In an unfavorable high deviation (see **Fig. 18**C), the septum deviates opposite to the side of intended nasal bone movement (similar to the preoperative dorsal deviation) and thereby limits how much the nasal bone can be medialized. A CHR (with effective medialization of the nasal bones) can be easily used in favorable high deviations, whereas a DPR procedure may be preferred in unfavorable high deviations.

LIGAMENTOUS ATTACHMENTS

The fibrous attachments of the nose maintain the structural integrity of the nose. They can be divided into longitudinal (along the nasal axis), transverse (across the midline) and vertical (between the nasal framework and STE) (**Fig. 19**). The transverse group fuses the 3 components of the LLC and can be subdivided as follows:

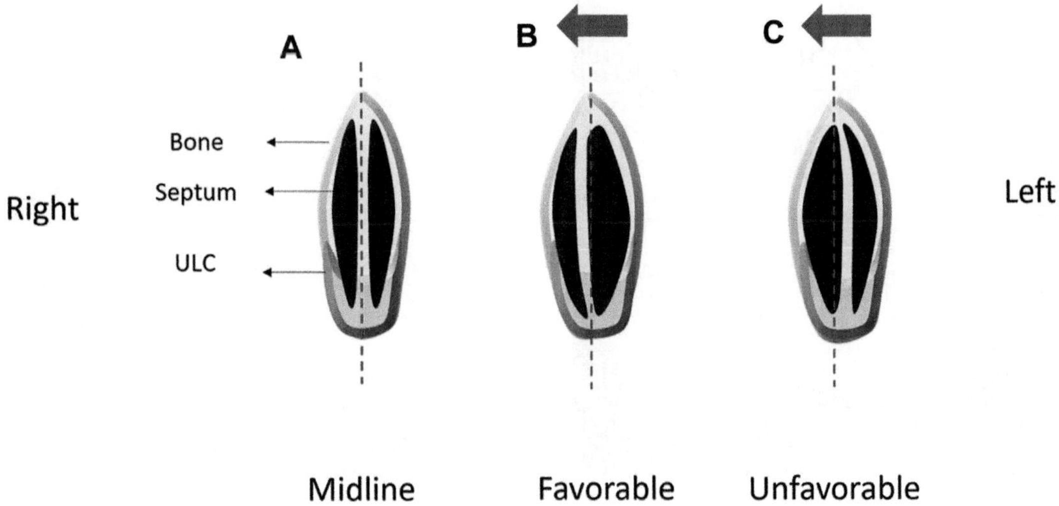

Fig. 18. High septal deviation after CHR. (*A*) A midline septum after hump resection. In a deviated dorsum to the left, (*B*) a favorable high deviation, and (*C*) an unfavorable high deviation. *Red arrow* (*to the right*) shows the intended direction for correcting the left sided dorsal deviation.

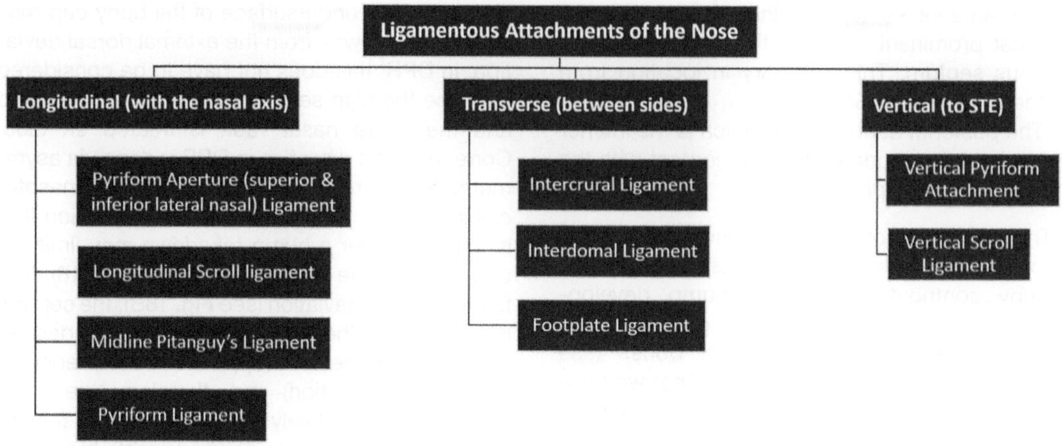

Fig. 19. Ligamentous attachments of the nose. A schema of ligaments longitudinal to the nasal axis, transverse to the axis, and vertical to the STE.

1. The intercrural ligament (ICL) is an attachment between the cephalic edge of the entire alar cartilage (lateral crura, intermediate crura, and medial crura). The component that extends between the lateral crura is known as the suspensory ligament of Converse and passes over the caudal portion of the dorsum and the ASA (**Fig. 20**).[46] The intermediate crura ICL component lies deeper to other ligaments (Pitanguy's ligament and interdomal ligament). The medial crura component accounts for the attachment between the medial crura and the caudal septum near the anterior nasal spine (**Fig. 21**).
2. The interdomal ligament (**Fig. 22**) lies anterior to the intermediate crura ICL and attaches the intermediate crura together at their caudal portion.[40]
3. The footplate transverse ligament lies superficial to the lowermost portion of the medial crura ICL.

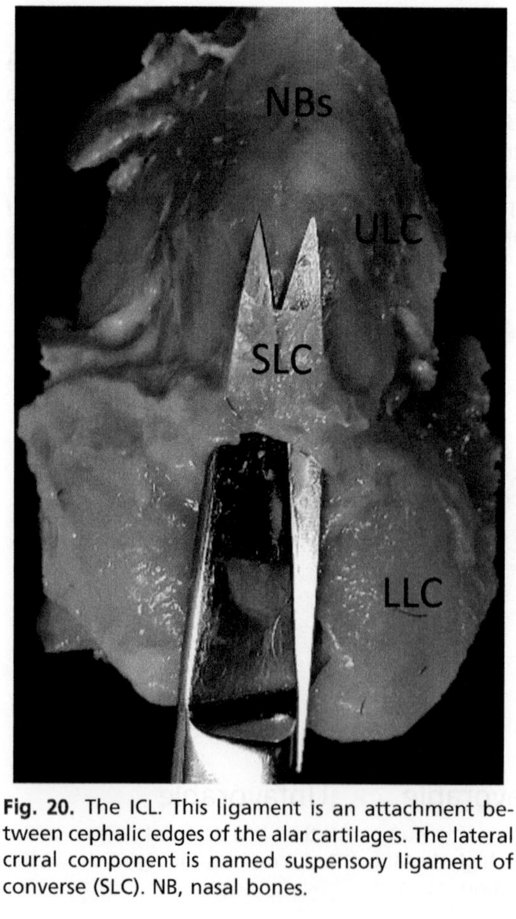

Fig. 20. The ICL. This ligament is an attachment between cephalic edges of the alar cartilages. The lateral crural component is named suspensory ligament of converse (SLC). NB, nasal bones.

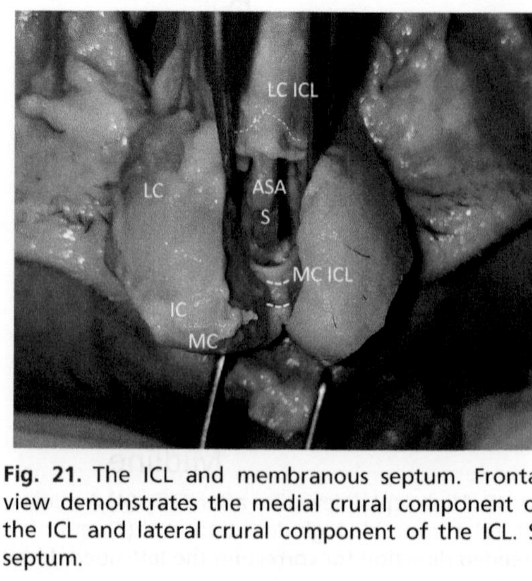

Fig. 21. The ICL and membranous septum. Frontal view demonstrates the medial crural component of the ICL and lateral crural component of the ICL. S, septum.

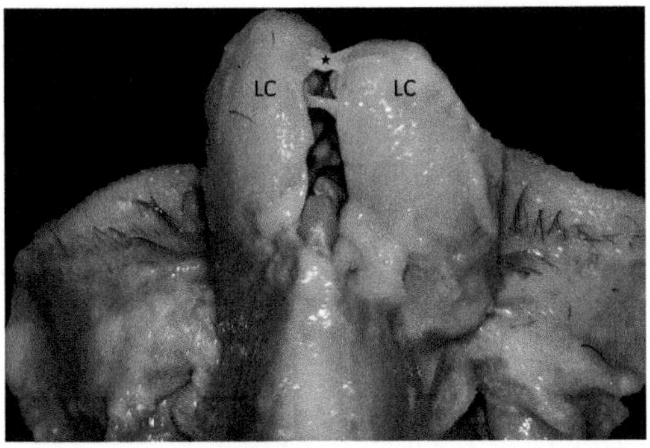

Fig. 22. Interdomal ligament. This ligament (*asterisk*) attaches the intermediate crura together at their caudal portion. LC, lateral crus.

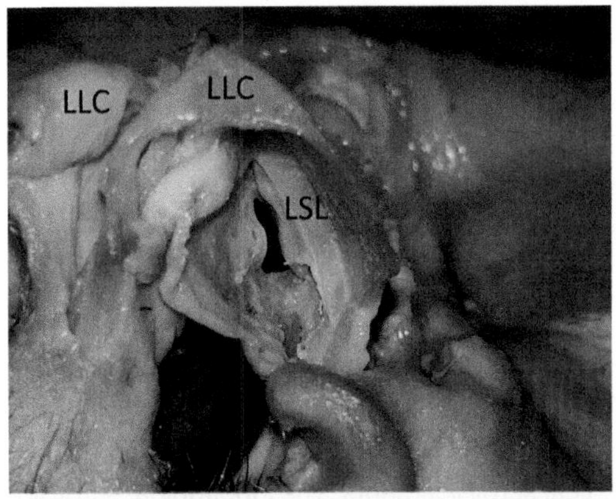

Fig. 24. Longitudinal scroll ligament. After dissecting vestibular skin, the longitudinal scroll ligament (LSL) is shown intranasally between the ULC and the LLC. LC, lateral crus.

Longitudinal fibers include the midline Pitanguy's ligament (MPL) complex[47] (formerly known as the dermatocartilaginous ligament; **Fig. 23**), the pyriform aperture ligament (or the superior and inferior lateral nasal ligaments; see **Figs. 11** and **17**) and the longitudinal scroll ligament (**Figs. 24** and **25**),[8,10,16,40] sometimes described as the intercartilagenous ligament.[48] The caudal segment of the MPL runs between the medial edges of both lateral crura and at the interdomal ligament divides into a superficial and deep layers (**Fig. 26**). Caudally, the superficial MPL continues as the superficial orbicularis oris nasalis and at the columella it runs immediately behind the skin, where it contains a pair of columellar arteries. An interdomal pad of fat lies superficial to the superficial MPL at the nasal tip, whereas the interdomal ligament sits deep to it. The deep MPL lies under the interdomal ligament but superficial to the ASA. Caudally, the deep MPL blends with the depressor septi nasalis and, therefore, has a role in tip movement with activation of this muscle (eg, smiling).[2,7,47,49] Importantly, the deep MPL contributes to the membranous septum and contributes to the attachment between the septum and columella. The scroll ligament complex consists of both longitudinal scroll ligament and

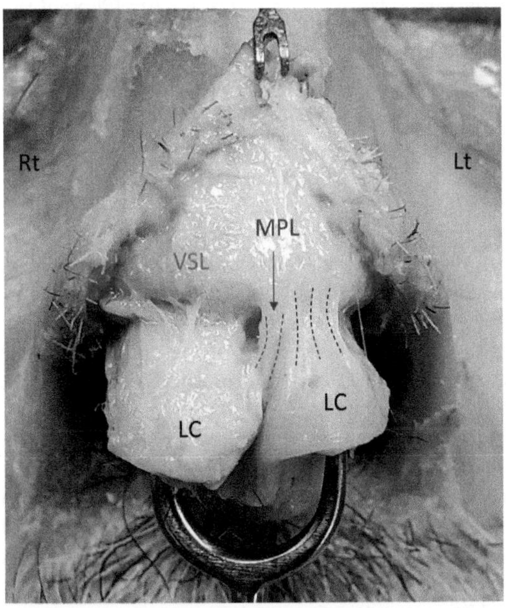

Fig. 23. Caudal extension of the SMAS. The midline SMAS continues as the MPL, and laterally splits into deep and superficial layers at the INV. The superficial layer on the left (Lt) is intact and continues over lateral crus. On the right (Rt) the superficial layer is cut showing the deeper layer that forms the vertical scroll ligament (VSL).

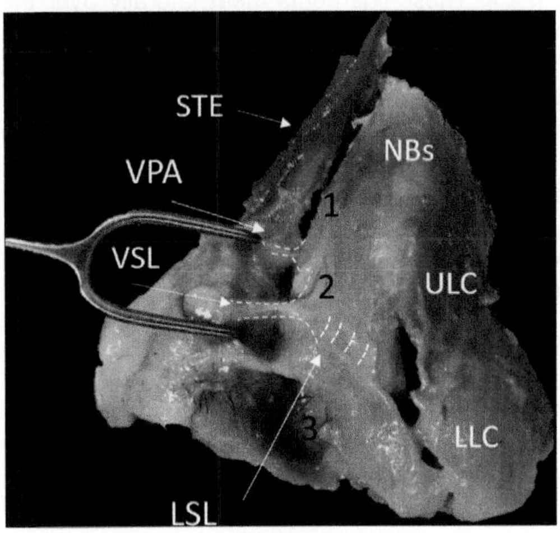

Fig. 25. Vertical ligamentous attachments. The vertical scroll ligament (VSL) is 1 of the 2 vertical attachments forming 3 compartments. LSL, longitudinal scroll ligament; VPA, vertical pyriform attachment.

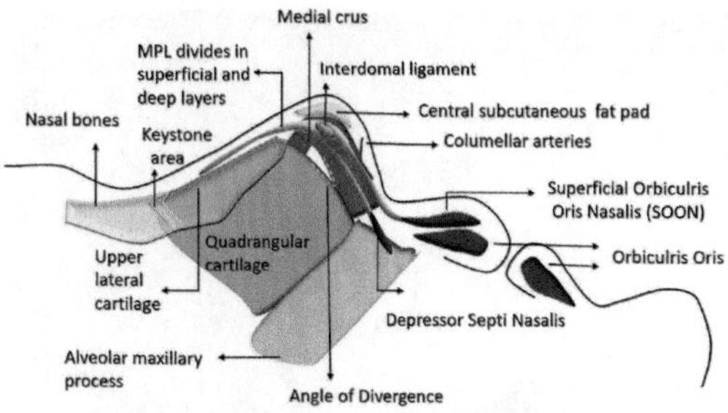

Fig. 26. MPL. An animation showing the MPL extension and division into a superficial and a deep layer.

vertical scroll ligaments. The longitudinal scroll ligament component extends between the edges of the ULC and LLC (see **Figs. 24** and **25**), may contain small sesamoid cartilages, and corresponds to the INV externally.

Similar to the division of MPL (medial SMAS),[7] the lateral SMAS divides into superficial and deep layers. The deep layer allows for vertical attachments between the framework and STE. At the INV, this vertical attachment appears more yellow relative to superficial layers forming the vertical scroll ligaments (see **Figs. 23** and **25**).[8] This ligament allows for motion transmission from the SMAS to the INV.[7] It was assumed that preserving (by subperichondrial dissection) or reattaching the vertical scroll ligaments may accentuate the alar groove, close the lateral dead space, and potentially minimize functional disruption of the airway.[10] A similar vertical attachment exists at the level of the pyriform aperture forming the vertical pyriform attachment (see **Fig. 25**). These 2 vertical attachments divide the nasal sub-SMAS layer (loose areolar plane) into 3 compartments (see **Fig. 25**). These ligaments meet laterally over the external lateral triangle that is devoid of any underlying cartilage.[10,38] These vertical attachments are rich in vessels from the overlying SMAS and require cautery for separation; thus, dissection in a subperichondrial plane would preserve their vascularity.[50] Caudal to the INV, the SMAS continues only as a superficial layer that continues over the perichondrium of the LLC to the skin of the alar margin (see **Fig. 23**).

MEMBRANOUS SEPTUM

The membranous septum lies between the cephalic edge of the medial crura and caudal septum.[51] It contains delicate fibers of the medial crura and intermediate crura components of the ICL (see **Fig. 21**) and deep MPL. Although debated by Daniel and Palhazi,[10] the ICL may also serve as a connection between the footplates of the medial crura and caudal septum creating the angle of divergence (see **Fig. 26**).[52] Iatrogenic closure of this angle can result in tip over-rotation; thus, careful restoration of this relationship is important.[53]

Anatomic relations between the medial crura and the septum include the following:

a. The ICL, which extends from the cephalic edge of the medial crura to the caudal septum. This attachment can be disrupted in a total transfixion incision.
b. The footplate transverse ligament, which creates a cephalocaudal attachment between the footplates and the caudal septum.
c. The deep MPL, which runs through the membranous septum and creates an attachment to the caudal septum.[10]

Surgically restoring this relationship is important when performing a tongue-in-groove procedure for tip stabilization. This procedure was described originally for columellar hanging by Kridel and colleagues,[54] and further elaborated by Most, who noted the angle of divergence (see **Fig. 26**)[52,53] Care must be taken to carefully place sutures at equal distances from the outer edge of both medial crura for adequate control of tip projection, rotation and stiffness.

SUMMARY

Herein we have reviewed in detail the relevant but somewhat complicated anatomy of the nose, as described by surgeon–anatomists, who we have referenced heavily. Our hope is that the reader may use this as a reference while reading the other papers in this issue and understanding the anatomic basis of both preservation and nonpreservation rhinoplasty. For further details regarding the anatomic descriptions reviewed here, the primary literature and textbooks referenced are an excellent resource, particularly the chapter on anatomy in the *Preservation Rhinoplasty* textbook, as well as the fine description of the nasal SMAS by Saban.[2,7] DPR is one of the critical components of preservation rhinoplasty that focuses on preserving the keystone area and the bony cartilaginous interface to provide a natural looking nose. However, not every dorsum can be managed with such techniques, and the versatility of an open structural CHR should be considered. These techniques require an in-depth understanding of the framework and its supporting ligaments.

CLINICS CARE POINTS

- Dorsal preservation rhinoplasty is one of the critical components of preservation rhinoplasty that focuses on preserving the keystone area and the bony cartilaginous interface to provide a natural looking nose.

- Preservation of the keystone area (divided into a dorsal and lateral components) contributes to the continuity of dorsal aesthetic lines.
- Not every dorsum can be managed with such techniques, and the versatility of an open structural dorsal resection should be considered.

DISCLOSURE

Cadavers were obtained through a grant from the Cultural & Educational Bureau of the Egyptian Embassy in Washington, DC.

REFERENCES

1. Saban Y, Daniel RK, Polselli R, et al. Dorsal preservation: the push down technique reassessed. Aesthet Surg J 2018. https://doi.org/10.1093/asj/sjx180.
2. Palhazi P, Daniel RK. Essential operative anatomy for preservation rhinoplasty. Preservation Rhinoplasty 2018.
3. Kosins AM, Daniel RK. Decision making in preservation rhinoplasty: a 100 case series with one- year follow-up. Aesthet Surg J 2019. https://doi.org/10.1093/asj/sjz107.
4. Neves JC, Arancibia Tagle D, Dewes W, et al. The split preservation rhinoplasty: "the Vitruvian Man split maneuver". Eur J Plast Surg 2020;43:323–33. https://doi.org/10.1007/s00238-019-01600-3.
5. Montes-Bracchini JJ. Nasal profile hump reduction using the let-down technique. Facial Plast Surg 2019;35(5):486–91.
6. Joseph J. The classic reprint: nasal reductions. Plast Reconstr Surg 1971;47(1):79–83.
7. Saban Y, Amodeo CA, Hammou JC, et al. An anatomical study of the nasal superficial musculoaponeurotic system surgical applications in rhinoplasty. Arch Facial Plast Surg 2008;10(2):109–15.
8. Saban Y, Polselli R. Atlas d'Anatomie Chrirurgicale de La Face et Du Cou. Firenze (Italy): SEE Editrice; 2009. p. 16. Available at: https://scholar.google.com/scholar?hl=en&as_sdt=0,44&lookup=0&q=Atlas+d%27Anatomie+Chirurgicale+de+la+Face+et+du+Cou.
9. Palhazi P, Daniel RK, Kosins AM. The osseocartilaginous vault of the nose: anatomy and surgical observations. Aesthet Surg J 2015. https://doi.org/10.1093/asj/sju079.
10. Daniel RK, Palhazi P. The nasal ligaments and tip support in rhinoplasty: an anatomical study. Aesthet Surg J 2018;38(4):357–68.
11. Patel PN, Abdelwahab M, Most SP. Invited commentary a review and modification of dorsal preservation rhinoplasty techniques. Facial Plast Surg Aesthet Med 2020;22(2):71–9.
12. BN E. Evaluation of the face. In: Fonseca RJ, Marciani RDTT, editors. Oral and maxillofacial surgery, vol. 2009, 2nd edition. Saunders Elsevier; 2009. p. 1–59.
13. Koury ME, Epker BN. Maxillofacial esthetics: anthropometrics of the maxillofacial region. J Oral Maxillofac Surg 1992. https://doi.org/10.1016/0278-2391(92)90270-A.
14. Drumheller GW. Topology of the lateral nasal cartilages: the anatomical relationship of the lateral nasal to the greater alar cartilage, lateral crus. Anat Rec 1973. https://doi.org/10.1002/ar.1091760307.
15. Bloom JD, Antunes MB, Becker DG. Anatomy, Physiology, and General Concepts in Nasal Reconstruction. Facial Plast Surg Clin North Am 2011;19(1):1–11.
16. Letourneau A, Daniel RK. The superficial musculoaponeurotic system of the nose. Plast Reconstr Surg 1988. https://doi.org/10.1097/00006534-198882010-00010.
17. Peck GC, Michelson LN. Anatomy of aesthetic surgery of the nose. Clin Plast Surg 1987;14(4):737–48.
18. Oneal RM, Beil RJ. Surgical anatomy of the nose. In: Advanced Aesthetic Rhinoplasty: Art, Science, and New Clinical Techniques. 2013. https://doi.org/10.1007/978-3-642-28053-5_4.
19. Jordan JR. Dallas rhinoplasty: nasal surgery by the masters. By Jack P. Gunter, Rod J. Rohrich, William P. Adams, Quality Medical Publishing, Inc. St Louis (MO), 2002, 1200 pp, 2 volume set. Gunter, J. P., Rohrich, R. J., & Adams WP, ed. Head Neck. 2003;25(6):511-511. https://doi.org/10.1002/hed.10248.
20. Rhinoplasty. the art and the science (vol I, II). J Oral Maxillofac Surg 1997. https://doi.org/10.1016/s0278-2391(97)90618-2.
21. Çakir B, Doğan T, Öreroğlu AR, et al. Rhinoplasty: surface aesthetics and surgical techniques. Aesthet Surg J 2013;33(3):363–75.
22. Lazovic GD, Daniel RK, Janosevic LB, et al. Rhinoplasty: the nasal bones-anatomy and analysis. Aesthet Surg J 2015. https://doi.org/10.1093/asj/sju050.
23. Lessard ML, Daniel RK. Surgical anatomy of septorhinoplasty. Arch Otolaryngol 1985. https://doi.org/10.1001/archotol.1985.00800030059006.
24. Hollingshead WH. Anatomy for surgeons. Head Neck 1982;1:497–8.
25. Toriumi DM, Johnson CM. Open structure rhinoplasty for precise control of nasal tip projection. Oper Tech Otolaryngol Head Neck Surg 1990. https://doi.org/10.1016/S1043-1810(10)80018-1.
26. Converse JM. XXV The cartilaginous structures of the nose. Ann Otol Rhinol Laryngol 1955. https://doi.org/10.1177/000348945506400125.

27. Saban Y. Rhinoplasty: lessons from "errors". HNO 2018;66(1):15–25.
28. Straatsma BR, Straatsma CR. The anatomical relationship of the lateral nasal cartilage to the nasal bone and the cartilaginous nasal septum. Plast Reconstr Surg 1951;8(6):433–55. Available at: http://www.ncbi.nlm.nih.gov/pubmed/14891393.
29. Abdelwahab MA, Neves CA, Patel PN, et al. Impact of dorsal preservation rhinoplasty versus dorsal hump resection on the internal nasal valve: a quantitative radiological study. Aesthetic Plast Surg 2020. https://doi.org/10.1007/s00266-020-01627-z.
30. Abdelwahab M, Yoon A, Okland T, et al. Impact of distraction osteogenesis maxillary expansion on the internal nasal valve in obstructive sleep apnea. Otolaryngol Head Neck Surg 2019. https://doi.org/10.1177/0194599819842808.
31. Fomon S, Gilbert JG, Caron AL, et al. Pathologic physiology and management. Arch Otolaryngol Head Neck Surg 1950. https://doi.org/10.1001/archotol.1950.00700020488001.
32. Byrd HS, Meade RA, Gonyon DL. Using the autospreader flap in primary rhinoplasty. Plast Reconstr Surg 2007. https://doi.org/10.1097/01.prs.0000259196.02216.a5.
33. Gruber RP, Park E, Newman J, et al. The spreader flap in primary rhinoplasty. Plast Reconstr Surg 2007. https://doi.org/10.1097/01.prs.0000259198.42852.d4.
34. Moubayed SP, Most SP. The autospreader flap for midvault reconstruction following dorsal hump resection. Facial Plast Surg 2016. https://doi.org/10.1055/s-0035-1570324.
35. Yoo S, Most SP. Nasal airway preservation using the autospreader technique: analysis of Outcomes Using a Disease-Specific Quality-of-Life Instrument. Arch Facial Plast Surg 2011. https://doi.org/10.1001/archfacial.2011.7.
36. Rudy S, Moubayed SP, Most SP. Midvault reconstruction in primary rhinoplasty. Facial Plast Surg 2017. https://doi.org/10.1055/s-0036-1598016.
37. Daniel RK, Letourneau A. Rhinoplasty: nasal anatomy. Ann Plast Surg 1988. https://doi.org/10.1097/00000637-198801000-00004.
38. Rohrich RJ, Hoxworth RE, Thornton JF, et al. The pyriform ligament. Plast Reconstr Surg 2008. https://doi.org/10.1097/01.prs.0000293880.38769.cc.
39. Clark MPA, Greenfield B, Hunt N, et al. Function of the nasal muscles in normal subjects assessed by dynamic MRI and EMG: its relevance to rhinoplasty surgery. Plast Reconstr Surg 1998. https://doi.org/10.1097/00006534-199806000-00027.
40. Janeke JB, Wright WK. Studies on the support of the nasal tip. Arch Otolaryngol 1971. https://doi.org/10.1001/archotol.1971.00770060704004.
41. Park SS. The flaring suture to augment the repair of the dysfunctional nasal valve. Plast Reconstr Surg 1998. https://doi.org/10.1097/00006534-199804040-00036.
42. Schlosser RJ, Park SS. Functional nasal surgery. Otolaryngol Clin North Am 1999. https://doi.org/10.1016/S0030-6665(05)70114-6.
43. Byrd HS, Andochick S, Copit S, et al. Septal extension grafts: a method of controlling tip projection shape. Plast Reconstr Surg 1997. https://doi.org/10.1097/00006534-199709001-00026.
44. Lee SK, Kim YS, Lim CY, et al. Prenatal growth pattern of the human maxilla. Cells Tissues Organs 1992. https://doi.org/10.1159/000147334.
45. Cottle MH. Nasal roof repair and hump removal. AMA Arch Otolaryngol 1954. https://doi.org/10.1001/archotol.1954.00720010420002.
46. Converse J. Reconstructive plastic surgery. Philadelphia: WB Saunders; 1977.
47. Pitanguy I. Surgical importance of a dermocartilaginous ligament in bulbous noses. Plast Reconstr Surg 1965. https://doi.org/10.1097/00006534-196508000-00014.
48. Han SK, Lee DG, Kim JB, et al. An anatomic study of nasal tip supporting structures. Ann Plast Surg 2004;52(2):134–9.
49. Pinto EBDS, Da Rocha RP, Queiroz Filho W, et al. Anatomy of the median part of the septum depressor muscle in aesthetic surgery. Aesthetic Plast Surg 1998. https://doi.org/10.1007/s002669900175.
50. Çakir B, Öreroğlu AR, Doğan T, et al. A complete subperichondrial dissection technique for rhinoplasty with management of the nasal ligaments. Aesthet Surg J 2012. https://doi.org/10.1177/1090820X12445471.
51. Stovin JS. The importance of the membranous nasal septum. AMA Arch Otolaryngol 1958;67(5):540.
52. Spataro EA, Most SP. Tongue-in-groove technique for rhinoplasty: technical refinements and considerations. Facial Plast Surg 2018;34:529–38.
53. Spataro EA, Most SP. Nuances of the tongue-in-groove technique for controlling tip projection and rotation. JAMA Facial Plast Surg 2019. https://doi.org/10.1001/jamafacial.2018.0948.
54. Kridel RW, Scott BA, Foda HM. The tongue-in-groove technique in septorhinoplasty. A 10-year experience. Arch Facial Plast Surg 1999. https://doi.org/10.1001/archfaci.1.4.257.

Dorsal Preservation Rhinoplasty

Method and Outcomes of the Modified Subdorsal Strip Method

Priyesh N. Patel, MD[a], Mohamed Abdelwahab, MD, MS[b,c], Sam P. Most, MD[b,*]

KEYWORDS

- Dorsal preservation rhinoplasty • Structural preservation • Septoplasty • Dorsal hump
- Patient-reported outcome measures

KEY POINTS

- Dorsal preservation rhinoplasty is divided into two related components: approaches to the bony nasal pyramid and management of the septum.
- Several approaches to the septum have been described in dorsal preservation surgery, each differentiated primarily by the location of septal cartilage excision: subdorsal, midseptal, and inferior septal.
- The modified subdorsal strip method (MSSM) allows for a segment of subdorsal cartilage and the entire caudal aspect of the cartilage to be maintained, thereby allowing a structural approach to external preservation rhinoplasty.
- Patient-reported measures suggest improved postoperative cosmetic and functional outcomes in those undergoing the MSSM dorsal preservation technique.

INTRODUCTION

There has been particular recent interest in dorsal preservation rhinoplasty techniques because of claims of superior functional and aesthetic results relative to conventional hump reductions.[1,2] Studies have suggested that rhinoplasty procedures manipulating the nasal dorsum, more so than the nasal tip, have a greater impact on social perception of the nose.[3] Therefore, although the classic Joseph technique of removing dorsal nasal bone and cartilage is a hallmark of rhinoplasty, alternative techniques that avoid dorsal resection have been more recently advocated because of potentially improved functional and cosmetic outcomes.[2,4] The concept of preserving the dorsal nasal architecture was introduced in 1899 by the otolaryngologist Goodale and subsequent technical modifications have since been introduced.[5–11] International rhinoplasty experts published a book in 2018 entitled "Preservation Rhinoplasty" based on this philosophy.[12] This comprehensive text highlights many of the anatomic and technical considerations of preservation rhinoplasty. Fundamentally, dorsal preservation techniques have two related components: approaches to the bony nasal pyramid and management of the septum. This article reviews the

[a] Division of Facial Plastic and Reconstructive Surgery, Department of Otolaryngology, Vanderbilt University Medical Center, 1215 21st Avenue, South Suite 7209 Medical Center East, South Tower, Nashville, TN 37232, USA; [b] Division of Facial Plastic and Reconstructive Surgery, Stanford University School of Medicine, 801 Welch Road, Stanford, CA 94304, USA; [c] Department of Otolaryngology–Head & Neck Surgery, Division of Facial Plastic and Reconstructive Surgery, Mansoura University, Faculty of Medicine, 25 El Gomhouria St, Dakahlia Governorate 35516, Egypt
* Corresponding author.
E-mail address: smost@stanford.edu

Facial Plast Surg Clin N Am 29 (2021) 29–37
https://doi.org/10.1016/j.fsc.2020.08.004

approaches and technical considerations as they pertain to the septal work in dorsal preservation surgery, and incorporation of a modified method for dorsal preservation into structural rhinoplasty practices. In particular, the nuances and outcomes of the modified subdorsal strip method (MSSM), as described by the senior author, are discussed.[11]

THE BONY NASAL VAULT IN DORSAL PRESERVATION

Fundamental to the premise of dorsal preservation surgery is the maintenance of the bony nasal vault and ultimately the dorsal aesthetic lines. An understanding of septal techniques used in dorsal preservation surgery first requires an appreciation for how the bony pyramid is addressed. Although lateral and transverse osteotomies of the bony nasal vault are necessary to allow for lowering of the dorsum, two variations of this approach exist (**Fig. 1**).

The first, which was initially described by Goodale,[5,6] involves single bilateral lateral and transverse osteotomies (without any bone removal), subsequent disarticulation of the nasal-frontal junction, and lowering of the pyramid into the nasal cavity. This technique was further advocated by Cottle and Loring[9] and has become known as the push-down (PD) technique. In comparison, the let-down (LD) technique, first described by Lothrop[13] in 1914, involves similar osteotomies but with the additional resection of bilateral bony wedges along the nasal side wall. The nasal pyramid is lowered and rests on the maxilla as opposed to being advanced into the nasal cavity as in the PD technique. Descent of the nasal bones with the PD technique is limited by the bony attachment of the inferior turbinate to the lateral wall of the nose, and therefore the LD technique has been advocated for humps that are greater than 4 mm in size.[14] The LD procedure can also allow for correction of nasal deviations because an asymmetric wedge of bone is removed between sides. A recent cadaveric study from our group suggests that the PD can cause internal valve narrowing as the bone is forced medially, whereas the LD preserves the nasal valve.[15]

APPROACHES TO THE SEPTUM IN DORSAL PRESERVATION

Both the bony and cartilaginous septum provide support and attachments to the overlying nasal bone and lateral cartilage. Therefore, regardless of whether the LD or PD technique is used, lowering of the dorsum requires some form of excision and further manipulation of the septum. Two anatomic considerations are important in understanding the movement of the septum in reduction of a dorsal hump using preservation techniques. First, the perichondrium of the cartilaginous vault fuses with the periosteum of the nasal bones over the dorsum, and this junction is flexible.[16] Second, septal cartilage extends subdorsally under the nasal bones such that the bony cap sits above cartilage and not septal bone. Therefore, when a portion of the cartilaginous septum is removed, the dorsum, extending from a point cephalic to the nasal bone–cartilaginous vault junction to the anterior septal angle, descends. Also, the flexibility of the dorsum allows the convexity associated with a hump to be reduced during its decent.[1] Importantly, this process results in not only a lowering effect of the dorsum, but also increased rotation at the anterior aspect of the septum and the nasal tip.

Several approaches to the septum have been described in dorsal preservation surgery, each differentiated primarily by the location of septal cartilage excision (see **Fig. 1**; **Fig. 2**). These include a subdorsal excision, midseptal excision, inferior septal excision, and an MSSM developed by the senior author.

Subdorsal Septal Excision

In Goodale's[5,6] original description of his dorsal preservation technique, he accomplished lowering of the septum by removing a segment of cartilage immediately under the dorsum in a PD procedure (see **Figs. 1** and **2A**). Similarly, Lothrop[13] described using subdorsal cartilage resection in an LD procedure. In this approach, which has been championed by several dorsal preservation experts including first Gola and then Saban, an incision is first made along the contour of the dorsal hump immediately under the dorsum and extends to the anterior septal angle.[1,17,18] Minimal to no septal cartilage remains superior to this incision. A more inferior linear cut is made at a location several millimeters below the dorsal cut. The segment of cartilage between these two incisions is removed and represents the amount of desired dorsal reduction.[1,14] As such, the lower incision represents the new dorsal height and corresponds to the intended contour of the nasal profile. Proponents of this technique highlight the control in the design of the lower incision and thereby the ultimate shape of the dorsum. To allow for successful descent of the dorsum, a portion of the subdorsal ethmoid bone parallel to the excised cartilage is also resected. Although a minimal amount of cartilage should remain on the undersurface of the

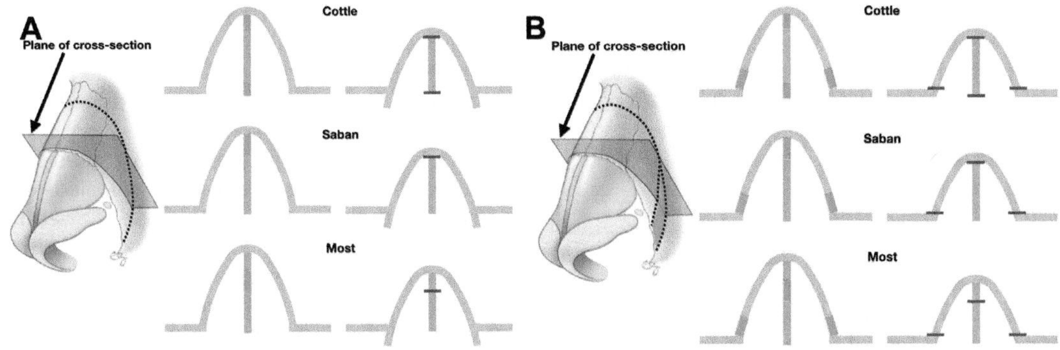

Fig. 1. A three-quarter view of the nose demonstrates the osteotomy sites for a push-down (*A*) and let-down procedure (*B*). Areas of bony resection are indicated in *green*. In each figure, the cuts made into the septum in the subdorsal resection (Saban method), inferior cartilage resection (Cottle method), and modified subdorsal resection (Most method) are schematically depicted. *Green marks* on *left column* indicate areas of septal and bony resection. *Red lines* on *right column* indicate corresponding junctions after inset of nasal pyramid in the push-down (*A*) and let-down (*B*) techniques.

dorsum with this technique, any remaining septum under the osseocartilaginous vault is scored to release tension that may prevent dorsal flattening. Ultimately, the dorsum is sutured to the underlying septum in its lowered position.[17]

Midseptal Excision

An excision in the midaspect of the cartilaginous septum has been advocated for by Ishida and colleagues[19] and Neves and coworkers.[20] With this technique, the subdorsal cartilage is not disrupted and no part of the osseous aspect of the septum is resected. The excision starts from the bony cartilaginous junction and extends anteriorly into the caudal aspect of the septum inferior to the anterior septal angle. In the description by Ishida and colleagues,[19] whereas the septal excision allows for lowering of the cartilaginous nasal vault, the nasal bones are reduced using an osteotome or rasp in a more classic fashion. As such, this is distinct from true dorsal preservation techniques that maintain the dorsal keystone area and where the nasal

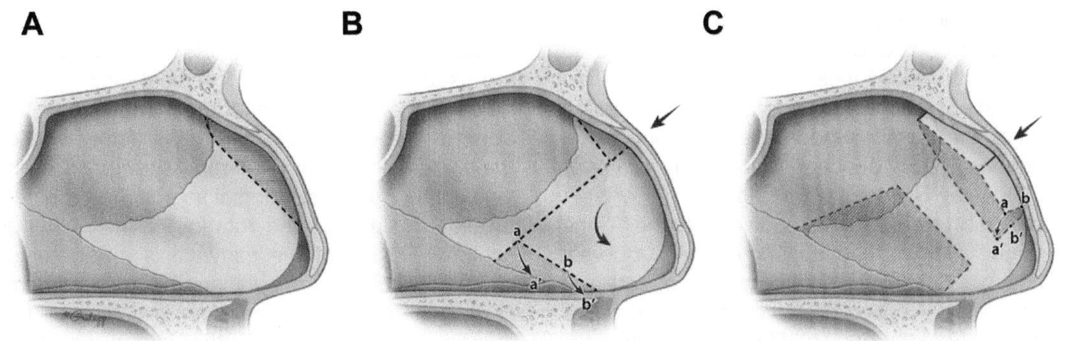

Fig. 2. Approaches to the septum in dorsal preservation rhinoplasty. (*A*) Subdorsal cartilage resection (Saban method). An incision is made immediately under the dorsum following the contour of the dorsal hump. It extends to the anterior septal angle. A lower cut corresponds to the new height and contour of the intended profile. A small amount of ethmoid bone is resected. (*B*) Inferior cartilage resection (Cottle method). Resection of a vertical segment at the bony cartilaginous junction (from the keystone to the vomer) is followed by a triangular resection of the ethmoid bone under the nasal bone. Along the maxillary spine, an inferior strip of cartilage is resected and this corresponds to the degree of desired dorsal lowering. Descent and rotation of the anterior septum allows for flattening of the dorsal convexity (a to a′, b to b′). (*C*) Modified subdorsal resection (Most method). A subdorsal septal resection is performed, but with preservation of a 3- to 5-mm subdorsal strut of cartilage. As the cut is started posterior to the anterior septal angle, a 1- to 1.5-cm caudal strut is maintained. At the apex of the dorsal hump, one or two vertical incisions are made into the subdorsal cartilage. This allows flexion of the overlying concavity. Anterior to the preserved subdorsal cartilage, a vertical resection of cartilage is performed to allow for flexion (and anterior rotation) of the cartilage (a to a′, b to b′).

bones and midvault are treated as a single entity. Nonetheless, a midseptal excision of cartilage, and possibly some bone, could be used to eliminate a dorsal hump while keeping the nasal bones and osseous midvault intact similar to the subdorsal techniques described previously.

Inferior Septal Excision

In 1946, Cottle and Loring[9] described the excision of septal cartilage at the premaxilla in the setting of nasal fractures to allow for adequate mobilization after down-fracture of the nasal bones (see **Figs. 1** and **2B**). When applied to rhinoplasty, they found that a similar resection of a strip of cartilage at the maxillary spine allowed for descent of the dorsum. The amount of cartilage removed corresponds to the amount of desired dorsal reduction. To allow for complete removal of a dorsal hump, this inferior cartilage excision is combined with a resection of a vertical 4-mm segment at the bony cartilaginous junction (from the keystone to the vomer) and a resection of the ethmoid bone under the nasal bone. Similar to other techniques, the remaining septal cartilage and thereby the dorsum is stabilized into position via sutures. The complex cuts within the septum and difficulty with anchoring the septal cartilage to the maxillary spine leading to increased operative times have been cited as challenges with this technique.[1]

MODIFIED SUBDORSAL STRIP METHOD

Technical Considerations

The senior author (SPM) has developed a septal approach to dorsal preservation surgery, termed herein as an MSSM (see **Figs. 1** and **2C**).[11] This structural approach is considered an intermediate between the classic subdorsal and inferior septal resections. This concept has been similarly described by Neves and colleagues[20] as a "split preservation method" and modified into the "Tetris concept." Rather than an immediate subdorsal resection, a 3- to 5-mm subdorsal strip of cartilage is maintained. A cut parallel to the dorsum is made extending from the bony cartilaginous junction toward the caudal septum, but unlike other techniques, this cut terminates posterior to the anterior septal angle. As such, a 1- to 1.5-cm caudal strut of septal cartilage is maintained. The paraseptal cleft, consisting of fibrous attachments between the upper lateral cartilages at the anterior septum, is released to allow for improved visualization of the septum. Importantly, this also allows for unimpacted descent of the dorsum despite the presence of a caudal strut in place. Because the entire caudal aspect of the septum remains intact, it can be used to attach the tripod complex in any desired projected or rotated position. It can also be trimmed secondarily if needed. Although the other aforementioned dorsal preservation septal techniques have been largely performed in a closed or endonasal fashion (with or without endoscopic assistance), an external approach has been implemented at our center for the modified subdorsal septal excision.[1,14,17] This has allowed for the needed exposure to modify the tip with previously used strategies, such as suture modification of the domes, alar spanning sutures, and cephalic turn-ins.[21] Thus, this method fits the category of "structural preservation" rhinoplasty (a combination of dorsal osseocartilaginous preservation and structural external approach techniques to the tip/tripod complex).

Although a triangular segment of ethmoid bone is classically removed in other techniques, the senior author prefers creating a longitudinal cut into the bony septum such that there is slight side-to-side overlap between bone once there is descent of the dorsum. This can only be performed when the bone is thin, or else axis deviation of the bony vault may occur. This method helps limit overdisplacement of the disarticulated nasal vault into the nose with the open approach in which overlying periosteal attachments have been released. If overmobilization of the nasal bones posteriorly occurs, a radix graft using soft tissue or morselized cartilage may be needed.

Eliminating a dorsal hump, much like in the classic subdorsal resection technique, involves a combination of descent and flexion of the dorsum. This corresponds to lowering and anterior rotation of the septum. To allow for this, several strategies are used. First, one or two vertical incisions are made in the remaining subdorsal cartilage at the apex of the dorsal hump to allow for flexion of the dorsum. In addition, a vertical segment of cartilage anterior to the subdorsal segment is resected to allow for unhindered rotation of the posterior septum. Flexion of the midvault is made easier by cephalically disarticulating the upper lateral cartilages from the ascending process of the maxilla (without violating the lateral keystone area). When done in combination, these maneuvers allow for the subdorsal cartilage to be flexed and ultimately anchored to the remaining inferior cartilage.

A particular benefit of this method, as compared with the Cottle method, is that it allows for resection of the lower and posterior septum. As such, septal deviations are corrected, and cartilage is harvested for grafting purposes. Also, because a caudal strut is maintained without disarticulating it from the maxillary spine, there is no need to stabilize the septum to bone. The stable strut, as previously mentioned, allows repositioning of the nasal tip to the desired position. In addition, if the caudal strut has to be removed because of significant anterior septal deviation, it is replaced and stabilized to the subdorsal strut of cartilage that remains attached to the overlying dorsum and keystone region.[22–24] For example, anterior septal reconstruction (ASR), a modified extracorporeal septoplasty technique, has been used with success at our center in conjunction with the modified subdorsal resection.[22,23] In this technique, an ASR graft is fashioned from septal or rib cartilage and anchored to the subdorsal strut with three 5-0 nonabsorbable monofilament sutures and positioned to sit in a groove created in the maxillary spine. If no suitable groove can be created, the ASR graft is stabilized to the premaxilla using a miniplate.[25]

Surgical Outcomes

To evaluate outcomes with the MSSM, after institutional review board approval, retrospective chart review was performed on patients undergoing septorhinoplasty with this structural dorsal preservation technique. Patients undergoing surgery between June and December 2019 for dorsal hump reduction were included. The Standardized Cosmesis and Health Nasal Outcomes Survey (SCHNOS), a validated patient-reported outcome measure, was recorded preoperatively and postoperatively.[26,27] The SCHNOS survey consists of obstructive (SCHNOS-O) and cosmetic (SCHNOS-C) domains (scores ranging from 0 to 100, with 0 being no obstruction or no aesthetic concerns). Descriptive statistics were calculated for the patient population and preoperative and postoperative SCHNOS scores at most recent postoperative follow-up. A paired Student *t* test was used to compare the mean postoperative SCHNOS-O and SCHNOS-C scores with mean preoperative scores. Similar comparisons were made in patient visual analog scale (VAS) results including a functional scale (VAS-F; 0–10, with 0 being no nasal obstruction) and a cosmetic scale (VAS-C; 0–10, with 0 being no satisfaction with nasal appearance).

During this period, 22 patients underwent MSSM dorsal preservation rhinoplasty at our center and completed the SCHNOS and VAS surveys during the study period; 19 were female and three were males. Mean $\pm$ standard deviation (SD) age was 32.1 $\pm$ 11.2. No patient had undergone prior nasal surgery. Ten patients had functional breathing complaints with anatomic obstruction noted on preoperative examination. Of these patients, nine underwent turbinate reduction, nine underwent septoplasty (including three patients who underwent resection of the caudal septum with ASR), and two underwent placement of lateral crural strut grafts. Twelve patients underwent cosmetic surgery alone without any functional elements. Eight patients underwent a PD procedure and 14 underwent an LD operation. Mean $\pm$ SD follow-up was 108 $\pm$ 56 days. **Fig. 3** demonstrates a preoperative, 1-week, and 4-month postoperative example of a patient who underwent a structural dorsal preservation surgery with MSSM. Of note, a structural approach was used for stabilizing and shaping the nasal tip. Namely, tongue-in-groove was used to set tip rotation and projection, and a small cap graft. Bilateral minilateral crural strut grafts, as described by the senior author, were also used.[28]

The patient-reported outcomes of all 22 patients are summarized in **Table 1**. Outcomes are further stratified by the nature of surgical interventions: cosmetic only versus combined functional and cosmetic surgery. Overall, the mean $\pm$ SD preoperative SCHNOS-O and -C scores were 41.6 $\pm$ 31.1 and 62.1 $\pm$ 21.1, respectively. Postoperatively, these scores were 21.8 $\pm$ 17.8 (P = .009) and 6.9 $\pm$ 11.4 (P<.001), respectively. The mean $\pm$ SD preoperative VAS-F and VAS-C scores were 4.1 $\pm$ 2.9 and 2.7 $\pm$ 1.7, respectively. Postoperatively, the mean $\pm$ SD VAS-F and VAS-C scores were 1.82 $\pm$ 1.8 (P = .003) and 9.0 $\pm$ 1.1 (P<.001), respectively. In the patients who underwent a combined functional and cosmetic operation, the SCHNOS and VAS scores improved postoperatively for all functional and aesthetic domains (P<.001). For patients who underwent cosmetic operations alone, the VAS-C and SCHNOS-C significantly improved postoperatively. The VAS-F and SCHNOS-O did not change significantly in this group (see **Table 1**).

No complications including epistaxis, infection, or aesthetic deformity (ie, residual hump) were noted postoperatively. On examination, no patient had evidence of septal deformity, lateral wall insufficiency, or nasal valve stenosis at follow-up. In all patients, including the two who underwent ASR, nasal tip support was deemed to be excellent.

DISCUSSION

Dorsal preservation surgery prevents the irregularities and inconsistencies that may arise with standard Joseph-type hump reductions and the subsequent need for osteotomies to close open roof defects and midvault reconstruction. Success of these techniques requires a combination of mobilization of the bony vault with either the LD or PD maneuver and partial resection of the

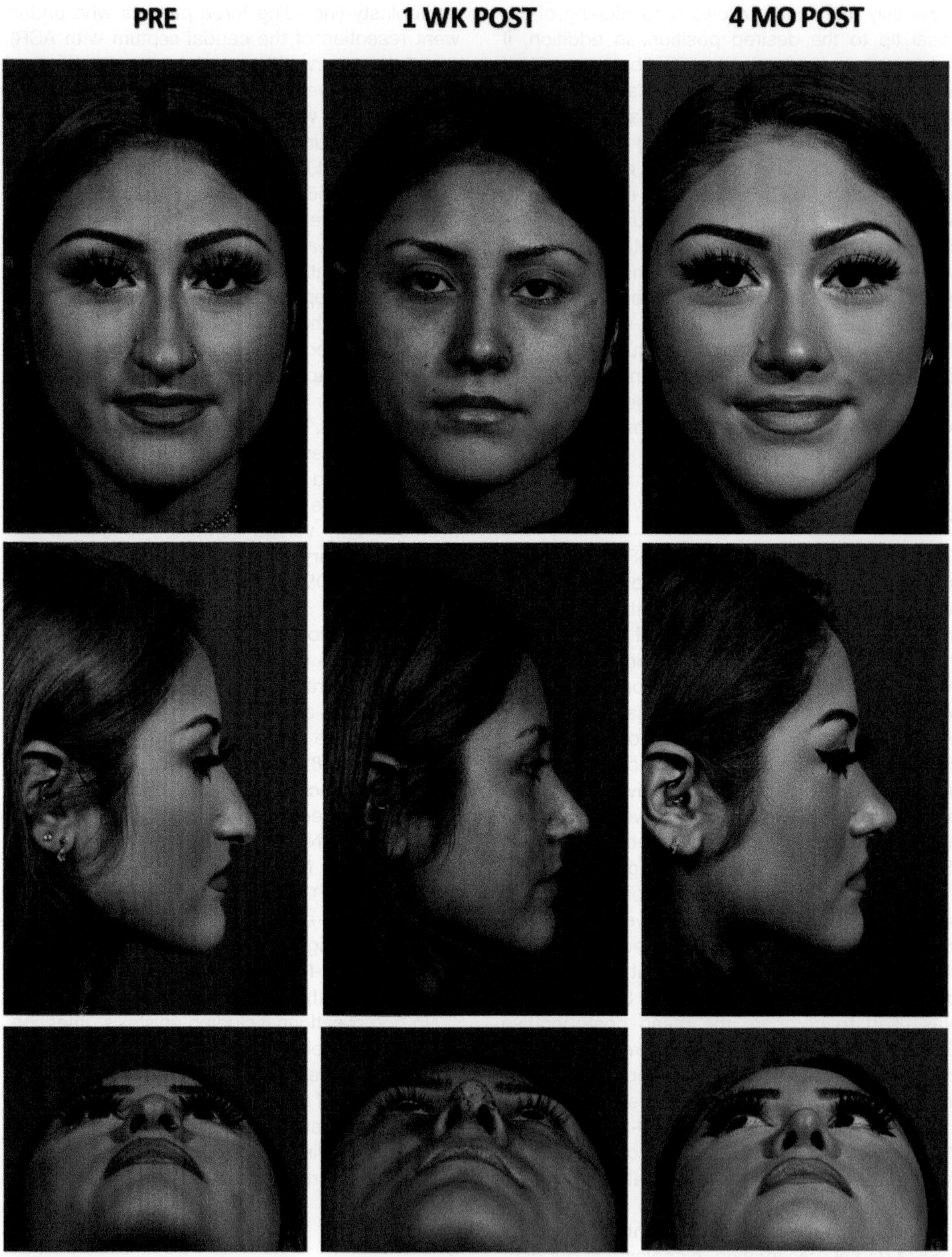

Fig. 3. Representative photographs of a patient undergoing a push-down procedure with a modified subdorsal resection technique. In this structured preservation operation, adjustments to the nasal tip were accomplished with cephalic trims, mini lateral crural strut grafts, tip grafts, and a tongue-in-groove technique. Improvements in external nasal contour with dorsal reduction and improvement in tip aesthetics is noted when comparing preoperative and 1-week and 4-month postoperative images.

Table 1
Patient-reported outcomes with the modified subdorsal strip method of dorsal preservation rhinoplasty

	VAS-F	VAS-C	SCNHOS-O	SCNHOS-C
All patients (n = 22)				
Preoperative, mean ± SD	4.05 ± 2.94	2.68 ± 1.70	41.59 ± 31.11	62.12 ± 21.14
Postoperative, mean ± SD	1.82 ± 1.82	8.95 ± 1.13	21.82 ± 17.83	6.96 ± 11.35
P value	0.003	<0.001	0.009	<0.001
Cosmetic only (n = 12)				
Preoperative, mean ± SD	2.17 ± 2.48	1.75 ± 1.48	20.83 ± 22.45	68.33 ± 15.92
Postoperative, mean ± SD	2.08 ± 2.02	9.25 ± 0.97	24.95 ± 20.56	3.33 ± 4.26
P value	0.463	<0.001	0.314	<0.001
Functional and cosmetic (n = 10)				
Preoperative, mean ± SD	6.30 ± 1.49	3.80 ± 1.23	66.50 ± 19.44	54.67 ± 24.91
Postoperative, mean ± SD	1.50 ± 1.58	8.60 ± 1.27	18.0 ± 13.98	11.33 ± 15.49
P value	<0.001	<0.001	<0.001	<0.001

Abbreviations: VAS-C, cosmetic VAS domain; VAS-F, functional VAS domain.

septum to allow for dorsal lowering. Management of the septum is a challenging aspect of dorsal preservation rhinoplasty and a variety of previously mentioned septal techniques have been used with success.

Several methods for addressing the septum exist, as described previously. Herein we present our preferred method, the MSSM. This differs from other techniques largely in the location of septal excision performed. It varies from Neves' Tetris concept the shape of the cartilaginous cut along the septal quadrangular cartilage bony junction and the bone cuts posterior to this. Like other methods, it allows for a segment of subdorsal cartilage and the entire caudal aspect of the cartilage to be maintained, thereby allowing these structures to be used for attachment of a neocaudal strut and the nasal tip, respectively. In this structural approach to dorsal preservation rhinoplasty, the open technique allows for further modification of the nasal tip. Because there is no disruption of lower portions of the septum posteriorly, septal deviations are removed in the event of nasal obstruction, or cartilage removed for the purposes of grafting. Importantly, we find that the MSSM with either an LD or PD maneuver yields excellent cosmetic results with particular preservation of dorsal aesthetic lines in a small initial cohort. Patient-reported measures similarly suggest excellent cosmetic and functional outcomes with this technique.

The success of other dorsal preservation septal techniques have been reported, although there is a lack of patient-reported or objective measurements in many of these studies. Saban and colleagues[1] describe excellent results in a series of 320 patients who underwent a subdorsal resection technique with endoscopic visualization and either the PD or LD procedure. Thirty patients were given the Nasal Obstruction Symptom Evaluation (NOSE) questionnaire and 90% of these patients reported improvements in nasal obstruction. No objective or patient-reported assessment of aesthetic outcomes was reported. Similarly, the subdorsal resection technique has been used by Gola[18] (n = 1000) and Tuncel and Aydogdu[14] (n = 520) with reports of great functional and aesthetic success but without any objective or patient subjective measures. Ishida and colleagues[19] describe satisfactory functional and aesthetic results in a series of 120 patients undergoing the midseptal cartilage strip resection technique. Again, no patient assessment tool is used in this study and disruption of the keystone area in their technique departs from dorsal preservation ideology. Santos and colleagues,[29] in a cohort of 100 patients who underwent a cartilaginous preservation surgery (spare roof technique), found there was an improvement in aesthetic and functional scores postoperatively. At 12 months postoperatively, mean aesthetic VAS scores showed a significant improvement from 3.67 to 8.44 ($P<.001$), and mean aesthetic scores from a five-question Likert scale (Utrecht Questionnaire for Outcome Assessment in Aesthetic Rhinoplasty) also showed improvement (13.9–7.08; $P<.001$). Mean VAS-F scores improved on the right side (5.13–8.62; $P<.001$) and left side (4.49–8.72; $P<.001$) 12 months postoperatively. Although patient-reported outcome measures are used in this study, this technique does not preserve the bony dorsum and is thus differentiated from other osseocartilaginous dorsal preservation surgery.

A potential concern with dorsal preservation surgery, particularly with long-term follow-up, is the possibility of recurrence of a dorsal hump. Because the dorsal hump is not excised and instead lowered and stabilized to a new position, there is a theoretic risk of a remaining residual hump or the recurrence of a hump with time. No patients undergoing MSSM in the current cohort experienced these complications, although it is unclear if this would change with longer follow-up. Ishida and colleagues[19] report a 15% partial hump recurrence rate in patients who underwent a midlevel septal strip resection. Saban and coworkers,[1] however, report only a 3.4% hump recurrence rate with the subdorsal resection technique. They propose that maintaining any subdorsal cartilage increases the risk of hump recurrence because it makes the precise evaluation of the amount of dorsal lowering required more difficult. In addition, they suggest that the residual cartilage prevents the shape of the dorsum from changing.[1] Tuncel and Aydogdu[14] report a higher (12%) rate of hump recurrence with the same subdorsal resection technique. As such, it remains unclear if there is a discrepancy between techniques with regard to hump recurrence. Tuncel and Aydogdu[14] recommend several strategies to help minimize hump relapse including: (1) scoring any small amount of the septum remaining at the keystone area, (2) performing a lateral keystone dissection, and (3) performing the LD over the PD operation. In the MSSM, a lateral keystone dissection is performed as the upper lateral cartilages are disarticulated from the nasal bones. Rather than scoring the remaining subdorsal cartilage, vertical cuts performed in this cartilage at the apex of the hump allow for adequate flexion and flattening of the dorsum. Finally, multiple sutures placed between the dorsum and lower septum and between the subdorsal strut and lower septum should help minimize the unwanted recurrence of a dorsal hump.

SUMMARY

Dorsal preservation surgery involves manipulation of the bony vault and the septum. Management of the septum represents an integral and somewhat challenging aspect of dorsal preservation surgery with several prior techniques described. These techniques largely differ in the location of cartilage excision performed (subdorsal resection, midseptal resection, and inferior septal resection). The MSSM and Tetris methods allow for the maintenance of a stable caudal strut and a subdorsal segment of cartilage without disruption of lower portions of the septum. Functional procedures, including septoplasty and ASR, and modification of tip position, can thereby be performed effectively. Patient-reported measures suggest significant improvement in functional and aesthetic outcomes after the MSSM.

CLINIC CARE POINTS

- Septal approaches to dorsal preservation surgery are variable, and each have been reported to yield good functional and aesthetic results.
- In the MSSM technique, a subdorsal strut of cartilage is maintained and the cartilage cut terminates posterior to the anterior septal angle, thereby preserving the entirety of the caudal strut.
- To limit overdisplacement of the disarticulated nasal vault into the nose with the open approach, a longitudinal cut into the bony septum is made instead of resecting a wedge of ethmoid bone.

REFERENCES

1. Saban Y, Daniel RK, Polselli R, et al. Dorsal preservation: the push down technique reassessed. Aesthet Surg J 2018;38:117–31.
2. Daniel RK. The preservation rhinoplasty: a new rhinoplasty revolution. Aesthet Surg J 2018;38:228–9.
3. Kandathil CK, Saltychev M, Moubayed SP, et al. Association of dorsal reduction and tip rotation with social perception. JAMA Facial Plast Surg 2018;20: 362–6.
4. Joseph J. The classic reprint: nasal reductions. Plast Reconstr Surg 1971;47:79–83.
5. Goodale JL. A new method for the operative correction of exaggerated roman nose. Boston Med Surg J 1899;140:112.
6. Goodale JL. The correction of old lateral displacements of the nasal bones. Boston Med Surg J 1901;145:538–9.
7. Maurel G. Chirurgie maxilla-faciale. Paris: Le François; 1940. p. 1127–33.
8. Sebileau P, Dufourmentel L. Correction chirurgicale des difformités congénitales et acquises de la pyramide nasale. Paris: Arnette; 1926. p. 104–5.
9. Cottle MH, Loring RM. Corrective surgery of the external nasal pyramid and the nasal septum for restoration of normal physiology. Ill Med J 1946;90: 119–35.
10. Rohrich RJ, Muzaffar AR, Janis JE. Component dorsal hump reduction: the importance of maintaining

dorsal aesthetic lines in rhinoplasty. Plast Reconstr Surg 2004;114:1298–308 [discussion: 1309–12].
11. Patel PN, Abdelwahab M, Most SP. A review and modification of dorsal preservation rhinoplasty techniques. Facial Plast Surg Aesthet Med 2020;22: 71–9.
12. B Ç, Saban Y, Daniel RK, et al. Preservation rhinoplasty book. Istanbul: Septum Publishing; 2018.
13. Lothrop O. An operation for correcting the aquiline nasal deformity; the use of new instrument; report of a case. Boston Med Surg J 1914;170:835–7.
14. Tuncel U, Aydogdu O. The probable reasons for dorsal hump problems following let-down/push-down rhinoplasty and solution proposals. Plast Reconstr Surg 2019;144:378e–85e.
15. Abdelwahab M, Most SP, Patel PN. Impact of dorsal preservation rhinoplasty versus dorsal hump resection on the internal nasal valve: a quantitative radiological study. Aesthet Plast Surg 2019;44(3):879–87.
16. Palhazi P, Daniel RK, Kosins AM. The osseocartilaginous vault of the nose: anatomy and surgical observations. Aesthet Surg J 2015;35:242–51.
17. Kosins AM, Daniel RK. Decision making in preservation rhinoplasty: a 100 case series with one-year follow-up. Aesthet Surg J 2020;40(1):34–48.
18. Gola R. Functional and esthetic rhinoplasty. Aesthet Plast Surg 2003;27:390–6.
19. Ishida J, Ishida LC, Ishida LH, et al. Treatment of the nasal hump with preservation of the cartilaginous framework. Plast Reconstr Surg 1999;103:1729–33 [discussion: 1734–5].
20. Neves JC, Arancibia Tagle D, Dewes W, et al. The split preservation rhinoplasty: "the Vitruvian Man split maneuver". Eur J Plast Surg 2020;43:323–33.
21. Murakami CS, Barrera JE, Most SP. Preserving structural integrity of the alar cartilage in aesthetic rhinoplasty using a cephalic turn-in flap. Arch Facial Plast Surg 2009;11:126–8.
22. Spataro E, Olds C, Nuyen B, et al. Comparison of primary and secondary anterior septal reconstruction: a cohort study. Facial Plast Surg 2019;35:65–7.
23. Surowitz J, Lee MK, Most SP. Anterior septal reconstruction for treatment of severe caudal septal deviation: clinical severity and outcomes. Otolaryngol Head Neck Surg 2015;153:27–33.
24. Patel PN, Kandathil CK, Most SP. Outcomes of combined anterior septal reconstruction and dorsal hump reduction. Laryngoscope 2020. https://doi.org/10.1002/lary.28611.
25. Mittermiller PA, Sheckter CC, Most SP. Efficacy and safety of titanium miniplates for patients undergoing septorhinoplasty. JAMA Facial Plast Surg 2018;20: 82–4.
26. Moubayed SP, Ioannidis JPA, Saltychev M, et al. The 10-item Standardized Cosmesis and Health Nasal Outcomes Survey (SCHNOS) for functional and cosmetic rhinoplasty. JAMA Facial Plast Surg 2018;20:37–42.
27. Saltychev M, Kandathil CK, Abdelwahab M, et al. Psychometric properties of the Standardized Cosmesis and Health Nasal Outcomes Survey: item response theory analysis. JAMA Facial Plast Surg 2018;20:519–21.
28. Abdelwahab M, Most SP. The miniature lateral crural strut graft: efficacy of a novel technique in tip plasty. Laryngoscope 2020. https://doi.org/10.1002/lary.28530.
29. Santos M, Rego AR, Coutinho M, et al. Spare roof technique in reduction rhinoplasty: prospective study of the first one hundred patients. Laryngoscope 2019;129:2702–6.

Key Points in Subperichondrial-Subperiosteal Dissection

Bülent Genç, MD[a,*], Ali Murat Akkuş, MD[b], Barış Çakır, MD[c]

KEYWORDS

• Preservation rhinoplasty • Subperichondrial dissection • Subperiosteal dissection

KEY POINTS

- Subperichondrial-subperiosteal dissection in rhinoplasty ensures minimal trauma to soft tissues.
- This plane of dissection provides better healing by avoiding fibrosis and preserving the important ligament system of the nose.
- It generates a cover over the reconstructed osseocartilaginous framework.
- The learning curve may seem steep but, once mastered, this technique is faster compared to sub-SMAS plane.
- Respecting the key points in dissection and appropriate instrumentation are important.

INTRODUCTION

The subperichondrial-subperiosteal technique (SSDT) has started to gain popularity after the year 2013.[1] In SSDT, the perichondrium and periosteum protect the adipomuscular layer of the nose from dissection and retraction trauma, and thereby minimizes soft tissue injury.[2] Faster healing can be achieved in primary rhinoplasty patients. The 20-day postoperative result of a primary rhinoplasty with SSDT can be seen as an example (**Fig. 1**). Preservation of the scroll and Pitanguy ligaments was achievable with the dissection of the perichondrium.[1] The positive effect of the Pitanguy and scroll ligaments on projection and definition of the nasal tip has started to gain acceptance in the scientific arena.[3–5] By means of the preservation of the ligaments, the need for soft tissue resections or onlay tip grafts is rare. It is possible to achieve satisfying results in the long term with the SSD technique. The postoperative 7-year result of a patient with SSDT can be seen in **Fig. 2**.

There is a learning curve of SSDT. Especially the dissection of the perichondrium of the nasal tip cartilages is not easy. Cartilages can be injured if dissection is not commenced at the correct location.[2] Many surgeons have reported feedback such as "I have difficulty in getting under the perichondrium over the nasal dorsum and lateral crura" or "the perichondrium gets torn." The localizations where it is easier to dissect the perichondrium and periosteum and the surgical instrumentation have been noted down. By way of this article, the authors attempt to see that the SSDT that they have been using since 2008 is used by more surgeons.

PATIENTS AND TECHNIQUE

The aforementioned surgeons have routinely used the SSDT between the years 2008 and 2019 in more than 4000 rhinoplasties.

[a] Caddebostan Mah. Çam Fıstığı Sk No:1 A Blok D:3 Kadıköy, Istanbul; [b] Abdi İpekçi Caddesi No:39, Hayal Apt. D:2, Nişantaşı Şişli, Şişli, Istanbul 34800, Turkey; [c] Abdi İpekçi No 53 Side Apt., Şişli, Istanbul, Turkey
* Corresponding author.
E-mail address: bulentgencmd@gmail.com

Facial Plast Surg Clin N Am 29 (2021) 39–45
https://doi.org/10.1016/j.fsc.2020.09.002

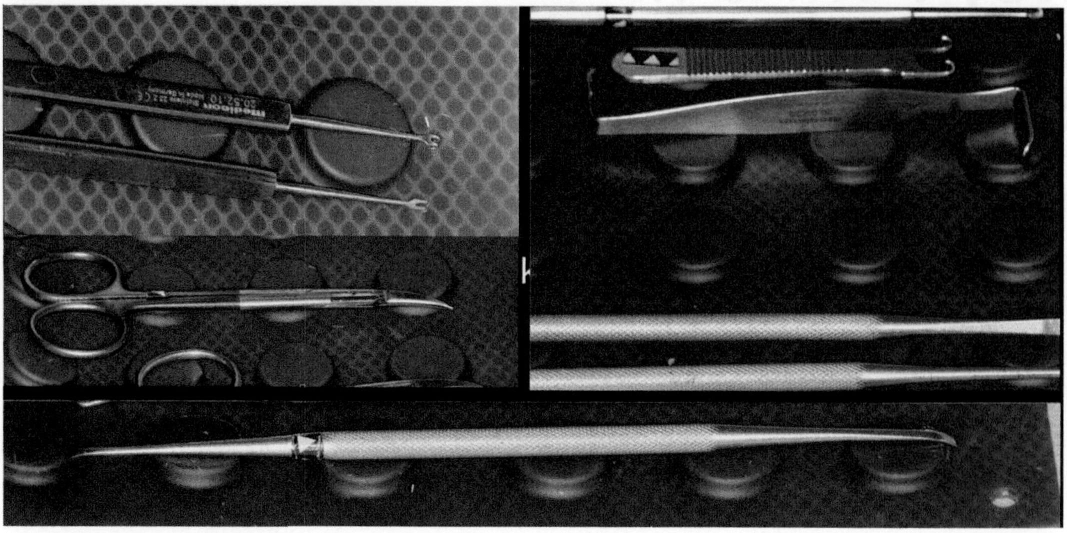

Fig. 1. Key points of SSDT.

SURGICAL INSTRUMENTATION NECESSARY FOR SUBPERICHONDRIAL-SUBPERIOSTEAL DISSECTION TECHNIQUE

It is troublesome to apply SSDT without using the right instruments in the right order. It is almost impossible to perform the technique with traditional elevators or thick-tipped scissors. The instruments required for SSDT are Crile retractor (Medicon, Germany), Daniel-Cakir elevator (Medicon, Germany), Çerkeş scissors (Marina Medical, USA), double hook retractor (Medicon, Germany) (**Fig. 3**).

Five principal key points have been identified for SSDT (**Fig. 4**).

1. *Posterior septal angle:* the septum is thicker close to the maxillary spine. It is not rare to encounter more than one layer of perichondrium in the floor of the septum. Dissection at the anterior septal angle is difficult because the cartilage is thin and there is a single layer of perichondrium. The septum is reached through a transfixion incision made on the caudal septum (**Fig. 5**A). The caudal septum becomes visible after mucosa is cut at a depth of 1 to 2 mm. The caudal septum is incised so that a 0.5 to 1 mm strip of cartilage is left attached to the Pitanguy ligament that courses along the membranous septum (**Fig. 5**B). The strip of cartilage left attached to the Pitanguy ligament is called "the posterior strut."[1] After septal caudal resection is finished, projection is controlled by suturing the posterior strut cartilage back to the septum at a desired level. The perichondrium on both sides of the posterior septal angle is scratched with a number 15 blade. This maneuver creates a plane for the elevator to get under the perichondrium. Thin and moderately sharp elevators need to be used at this location. The most convenient instrument is the perichondrial tip of the Daniel-Cakir elevator (**Fig. 5**C). The perichondrium of the posterior septal angle is dissected 3 to 4 mm posteriorly. The elevator is moved toward the anterior septal angle, and the caudal septum is easily revealed (**Fig. 5**D).
2. *W point:* the area where the dorsal septum unites with the upper lateral cartilages is named as the W point by Saban and Palhazi, as it resembles the letter W.[6] The caudal septum should be dissected first to reach the W point. The Crile retractor and the Cerkes scissors (Marina Medical) are indispensable at this stage. The thin end of the Crile retractor is advanced until the internal valve level and the tissues are retracted anteriorly (**Fig. 6**A). The blades of the scissors

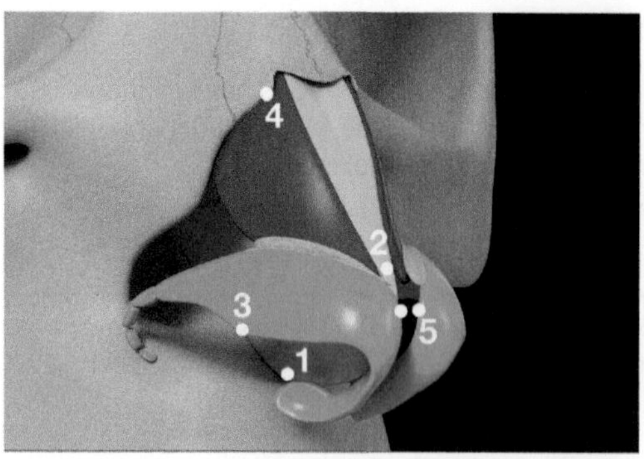

Fig. 2. Five principal key points for SSDT.

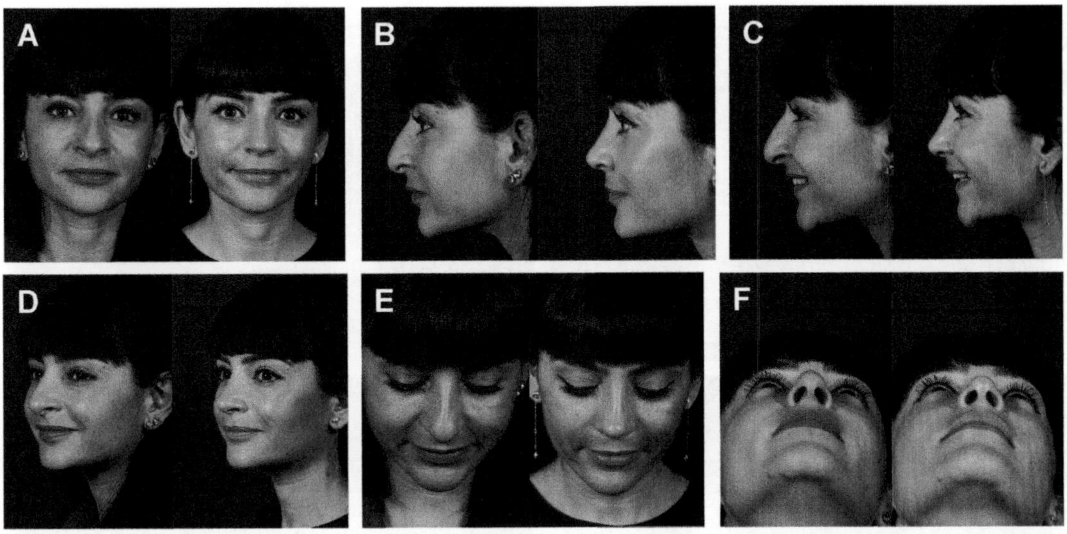

Fig. 3. (*A–F*) Standard before and after studio photographs of a patient's 7 years postoperative follow-up after rhinoplasty with SSDT.

are held so that they are parallel to the nasal dorsum. The blades of the scissors are opened 3 to 4 mm and closed, and the upper lateral cartilages are reached. Dorsal perichondrium starts from the W point. It is more difficult to find the dorsal perichondrium from the scroll region. The perichondrium is dissected for 1 to 3 mm over the W point with the sharp tips of the scissors (**Fig. 6**B). Dissection is carried out dorsally for 4 to 5 mm with Daniel-Cakir elevator (**Fig. 6**C). The perichondrium of the upper lateral cartilages is dissected until the scroll ligament is encountered with a sweeping movement to the right and left (**Fig. 6**D).

3. *Lateral crural turning point:* this is one of the regions where the lateral crus is the thickest. Rim flap technique, as the posterior strut, facilitates subperichondrial dissection[7] (**Fig. 7**A). After the incision, small double hooks are placed to the mucosa of the lower lateral cartilage, and care is given not to pierce the cartilage. The assistant is asked to pull the hooks inferiorly. The skin is elevated with microforceps. Perichondrium is rendered visible along the caudal edge using the reverse side of number 15 blade (**Fig. 7**B). A pocket big enough for the Daniel elevator is created with Cerkes scissors

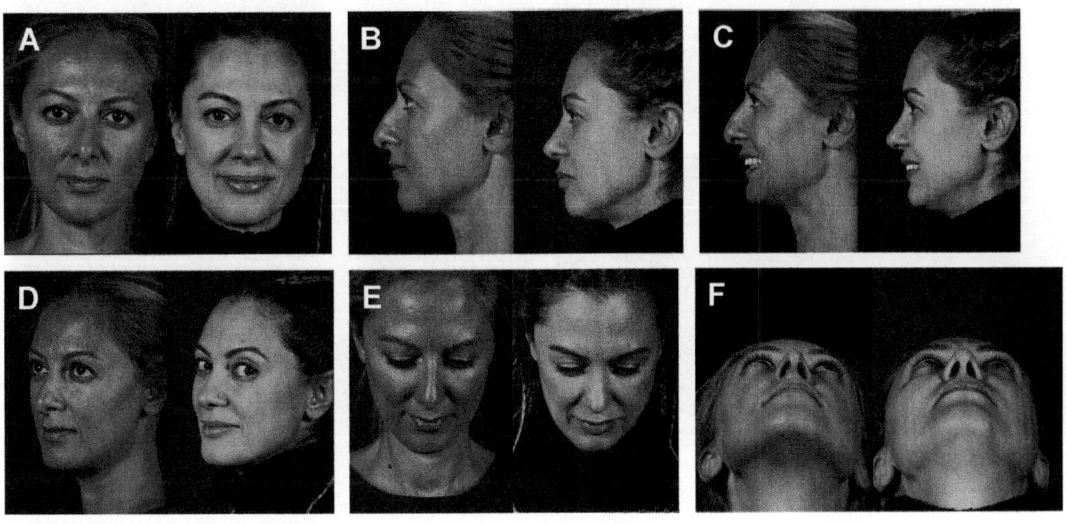

Fig. 4. Instruments used for SSDT.

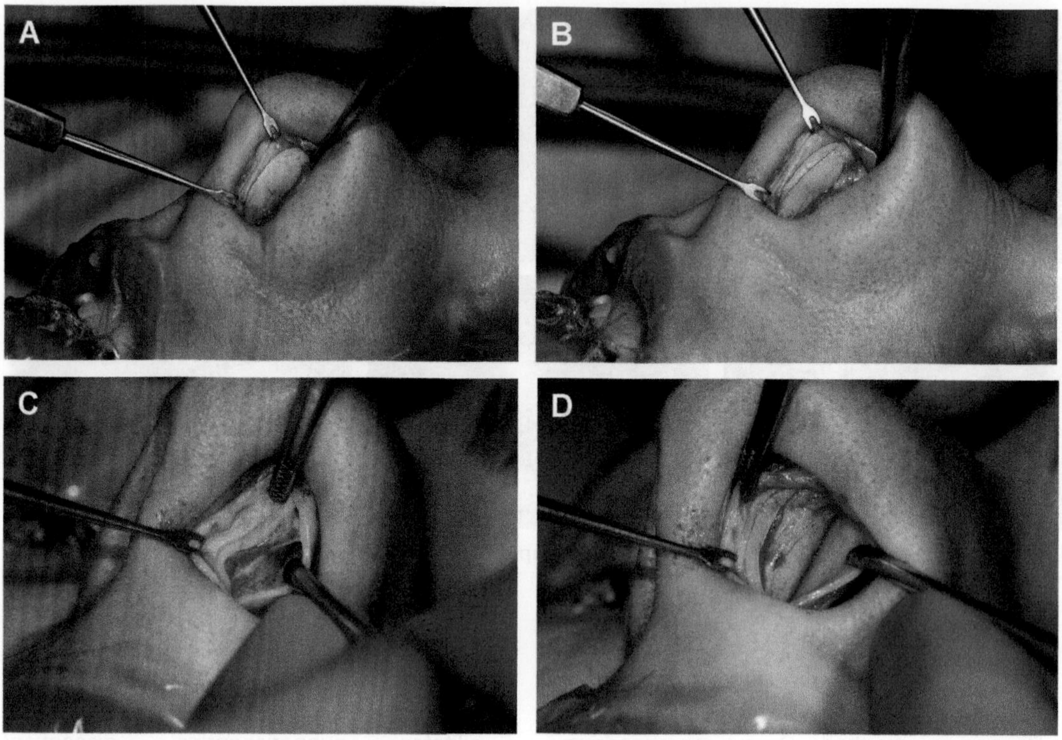

Fig. 5. (*A–D*) SSDT first key point. Posterior septal angle.

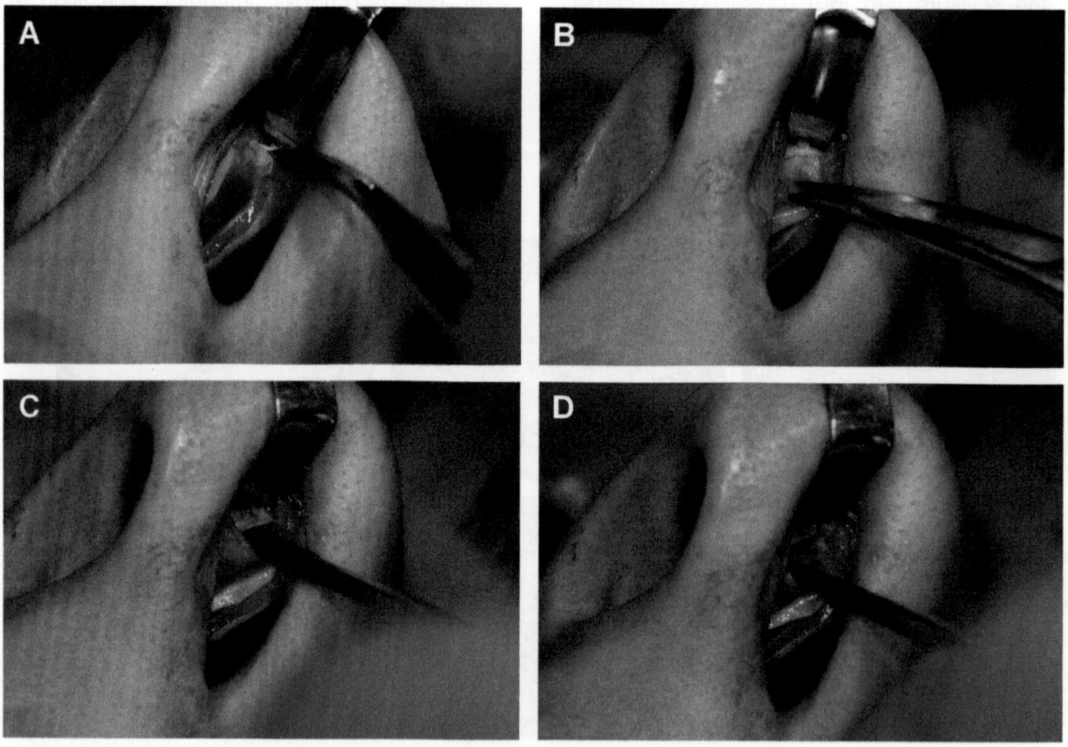

Fig. 6. (*A–D*) SSDT second key point. Anterior septal angle.

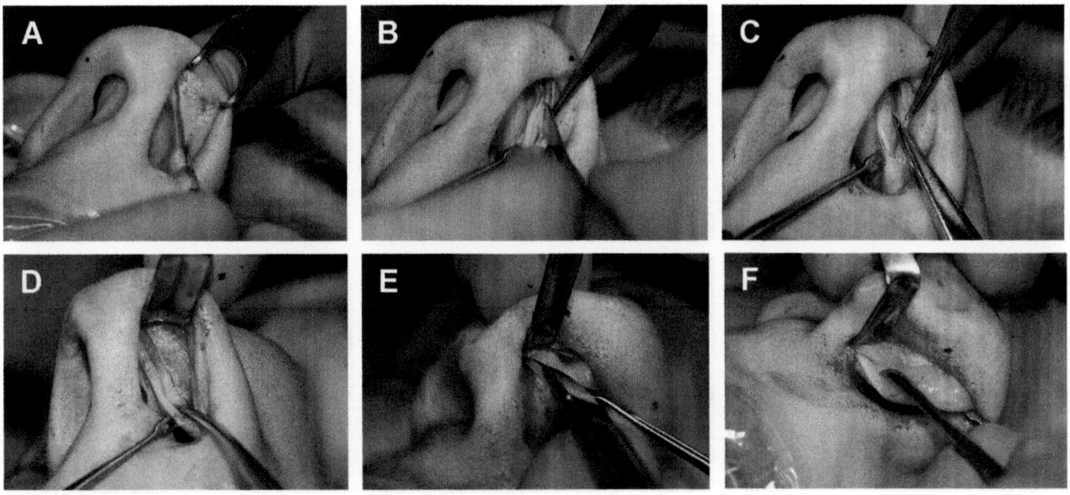

Fig. 7. (*A–F*) SSDT third key point. Lateral crural turning point.

(**Fig. 7**C). The Crile retractor is placed, and the perichondrium is dissected 2 to 3 mm with the Daniel elevator. The thin end of the Crile retractor is placed into the pocket formed with the Daniel elevator. Although the Crile retractor is held with the thumb and index finger, the middle finger pushes on the skin. The lateral crural perichondrium is squeezed between the skin and elevator and pulled to the side. This maneuver facilitates and speeds up the dissection of the lateral crus (**Fig. 7**D). When the dissection reaches the dome, the hooks are placed right under the dome and pulled downwards (**Fig. 7**E). When the dome is passed, the assistant pulls the hooks cranially and the medial crura are dissected (**Fig. 7**F).

4. Lateral keystone: the cartilaginous dorsum and upper lateral cartilages have been dissected from the W point. The lateral crus is pushed posteriorly, the vertical scroll ligament is dissected off the SMAS and the upper lateral cartilage plane is reached (**Fig. 8**A). Dissecting the bony dorsum from the midline is more difficult. Dissecting the sides is easier. The caudal edge of the bone is encountered with subperichondrial dissection as the upper lateral cartilages go under the bone (**Fig. 8**B). The caudal edge of the bone has a sharp structure. The sharp periosteum tip of the Daniel-Cakir elevator is used to scratch the caudal edge of the bone and the periosteum is easily cut between the sharp edge of the bone and the sharp tip of the elevator (**Fig. 8**C). Tightening up the

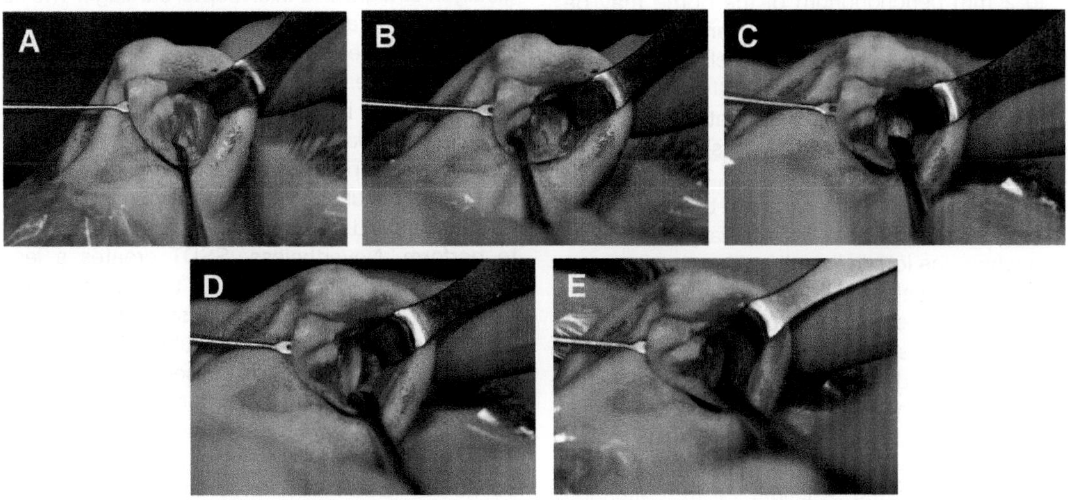

Fig. 8. (*A–E*) SSDT fourth key point. Lateral keystone.

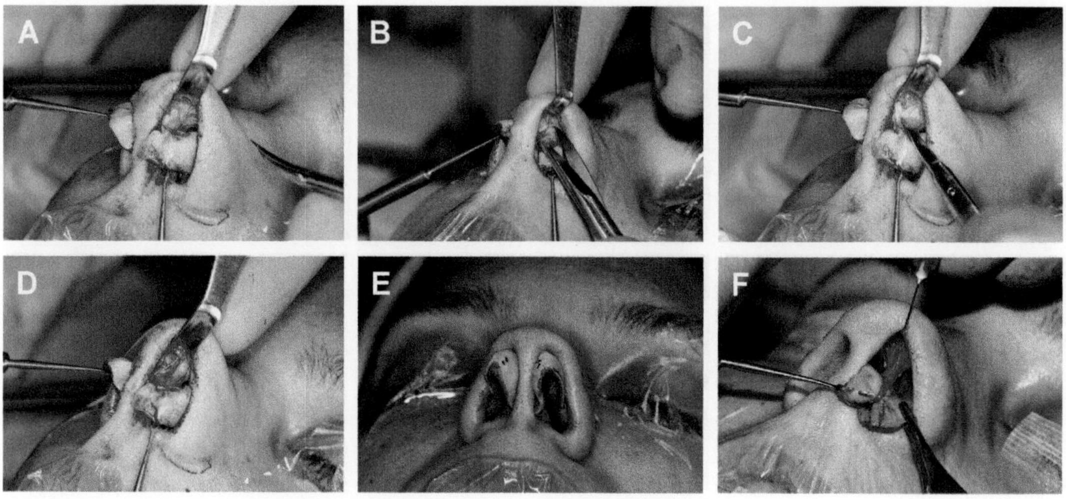

Fig. 9. (*A–F*) SSDT fifth key point. Medial perichondrium of the domes.

skin of the upper lateral cartilages with a Crile retractor aids periosteal dissection. Limited or wide dissection is carried out according to the planned nasal dorsum technique (**Fig. 8**D). After the contralateral side is dissected, the periosteum of the bony cap is cut with a periosteal elevator. The midline is dissected, and the dissected right and left sides are united.

5. *The medial perichondrium of the domes:* a window is created between the 2 layers of the Pitanguy ligament to deliver and suture the nasal tip cartilages. In this way, the Pitanguy ligament is preserved. For this procedure, small hooks are placed under both domes and pulled laterally and handed to the assistant. The nostril apex is retracted with a Crile retractor. Scissors are used to dissect 1 to 2 mm from where the perichondrium of both domes end (**Fig. 9**A). In cases where the tip needs to be narrowed, 1 to 2 mm perichondrium of the dome may be left attached to the deep Pitanguy ligament (**Fig. 9**B). This 1 to 2 mm perichondrium may be resected. Approaching from the nostril close to the surgeon, a window is created using scissors, with the blades of the scissor's vertical to the face (**Fig. 9**C, D). In this way, the deep layer of the Pitanguy ligament is left below and the superficial layer above. Especially in patients in whom the lobule is to be elongated, dissection is continued superiorly to create a big enough space. Supratip breakpoint will form where the dissection ends. Marking the projection of the end of the dissection helps the surgeon and roughly shows the breakpoint. Supratip breakpoint is approximately in the middle between the tip and K point.[3] The window between the 2 layers of the Pitanguy ligament is widened until the footplates to allow for the delivery of the domes (**Fig. 9**E). Tip surgery can easily be performed by preserving the Pitanguy ligament (**Fig. 9**F). When the tip surgery is finished, if the supratip breakpoint is prominent more than necessary, the dissection is continued cranially. If this is not sufficient, the lateral crural cephalic resection cartilages can be crushed and placed over the Pitanguy ligament. The Pitanguy ligament may be needed to be cut in patients with thin skin and over projection.

DISCUSSION

Subperichondrial dissection is gold standard in septoplasty surgery because bleeding and fibrosis are less. Subperichondrial dissection is easier surgically in straight and thick septal cartilage. The tip and upper lateral cartilages are not straight as the septum and neither are they as strong as the septal cartilage. Therefore, entering the subperichondrial plane is more difficult. But once the subperichondrial plane is reached, dissection is easier and faster compared with the submuscular plane. The submuscular plane has been the most commonly used plane in rhinoplasty, as it is easier to perform. Nevertheless, SSDT creates a less bloody plane compared with the submuscular dissection and may decrease tissue injury. The advantages of SSDT over the submuscular plane have extensively been discussed.[1] The authors hope to make SSDT easier for rhinoplasty surgeons with the method described herein.

Making use of the right instrumentation and key points for SSDT facilitates the technique. To achieve an easier dissection,

a. One needs to start the dissection at the right localization. This is usually where the cartilage is the thickest.
b. The cartilage needs to be pulled in the right direction.
c. The right instruments should be used (see **Fig. 4**).
d. A bloodless field is mandatory. Intermittent infiltration of 5 cc of 1/80,000 adrenaline-containing solution for more than 10 minutes to the incision sites after systolic blood pressure drops less than 90 mm Hg is enough to create a bloodless surgical field.[3]

RESULT

SSDT is being used by more surgeons every passing year. Preservation of soft tissues in rhinoplasty has gained importance in recent years. The authors believe that the number of surgeons using SSDT will increase with the use of the key points in dissection and correct instruments.

DISCLOSURE

Dr Çakır receives royalty from Daniel Çakır elevators.

REFERENCES

1. Cakir B, Oreroğlu AR, Dogan T, et al. A complete subperichondrial dissection technique for rhinoplasty with management of the nasal ligaments. Aesthet Surg J 2012;32(5):564–74.
2. Patron V, Hitier M, Gamby R, et al. How to perform subperichondrial and subperiosteal rhinoplasty. Eur Ann Otorhinolaryngol Head Neck Dis 2019;136(4):325–9.
3. Cakir B. Aesthetic septorhinoplasty. Cham, Springer; 2016.
4. Daniel RK. The Preservation Rhinoplasty: A New Rhinoplasty Revolution. Aesthet Surg J 2018;38(2):228–9.
5. Kosins AM, Daniel RK. Decision Making in Preservation Rhinoplasty: A 100 Case Series With One-Year Follow-Up. Aesthet Surg J 2019;107.
6. Cakir B, Saban Y, Palhazi P, et al. Preservation Rhinoplasty. Istanbul, Septum, 2019.
7. Cakir B, Kucuker I, Aksakal IA, et al. Auto-Rim Flap Technique for Lateral Crura Caudal Excess Treatment. Aesthet Surg J 2017;37(1):24–32.

Tip Ligament Preservation and Suspension
Why and How?

Jeffrey R. Marcus, MD, Analise B. Thomas, MD, Heather A. Levites, MD

KEYWORDS

• Ligament • Midvault • Reconstruction • Rhinoplasty • Surgery • preservation • interdomal • intercrural • projection • rotation • ala

KEY POINTS

- "Preservation" refers not only to the dorsum but to any structure preserved for advantage or to avoid an undesired effect.
- The interdomal and intercrural ligaments provide the mechanism by which the caudal septum influences tip rotation and projection.
- These ligaments also maintain the symmetry of the paired alar cartilages and dome-defining points.
- Preservation of the interalar ligaments helps to maintain symmetry of the alar cartilages.
- Ligament preservation facilitates tip suspension with control over rotation, projection, and columellar show.

INTRODUCTION

This article of *Clinics* explores the concept of "preservation" rhinoplasty. At present, this topic is gaining considerable attention. But what is meant specifically and generally by "preservation"? The term came to popularity with the specific descriptions of midvault structural preservation for dorsal hump reduction by the push-down and let-down techniques.[1,2] These techniques are well characterized in other chapters, but in brief, in these approaches, the interfaces of septum and upper lateral cartilages along the dorsum are maintained while the hump is reduced, thereby "preserving the midvault." Through this preservation of the dorsum, natural contours can be retained or enhanced, and the internal valves are left undisturbed. In contrast to humpectomy or component reduction of the dorsum, with preservation techniques, the potential sequelae of the act of opening the midvault and subsequently reconstructing it are avoided.[3,4]

"Preservation" does not necessarily apply exclusively to the dorsum though; in general terms, it may be viewed as maintaining a particular structure for a particular desirable advantage rather than deconstructing it.[5,6] Many of the most common maneuvers used in rhinoplasty surgery involve deconstruction of structures and relationships with their subsequent reconstruction. As proponents of preservation suggest, a great number of problems we encounter in rhinoplasty are problems that were not present before the surgery; therefore, they can often be attributed to the deconstruction and reconstruction that took place. Rhinoplasty has become confusing and difficult to teach for many reasons. Among them include the complex and intricate methods we use to reconstruct structures and relationships that we ourselves chose to take apart. And often secondarily, we are compelled to use aggressive and/or nonanatomic methods in order to treat iatrogenic problems. In some instances, deconstruction is required in order to make a change pursuant to a goal of the operation; but in other instances, we simply restore structures to their original

Division of Plastic, Maxillofacial and Oral Surgery, DUMC 3974 Baker House, 200 Trent Drive, Durham, NC 27710, USA

Facial Plast Surg Clin N Am 29 (2021) 47–58
https://doi.org/10.1016/j.fsc.2020.09.003

state. The latter questions the logic behind deconstruction. The concept of preservation suggests that we refrain from unnecessary deconstruction steps in primary rhinoplasty, thereby simplifying procedures to a certain extent and limiting the need for more complex secondary repairs.

Another example of preservation, described herein, pertains to the ligamentous anatomy that coalesces between the medial and middle crurae of the alar cartilages and the caudal septum. In open rhinoplasty, the lower lateral cartilages are routinely separated entirely from one another by dividing ligamentous structures in order to facilitate exposure for subsequent steps. The act itself of dividing the ligaments ("split tip approach") is a means rather than an end; that is, it is a process-related deconstructive step. In closed rhinoplasty, delivery of the lower lateral cartilages is often combined with full transfixion. In both the split tip and delivery with full transfixion, tip ligaments and their connection to the caudal septum are surgically released. Later, the lower lateral cartilages are reapproximated with sutures to reconstruct the unity of the tip previously provided by the ligaments. In addition, vertical support grafts (eg, columellar strut or septal extension) are placed between the medial crurae to restore, reduce, or enhance projection. In open rhinoplasty and in closed rhinoplasty with a full transfixion incision, there had been consensus that extrinsic structural support via grafting was obligatory because the natural ligamentous support of the tip had been eliminated. However, these particular ligaments—the interdomal and intercrural ligaments—may be kept intact preserved. In doing so, the relationship between the 2 sides is preserved benefiting maintenance of symmetry. The ligamentous construct may then be used to resuspend the tip construct to the caudal septum, recapitulating the natural supportive relationship between these structures. We will investigate the rationale, techniques, and utility for preservation of these ligamentous connections. For clarity, these ligaments will be referenced specifically by name or collectively as the "inter-alar ligaments."

DISCUSSION

Determinants of Success in Aesthetic Tip Surgery

Surgery of the nasal tip can be incredibly elegant. Baris Cakir, in his recent superb text, analyzes the nasal tip and characterizes it as a set of fine polygonal shapes that form aesthetic angles, contours, surface characteristics, and light reflections.[7] Advanced rhinoplasty surgeons may learn a great deal from these works to refine their techniques to achieve wonderful, artistic forms. However, basic tip surgery begins with only a few critical elements in order to get on base. In every rhinoplasty, the surgeon must deliver on 4 key structural relationships; shortcomings therein provide the basis of the most common causes for tip revision. The 4 critical elements are projection, rotation, dome symmetry, and proper columella show. The surgeon has control over these factors if he/she understands the anatomic influences on them. Typically, we intend to alter or adjust one or more of these structural relationships. In the normal nonoperated state, all of these aesthetic attributes are governed by the intrinsic integrity (including dimensions and strength) of the lower lateral cartilages and the interrelationship of the interdomal and intercrural ligaments with the caudal septum. The tip tripod described by Anderson characterizes tip rotation and projection based on the length and strength of the 2 lateral crurae and the paired medial crurae.[8] A "tripod" is understood conceptually to be a stable/rigid support. But the *tip tripod* is mobile, not static; in fact, the footplates themselves generally do not articulate with the anterior nasal spine (skeletal base) and neither do the lateral-most extents of the lateral crurae. Yet the tip tripod is not floating freely in space; it is supported, so clearly there is something more to this. As stated by Bitik and colleagues[9] "In the normal nasal anatomy, an anterior septal angle of sufficient height keeps the feet of the medial crua off the anterior nasal spine; the medial crura do not bear a significant load...". A nonoperated aesthetic tip is supported by ligamentous structures that maintain the relationship between the alar crurae and their positions relative to the caudal septum. These structures are nicely described by Daniel and Palhazi and are summarized to follow.

The Interdomal and Intercrurl Ligaments

Drs Rollin Daniel and Peter Palhazi published perhaps the most highly detailed monograph of nasal anatomy in rhinoplasty.[10] In it, they describe the form and purpose of the interdomal and intercrural ligaments (**Fig. 1**A-C). The interdomal ligament is a relatively discreet structure that connects the 2 middle crurae along the cephalic junction of the infralobular segment. It does not bind the domes themselves tightly together but maintains a close approximation of the *posterior* aspects of the middle crurae, permitting an open angle anteriorly to result in 2 separate, but generally aligned, dome-defining points. Therefore, the

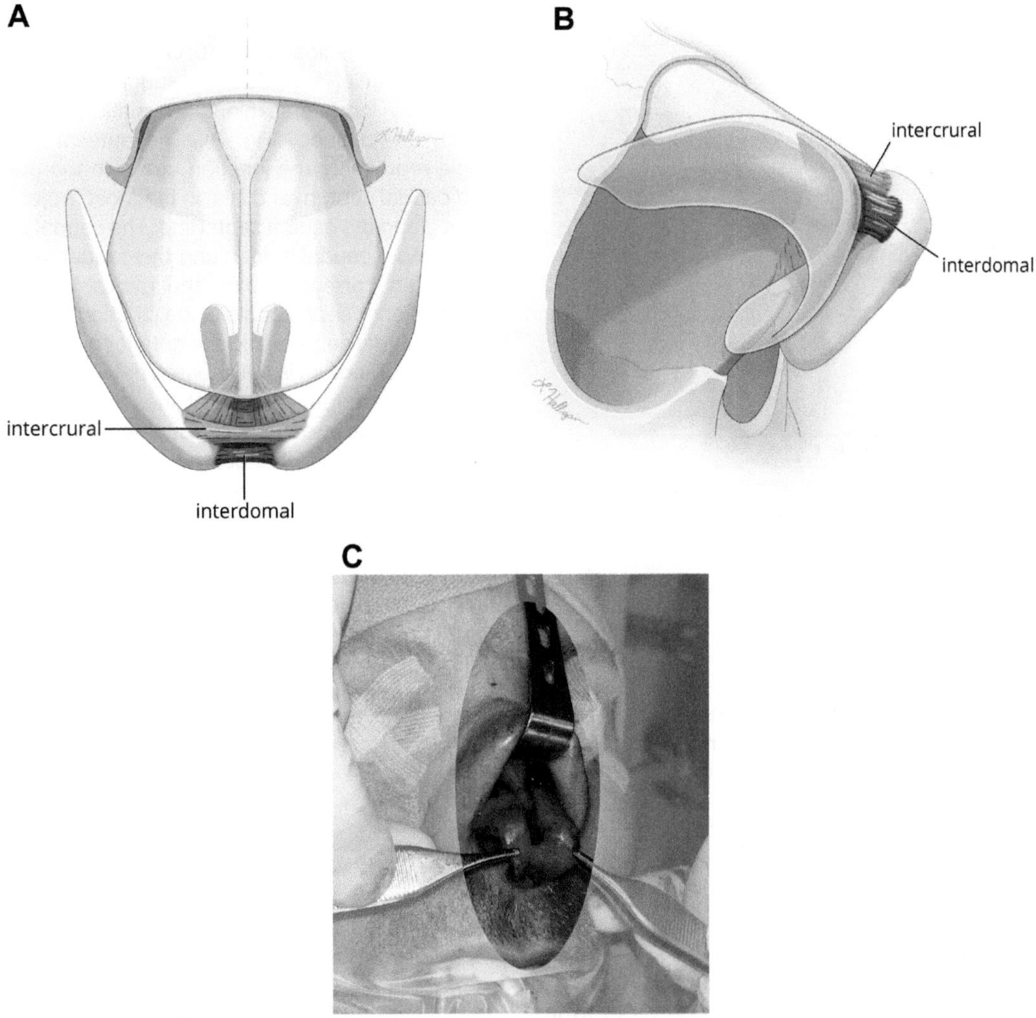

Fig. 1. (*A*) Oblique view of the interdomal and intercrural ligaments. The interdomal ligament runs between the cephalic borders of the lobular segment of the middle crurae. The interdomal ligament is a relatively discreet structure which binds the dome genu pair together. Deep to the interdomal ligament, the broader intercrural ligaments originate from the caudal septum and invest the posterior aspects of the middle and medial crurae. (*B*) Interdomal and intercrural ligaments depicted from a superior view. Note again that the interdomal ligament is relatively discreet and transversely oriented while the intercrural ligaments have both a transverse element and an AP oblique element. The transversely oriented fibers span between the posterior margins of the medial crurae, over the genu and also to a variable extent between the lateral crurae lateral to the genu. The AP oblique fibers span from the posterior alar margins to the caudal septum where they coalesce with the septal perichondrium. (*C*) Intraoperative view of the interdomal and intercrural ligaments from oblique perspective.

angle of divergence and the spatial symmetry of the domes are factors that depend on the presence of the interdomal ligament. When it is divided (along with the intercrural ligaments discussed later), as in "split tip" open rhinoplasty these important relationships are no longer supported and must be restored by a reconstructive technique. In order to reestablish the tip in space, the surgeon must reunite 2 separate structures and align the 2 properly not only with respect to the desired effect on projection and rotation, but to each other. Failure to do so would result in asymmetry of the domes (**Fig. 2**).

The intercrural ligaments are less frequently discussed, most frequently divided, and disproportionately important relative to our attention to

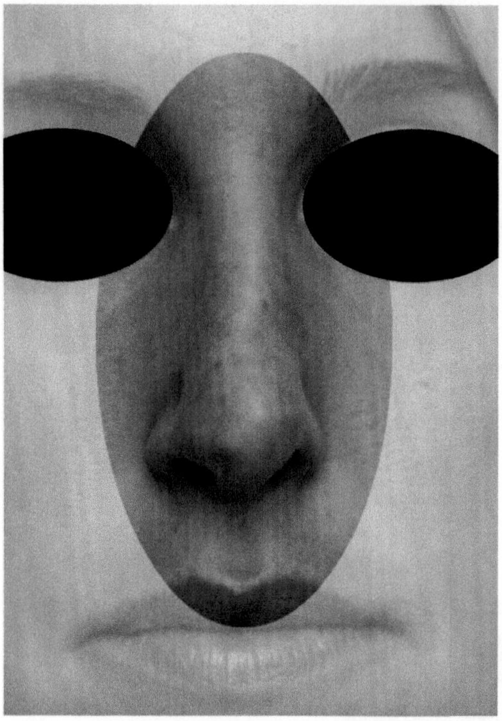

Fig. 2. A clinical example of a potential negative consequence of split tip open rhinoplasty. Division of the interdomal and intercrural ligaments in split-tip open rhinoplasty requires resetting of the dome position and can result in subsequent asymmetry. Note the position of the dome defining points; a vertical malalignment is present.

them. These ligaments are much broader than the interdomal ligament, and they reside deep to it. They invest the posterior aspects of the medial and middle crurae over a long segment, wherein the fibers run transversely between the right and left sides. In this fashion, they play a similar but perhaps an even more important role in maintaining the symmetric interdependence between the right and left alar cartilages. The intercrural ligaments also include fibers that run in the anteroposterior plane from the posterior edge of the crurae to coalesce with the mucoperichondrium on each side of the septum. It is this important observation that explains the support relationship of the caudal septal structures to tip projection, and it explains deprojection with a transfixion incision.

The Relationship of the Tip to the Caudal Septum

Daniel and Palhazi also characterized the spatial relationships between the alar cartilages and the caudal septum via their cadaveric dissections. Separately and unknowingly, we had undertaken a cadaveric study of 25 specimens to determine these relationships as well. Our studies, which support Daniel and Palhazi, suggest that there are 3 key landmarks along the caudal septum, which are defined (**Fig. 3**). The anterior septal angle represents the junction between the dorsal and caudal septum and is also the most projecting point along the caudal septal line. The caudal point is the most caudal point along the caudal septum and often corresponds to the midseptal angle. The posterior septal angle is the junction point between caudal septum and the anterior nasal spine. The caudal septum is not situated entirely between the medial crurae—except at the footplates. The medial crurae are normally situated in front of, behind, or abutting the caudal septum at each of the caudal septal landmarks. In our analysis, the posterior edges of the medial crurae were anterior to the caudal septum at the anterior septal angle, (less) anterior or abutting at the midseptal angle, and overlapping the caudal septum at the footplates.

The dimensions of the caudal septum affect rotation, projection, and columellar show. For

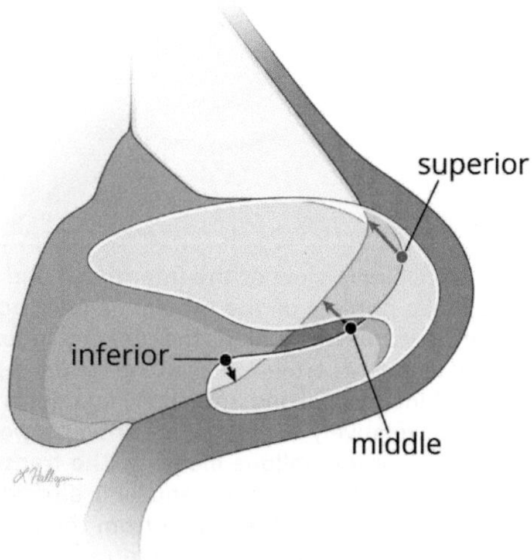

Fig. 3. The presenting relationship of the medial and middle crurae to the caudal septal edge is important to note in any rhinoplasty, but even more important if the caudal septum is to be used to provide extrinsic support. Based on cadaveric dissections, the footplates generally overlap the caudal septum, and the superior point is generally anterior to the anterior septal angle by several millimeters. The distance of the middle point to the middle septal angle is variable. The decision to augment, reduce, or maintain the caudal septum is based on an analysis of these relationships.

example, excess columellar show can be seen when there is excess at the midseptal angle. Another example is the "tension nose," in which general overgrowth of the septum drives the nose forward resulting in overprojection. Tip projection is determined in this instance by the position of the anterior septal angle. If the tip were independent, these conditions of excess septum would have no effect on tip dynamics. Tip projection, rotation, and columella show are passively influenced because ligamentous attachments cause the tip to follow the septum.

Contemporary Methods of Establishing Tip Projection and Rotation

Extrinsic projection (that is not naturally provided by the alar cartilages themselves and the ligamentous interfaces with the caudal septum) is provided by structural grafts. The most common are the columellar strut and the septal extension graft.

Columellar strut

In *Mastering Rhinoplasty*, Daniel, now a leading proponent of preservation techniques, wrote that, "The columellar strut is almost magical in its beneficial effects on the tip. The columellar strut and its suture serve three purposes: tip stability, tip projection, and columellar shape. Suturing the alars to the strut creates a unified tip complex and improves symmetry." After having released the interdomal and intercrural ligaments in a split tip approach, the columella strut is placed between the medial crurae and is secured in position,

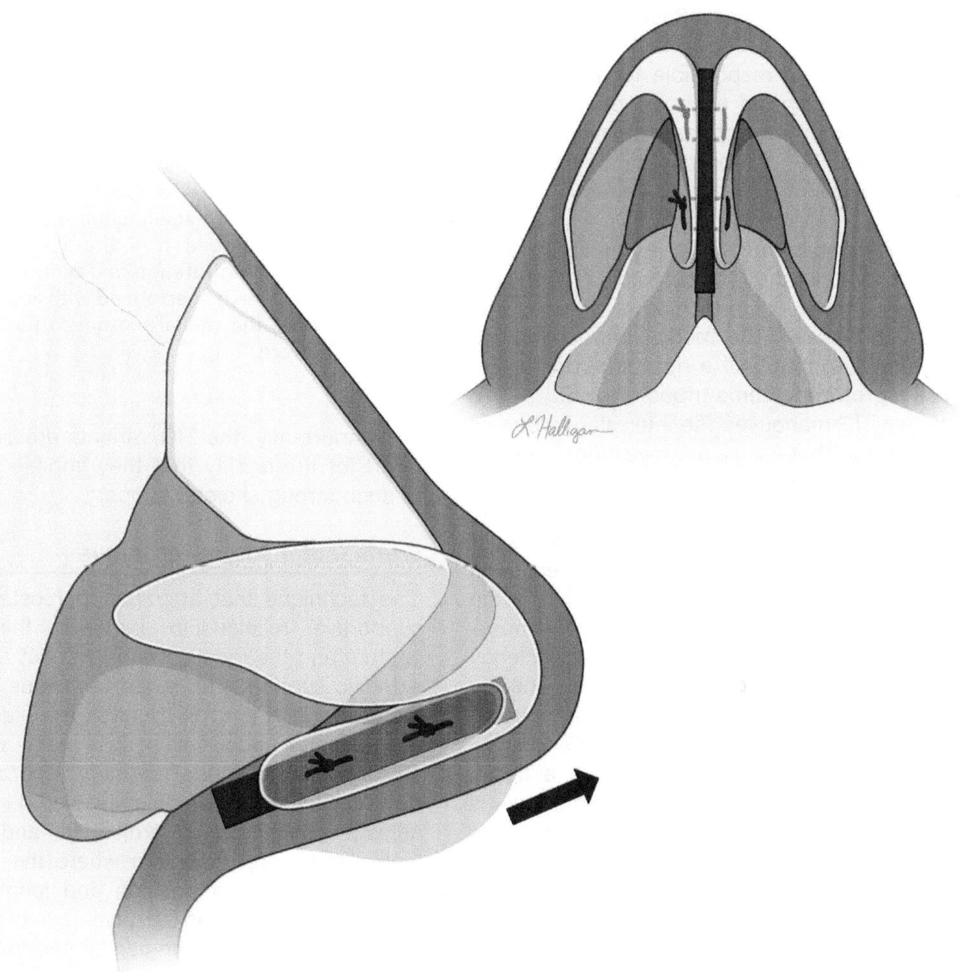

Fig. 4. A columellar strut is an extrinsic support graft which is placed and secured between the medial crurae. It requires that the alars are separated (dividing the interalar ligaments), and it reliably provides augmentation of projection. Note the sillouette in which projection as well as rotation are altered by the columellar strut. It does not, however, provide as reliable control over tip rotation.

taking care to reestablish the position of the alar cartilages symmetrically (**Fig. 4**).

There are disadvantages of columellar struts, and they are no longer ubiquitously applied as in the past. The deconstruction step of releasing the inter-alar ligaments introduces a risk of asymmetric dome position even in cases that began with symmetry. In addition, even though columellar strut replaces native septal support for the tip, the relationship of the medial crurae to the caudal septum is relevant. If there is any degree of caudal septal excess, one must resect caudal septum in order to make room for the columella strut. A common consequence of failure in this regard is excess columellar show, which did not exist preoperatively. Even in a "normal" relationship in which the medial crurae abut or overlap the caudal septum, placement of a columellar strut can result in excess columellar show or in a hinge effect at the edge-to-edge interface of the strut and caudal septal edge. The latter is responsible for tip deviation to one side, which did not exist preoperatively. Without a doubt, secondary operations have resulted from the use or misuse of columellar struts, especially when done universally.

Tongue-in-groove and septal extension grafts

Originally described by Russel Kridel in 1999, the tongue-in-groove (TIG) technique secures the septum *in between* the medial crurae, making the caudal septum itself a rigid support for the medial leg of Anderson's tripod (**Fig. 5**).[11–13] To perform a TIG maneuver, the inter-alar ligaments are divided so that each alar move independently as they are backed up to the caudal septum. It requires that caudal septum be centralized and secured perfectly, and it specifically allows for reduction of columellar show without resection of caudal septum. The native relationship of the medial crurae and caudal septum again is important with this technique; patients with deficiency of caudal septal length were not initially addressed, but later investigators advocated the use of a septal extension graft (SEG) to allow for the TIG method to be applied in a larger range of patients.[4,14,15] The TIG technique is the primary means of securing projection for some investigators, and the normal average caudal septal length is such that septal extension is required more often than not. The septal extension graft (SEG) interfaces edge to edge with the caudal septum because it is meant to be structurally in continuity with the septum. Therefore, it can also hinge at the interface and lead to asymmetry of the tip depending on the method and skill used to fixate the SEG. Finally, and importantly, the TIG variants are often criticized for the rigidity that they impose by virtue of such strong skeletal support.

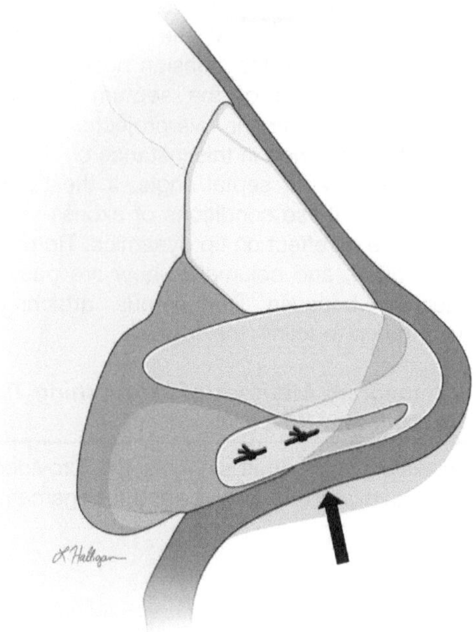

Fig. 5. When using a tongue-in-groove (TIG) technique in its original description, the medial crurae are backed up to overlap the caudal septum and secured to it. The caudal septum therefore is a sturdy extrinsic support which again requires that the interalar ligaments be divided. Note the silhouette, in this case TIG is providing rotation and reduction of columella show. TIG can be performed with augmentation or reduction of the caudal septum to further adjust rotational effects.

Crura-Septal Suture Technique

One technique that attempts to reestablish the supportive relationship between the caudal septum and the medial crurae without adding an extrinsic support graft is the technique of crura-septal suturing (**Fig. 6**). Sutures are placed from the posterior edge of each medial crus and secured to the caudal septum according to a desired vector that can be manipulated to achieve adjustment in rotation, projection, and/or columellar show depending on where the suture is placed. It relies on position and length of the caudal septum and has the advantage of versatility in that the caudal septum can be shortened when excessive. If the caudal septum is short, most would likely favor an SEG with TIG over crura-septal suturing, as strength is a premium. Crura-septal suturing can be done via transfixion in closed rhinoplasty but also has been described

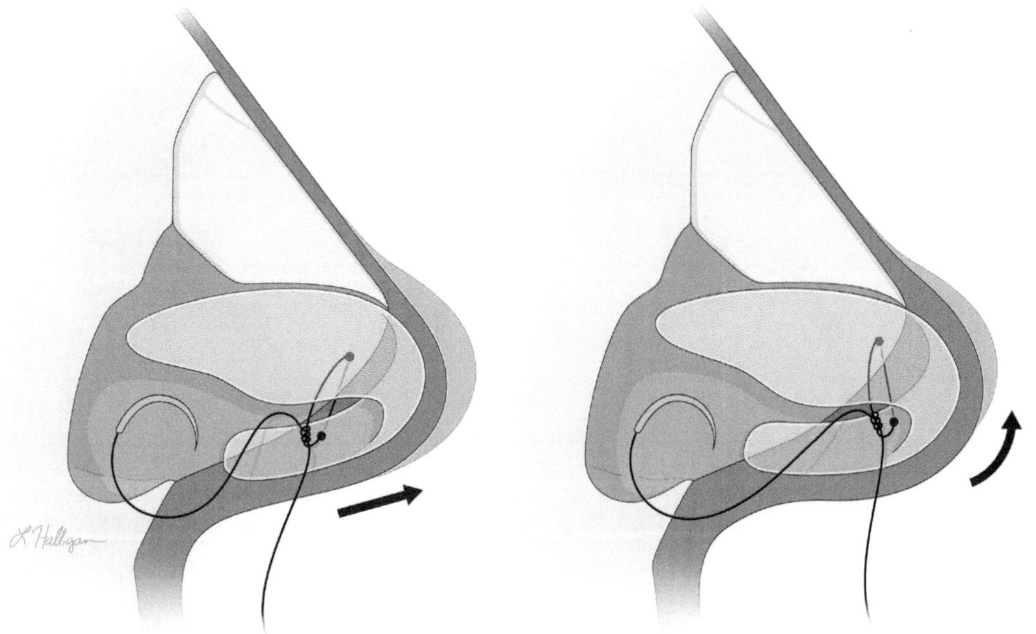

Fig. 6. The crura-septal suture: In this technique, a suture is placed from the medial crurae to the caudal septum. Depending on the vector chosen, this suture technique can deliver projection (left) or rotation (right) depending on where the suture is placed along the crurae and the caudal septum.

frequently in open rhinoplasty with a "split tip" such that each alar moves independently. Conceptually, crura-septal suturing is very appealing because it reconstitutes native relationships and generally avoids the aforementioned problems seen with extrinsic support grafts. However, division of the inter-alar ligaments means that the sutures not only restore suspension and support from septum to crurae but must also reunite the medial crurae and are responsible for recreating dome symmetry.

If the inter-alar ligaments are preserved from the beginning, these inter-alar relationships remain supported to a significant extent, and the ligamentous construct itself (which is robust) can be used to secure the conjoined middle leg of the tripod to the caudal septum. In doing so, this most closely recapitulates the natural support mechanism of the tip.

LIGAMENT PRESERVATION AND SUSPENSION

Preparation and Analysis

In every rhinoplasty case, preoperative analysis is critical. As stated, there are many nuances to a bespoke and sophisticated rhinoplasty, but there are core elements that must be addressed by all rhinoplasty surgeons from novice to expert. Among them are tip projection, tip rotation, and columellar show. The surgical goals relative to these elements must be achieved to near perfection. Because all 3 of these have a relationship to caudal septal dimensions, and the ligament suspension technique is based on the support of the caudal septum, we include the following in the analysis preoperatively:

1. Is the caudal septum in the midline?
2. At each level of the caudal septum (anterior, middle, and posterior), where are the medial crurae relative to the caudal septum? Do the crurae overlap/sandwich, abut, or stand in front of the caudal edge with a gap?
3. If a change in projection, rotation, or columella show is desired, are the positions of the caudal septal angles reasonable, or does the caudal septum need to be modified by reduction or extension?

Technique

With an open approach, the transcolumellar incision is made (**Fig. 7**). The columellar skin is elevated from the surface of the medial crurae in the subcutaneous plane up to the genu on each side. By focusing at this level on subcutaneous elevation, all ligamentous structures between the alars are preserved. Once the dissection is carried *over* the genu on each side, we then transition to a

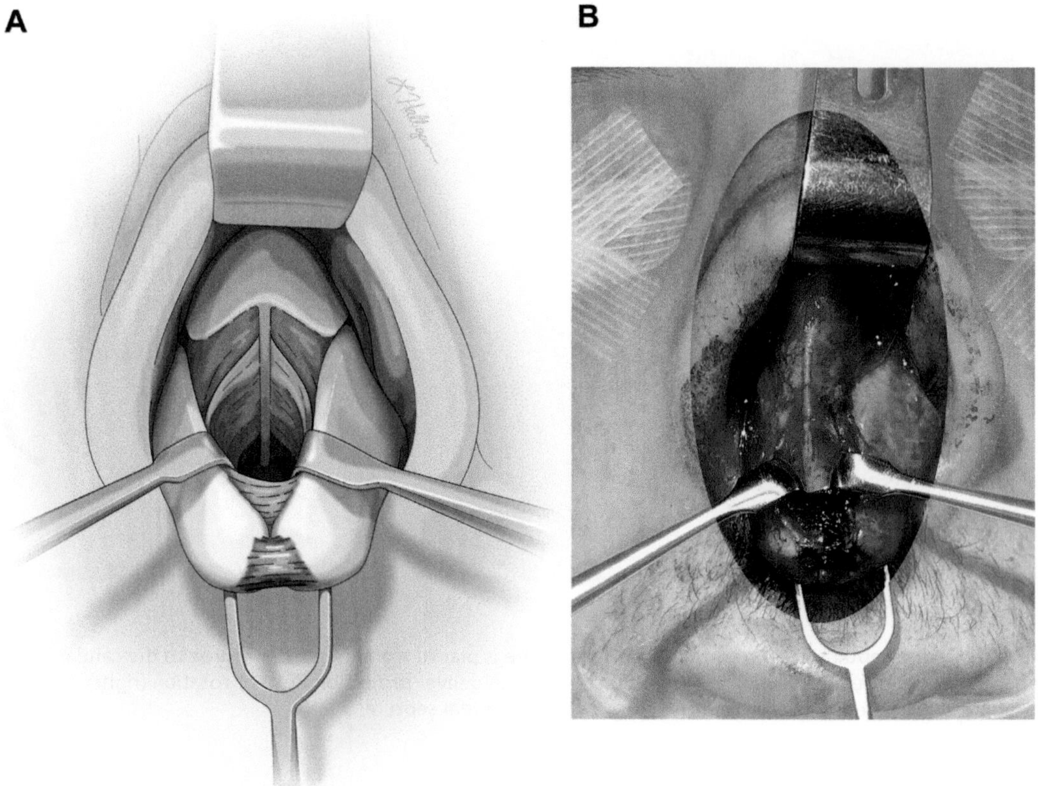

Fig. 7. (*A*) With preservation of the interalar ligaments, the midvault is accessed from above, retracting the tip inferiorly. There is an avascular plane between the medial crurae and the caudal septum. Fibers of the intercrural ligement from the posterior edges of the medial crurae to the caudal septum can be seen. (*B*) In this intraoperative view, the plane between the crurae and the caudal septum is demonstrated.

subperichondrial plane. After exposure of the lateral crurae on each side is completed, the Pitanguy ligament and scroll ligaments remain, attaching skin to structure. (Note: these ligaments may be managed in a variety of ways, but for purpose of this discussion, they are lysed for exposure). The anterior septal angle is palpated, and exposure is carried down to it, with the intent to further carry a subfascial or subperichondrial elevation over the midvault.

At this time, a variety of other maneuvers may be carried out to achieve the goals of the individual operation. The only difference between this technique and others is that the caudal septum will be exposed from above—preserving inter-alar ligaments but retracting the tip downward. A completely avascular plane exists between the caudal septal edge and the posterior aspects of the medical crurae. A gentle transverse spread of scissors opens this space all the way down to the anterior nasal spine in a narrow passage. In this passage the intercrural fibers are quite visible traversing from posterior edge of the medial crus to coalesce in the mucoperichondrium of the septum; it is not a subtle layer. Once the caudal septal edge is exposed, elevation of the septal mucoperichondrium can easily be carried out to facilitate septal work.

At the end of the operation, once all other steps have been carried out, the tip is addressed. Any variety of tip maneuvers can be performed without disturbing the inter-alar ligaments. In my practice, intradomal (dome defining) sutures are frequently used. Once these have been placed, all that remains is proper establishment of projection, rotation, and columellar show. If modification of the caudal septum was necessary, it would be accomplished. The unified tip complex is then positioned in relationship to the caudal septum (**Fig. 8**). A 4-0 clear nylon suture is passed from outside to inside through the intercrural ligament. It will then be placed just below the anterior septal angle. The level of the placement of the suture through the ligament depends on whether one wants to alter

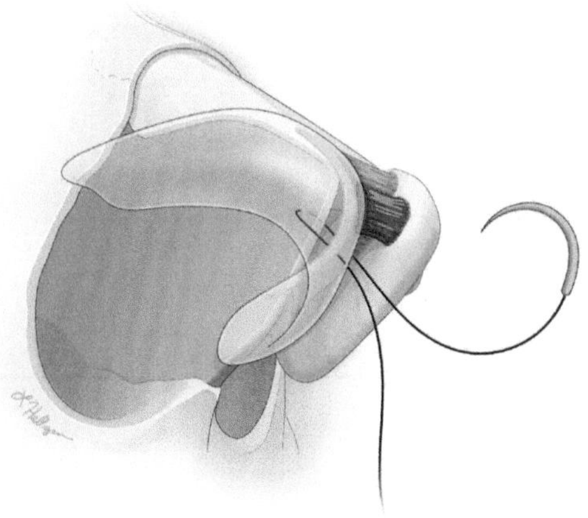

Fig. 8. Ligament suspension technique illustrated from the lateral view. The suture is placed through the inter-alar ligaments to the desired point on the caudal septum in order to reset the tip position with attention to how the vector can affect tip projection and rotation.

projection or rotation. If placed high (close to the genu), the tip will rotate as the suture is tied; if placed low, the tip will rise (project). The suture is tied differentially only to the point that it achieves its desired result. Most often a second suture is placed to further secure the construct, but usually without causing further change. In the final steps, an interdomal (dome binding) suture is placed to secure the apices of the domes and establish a proper angle of divergence and interdomal distance (**Figs. 9-12**).

Technical Points

1. Care must be taken during columella and tip exposure to preserve ligamentous structure.
2. Retraction on the tip should be gentle, as the retractor itself can attenuate ligaments.
3. The question has been raised: can ligament preservation be combined with a hemitransfixion approach to the septum rather than top-down as I perform? I believe it can, but I view

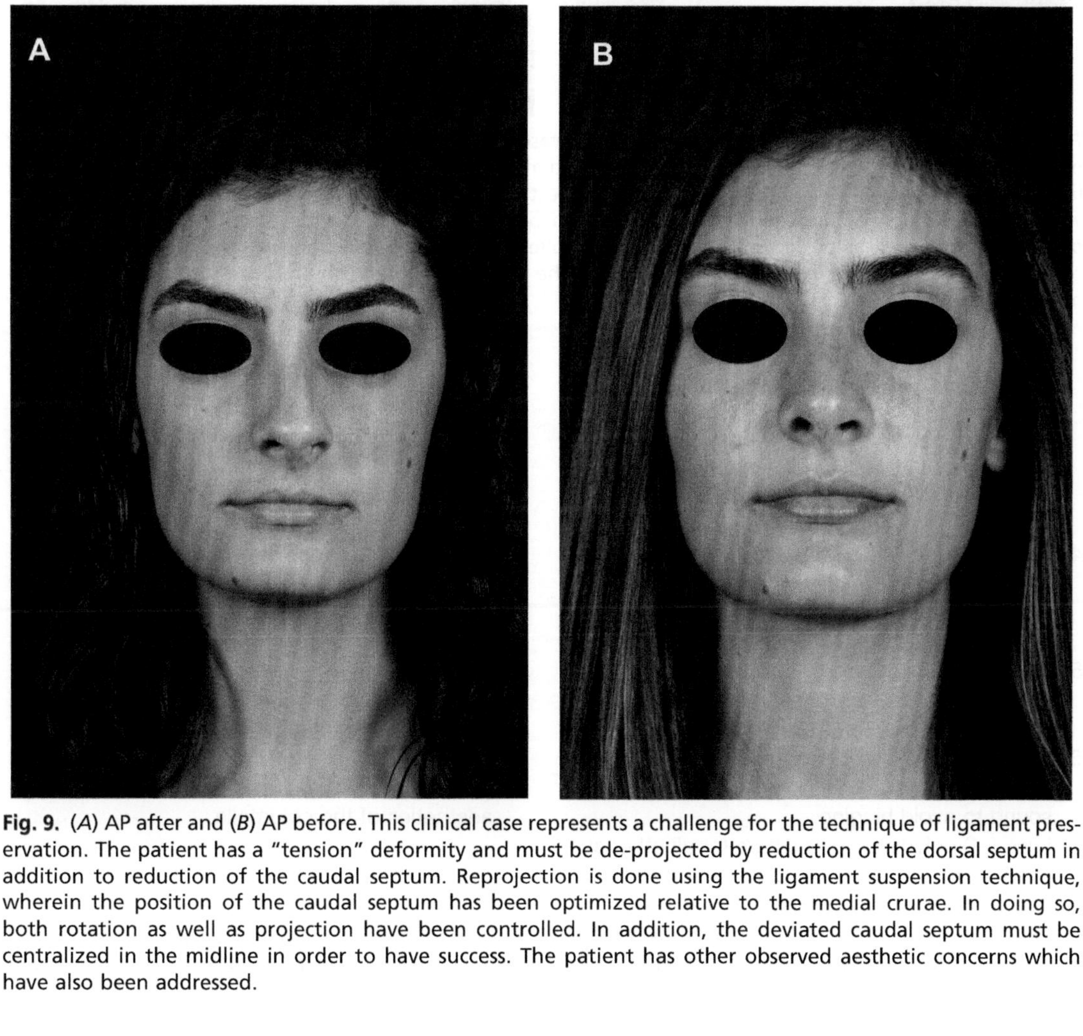

Fig. 9. (*A*) AP after and (*B*) AP before. This clinical case represents a challenge for the technique of ligament preservation. The patient has a "tension" deformity and must be de-projected by reduction of the dorsal septum in addition to reduction of the caudal septum. Reprojection is done using the ligament suspension technique, wherein the position of the caudal septum has been optimized relative to the medial crurae. In doing so, both rotation as well as projection have been controlled. In addition, the deviated caudal septum must be centralized in the midline in order to have success. The patient has other observed aesthetic concerns which have also been addressed.

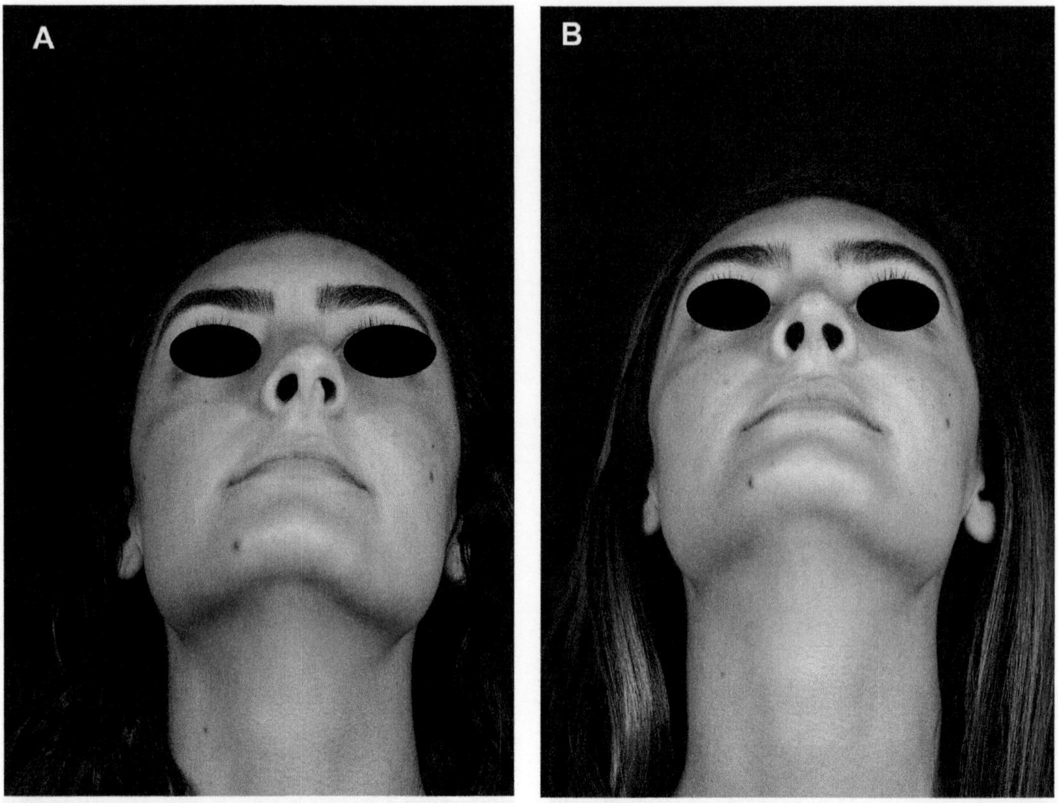

Fig. 10. (*A*) Base after and (*B*) base before. This clinical case represents a challenge for the technique of ligament preservation. The patient has a "tension" deformity and must be de-projected by reduction of the dorsal septum in addition to reduction of the caudal septum. Reprojection is done using the ligament suspension technique, wherein the position of the caudal septum has been optimized relative to the medial crurae. In doing so, both rotation as well as projection have been controlled. In addition, the deviated caudal septum must be centralized in the midline in order to have success. The patient has other observed aesthetic concerns which have also been addressed.

it as an additional and unnecessary incision that does not provide me any advantage and makes the suspension suture more difficult to place.

4. If the domes are significantly asymmetric to begin with, the benefits of this technique are somewhat diminished because ligaments may need to be released to modify the domes.
5. As with TIG technique or crural-septal suturing, caudal septal reduction or extension allows this technique to be applied broadly.
6. When septal extension is needed, the articulation of graft to septum must be structurally sound to avoid hinging.
7. I use 5-0 polydioxanone suture for all other sutures in rhinoplasty; the only exception is 4-0 clear nylon in this technique. The need for a permanent suture is not based in evidence, but rather preference. However, to date I have not encountered exposure or complication of this deep suture.
8. This technique relies on secure suspension of the ligaments to the septum and not the structural stability of the medial crurae, which can at times be weak or diminutive. If needed or desired to provide shape or structure to the columella, an intercrural (columellar) graft can be placed and secured between the medial crurae as a final step. A narrow graft such as this does not have the intent or design of a columellar strut but may help create or sustain the aesthetics of the columella.

SUMMARY

Preservation rhinoplasty should be viewed generally as a mindset to limit deconstructive steps in

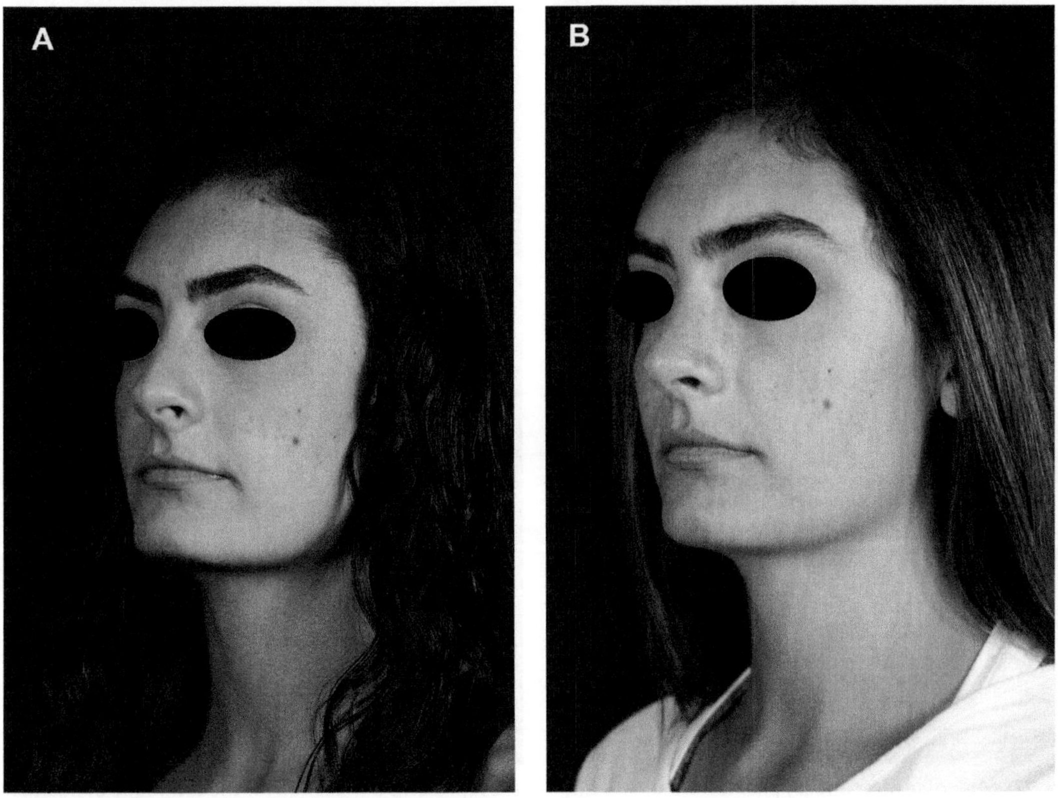

Fig. 11. (*A*) Oblique after and (*B*) oblique before. This clinical case represents a challenge for the technique of ligament preservation. The patient has a "tension" deformity and must be de-projected by reduction of the dorsal septum in addition to reduction of the caudal septum. Reprojection is done using the ligament suspension technique, wherein the position of the caudal septum has been optimized relative to the medial crurae. In doing so, both rotation as well as projection have been controlled. In addition, the deviated caudal septum must be centralized in the midline in order to have success. The patient has other observed aesthetic concerns which have also been addressed.

rhinoplasty when possible, understanding that these steps and those to later reconstruct provide the potential to create new problems that did not previously exist. If one considers the most popular techniques to control tip projection currently, it is clear that each and every one introduces potential new problems. The philosophy is not congruent with the preservation mindset. The most significant limitation of the proposed preservation proposition is that there exists no evidence yet of the long-term stability of this construct, whereas there exists robust literature on the stability of techniques such as TIG and columellar struts. However, in 8 years applying this technique thus far I have yet to perform revision for any of the key elements: projection, rotation, and columellar show. Conversely, like others, I have performed numerous secondary operations for the key elements (including dome symmetry as well) in which the more popular contemporary techniques have been used.

As with other preservation techniques, this approach further limits the need for graft material. In cosmetic rhinoplasty, my use of graft material has declined significantly along with septal exposure required to harvest, further reducing the variability and risk introduced by the surgeon. No technique or approach is perfect or fool-proof, and further evidence would be helpful to establish the merits of this or any newer technique.

DISCLOSURE

The authors have nothing to disclose.

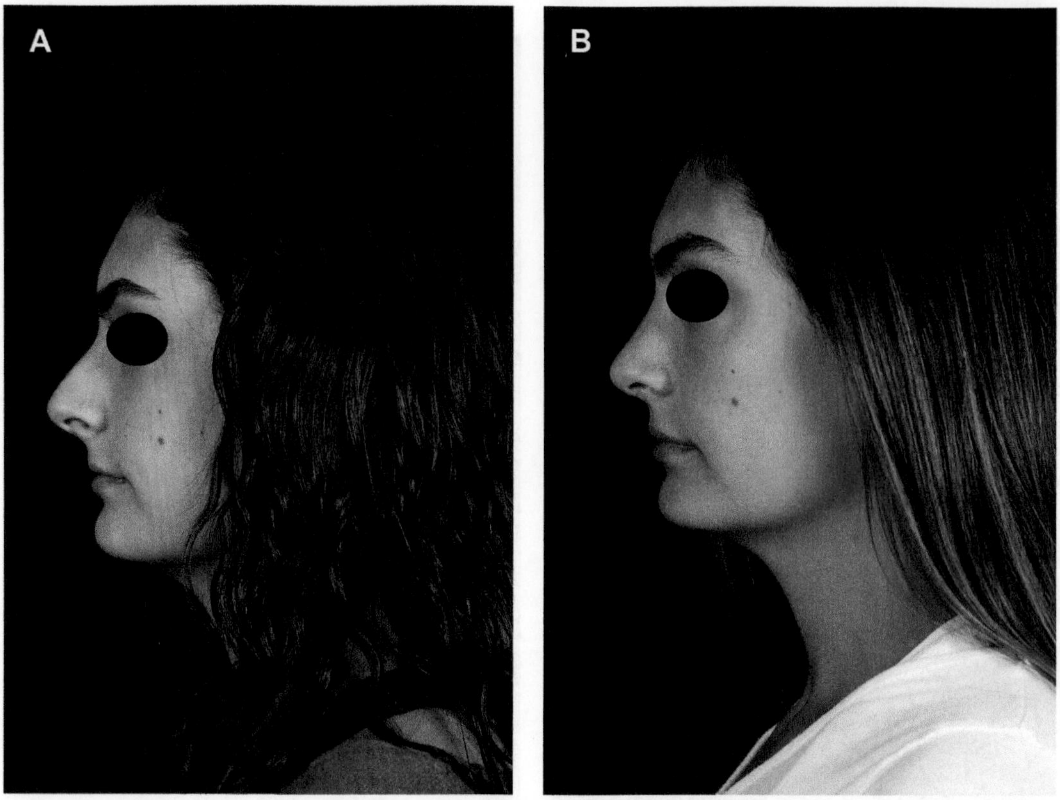

Fig. 12. (*A*) Profile after and (*B*) profile before. This clinical case represents a challenge for the technique of ligament preservation. The patient has a "tension" deformity and must be de-projected by reduction of the dorsal septum in addition to reduction of the caudal septum. Reprojection is done using the ligament suspension technique, wherein the position of the caudal septum has been optimized relative to the medial crurae. In doing so, both rotation as well as projection have been controlled. In addition, the deviated caudal septum must be centralized in the midline in order to have success. The patient has other observed aesthetic concerns which have also been addressed.

REFERENCES

1. Saban Y, Daniel RK, Polselli R, et al. Dorsal preservation: the push down technique reassessed. Aesthet Surg J 2018;38(2):117–31.
2. Barelli PA. Long term evaluation of "push down" procedures. Rhinology 1975;13(1):25–32.
3. Rohrich RJ, Muzaffar AR, Janis JE. Component dorsal hump reduction: the importance of maintaining dorsal aesthetic lines in rhinoplasty. Plast Reconstr Surg 2004;114(5):1298–308 [discussion: 1309-212].
4. Sheen JH. Spreader graft: a method of reconstructing the roof of the middle nasal vault following rhinoplasty. Plast Reconstr Surg 1984;73(2):230–9.
5. Regalado-Briz A. Aesthetic rhinoplasty with maximum preservation of alar cartilages: experience with 52 consecutive cases. Plast Reconstr Surg 1999;103(2):671–80 [discussion: 681-72].
6. Tebbetts JB. Shaping and positioning the nasal tip without structural disruption: a new, systematic approach. Plast Reconstr Surg 1994;94(1):61–77.
7. Cakir B, Oreroglu AR, Daniel RK. Surface aesthetics in tip rhinoplasty: a step-by-step guide. Aesthet Surg J 2014;34(6):941–55.
8. Anderson JR. A reasoned approach to nasal base surgery. Arch Otolaryngol 1984;110(6):349–58.
9. Bitik O, Uzun H, Kamburoglu HO, et al. Revisiting the role of columellar strut graft in primary open approach rhinoplasty. Plast Reconstr Surg 2015;135(4):987–97.
10. Daniel RK, Palhazi P. The nasal ligaments and tip support in rhinoplasty: an anatomical study. Aesthet Surg J 2018;38(4):357–68.
11. Kridel RW, Scott BA, Foda HM. The tongue-in-groove technique in septorhinoplasty. A 10-year experience. Arch Facial Plast Surg 1999;1(4):246–56 [discussion: 257-248].
12. Apaydin F. Projection and deprojection techniques in rhinoplasty. Clin Plast Surg 2016;43(1):151–68.
13. Daniel RK. Mastering rhinoplasty : a comprehensive atlas of surgical techniques with integrated video clips. 2nd edition. New York (NY): Springer; 2010.
14. Byrd HS, Andochick S, Copit S, et al. Septal extension grafts: a method of controlling tip projection shape. Plast Reconstr Surg 1997;100(4):999–1010.
15. Hubbard TJ. Exploiting the septum for maximal tip control. Ann Plast Surg 2000;44(2):173–80.

Preservation Rhinoplasty (Let-Down Technique) for Endonasal Dorsal Reduction

Jose Juan Montes-Bracchini, MD

KEYWORDS

• Preservation rhinoplasty • Let down • Biotensegrity • Dorsal reduction • Endonasal • Nasal valve

KEY POINTS

- The keystone area is the osseocartilaginous structure formed by the nasal bones and the upper lateral cartilages that constitutes a nonrigid structure beneath the nasal dorsum.
- The nasal dorsum is one that has rigid struts that bear tension and compression and a structure forms by the upper lateral cartilages that bear prestress.
- The differences between push-down and let-down maneuvers are how they can affect the nasal valve and hump removal.
- The push-down technique pushes the bones inside the nasal cavity, whereas the let-down technique preserves the nasal cavity area and the nasal valve.

INTRODUCTION

Management of the dorsum has always been a challenge in rhinoplasty. In most Caucasian noses, and even for those considered mestizo noses, reduction of the dorsum implies the resection of bone and cartilage, with the resulting disruption of the keystone area and the cartilages, requiring the placement of spreader grafts.[1]

Experience with rhinoplasty over time has shown that detailed anatomic analysis of the nose is an essential first step in achieving a successful outcome. Failure to recognize a particular anatomic feature preoperatively will often lead to a less than ideal long-term result.[2]

The analysis of a patient undergoing nasal surgery should not only be of the nose; it is important to consider race, perform an integral facial analysis, and determine the positive and negative facial characteristics to adequately diagnose the condition and take into account the technique to be used, which in addition to correcting the main problem, will give additional contributions to optimize the results.

In addition to considering the anatomic and functional concepts, the nose should be viewed as a comprehensive structure both functionally and aesthetically. It is important to consider that the concepts of form and function must not be separated; an esthetically pleasant nose is most likely to have an adequate functional state.[3]

ANATOMIC AND DYNAMIC CONSIDERATIONS OF THE NASAL DORSUM

Approaching the nasal dorsum, in particular, has become a very precise maneuver that requires a comprehensive knowledge of the anatomy as well as a properly trained surgeon to minimize complications.

To better understand the complexity of the dorsal structure of the nose, one must start by understanding the anatomy of the K-area. It is an osseocartilaginous structure formed by the nasal bones, the upper lateral cartilages, and the nasal septum beneath. Theses structures are not rigidly fused, they are joined together by a chondro-osseous joint.[4]

Private Practice, Cirugia Facial Polanco, Ejercito Nacional, 650-102, Polanco, Mexico City 11560, Mexico
E-mail address: jjuanmontes@me.com
Twitter: @jjcirugiafacial (J.J.M.-B.)

Facial Plast Surg Clin N Am 29 (2021) 59–66
https://doi.org/10.1016/j.fsc.2020.09.006

There is a portion of the cartilaginous septum that extends high cephalically to the K-area and almost no bony septum along this area, leaving the support of the bony cap to the quadrangular septum at his ventral portion and at the joint with the perpendicular plate of the ethmoid (**Fig. 1**). Taking this anatomic feature into consideration, one can understand that the nasal valve, a dynamic structure claimed to be the primary inflow regulator of air to the nose,[5] can be affected by a rhinologic surgery aimed to modify the dorsum. In fact, it is claimed to be the second most common cause of nasal valve abnormalities only after anterior deviation of the septum.[6]

Many investigators have pointed out the differences between push-down and let-down maneuvers with regards to how they can affect the nasal valve, as well as comparisons to hump removal.[7] The only study to date measuring the effect of the 3 techniques on the nasal valve is that of Most and colleagues[8] where they conclude after computed tomography measurements, that hump removal and let-down techniques do not impact the physiology of the nasal valve, whereas the push-down techniques does.

THE BIOTENSEGRITY CONCEPT APPLIED TO THE NASAL DORSUM

In 1998, Dr Donald E. Ingber[9] described that tensegrity structures are mechanically stable not because of the strength of individual members, but because of the way the entire structure distributes and balances mechanical stress. He emphasizes that there are 2 categories of structures: one is basically a framework made up of rigid struts that can bear compression or tension, and another stabilizes itself through a phenomenon known as prestress. These counteracting forces equilibrate throughout the structure, enabling it to stabilize itself.[9] Furthermore, as has been described by Dyer,[10] nasal tip support is a spring-loaded structure. He states that the difficulty of performing nasal tip surgery is the complex mechanism of support and the fact that surgeons are not used to think as engineers or architects while doing surgery in complex structures.[10]

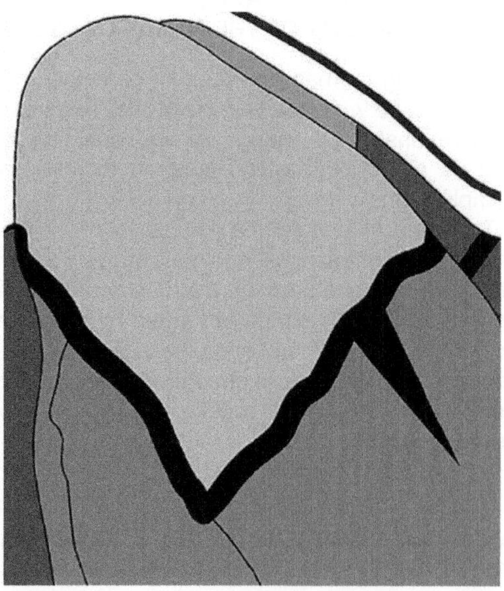

Fig. 1. Relationship between the quadrangular plate and the perpendicular plate of the ethmoid below the keystone area.

The structure of the nasal dorsum is one that has rigid struts that bear tension and compression (nasal bones) and a structure forms by the upper lateral cartilages that bear prestress, the 2 categories previously described, and they should be addressed separately during surgery. The 2 most common procedures performed in the nasal dorsum, hump removal and preservative surgery, should be analyzed regarding the anatomy and the dynamics of the structure that are to be modified. Although in hump removal the cartilaginous dorsum and the bony dorsum are addressed separately, the integrity of the two is compromised because the cap of bone is removed, and the structure formed by the upper lateral cartilages and the septum is removed and reconstructed, affecting the function of the nasal bones as struts, and the resistance of the nasal valve.

With the preservation technique, more precisely, with the let-down technique, the principle is to remove a portion of the cartilaginous septum below the Keystone area and of the nasal bones crating a gap that will be closed by letting the whole structure to come down preserving the support both internally and externally, while the cartilaginous dorsum suffers no disruption because the septum is repositioned at the nasal spine (**Fig. 2**).

SURGICAL TECHNIQUE

Dorsal preservation techniques are especially indicated in the following noses:

1. The straight nose with a moderate kyphotic hump.
2. The deviated nose with high dorsum.
3. The tension nose that often has elongated vertical nostrils and narrow internal nasal valves that tend to collapse.[11]

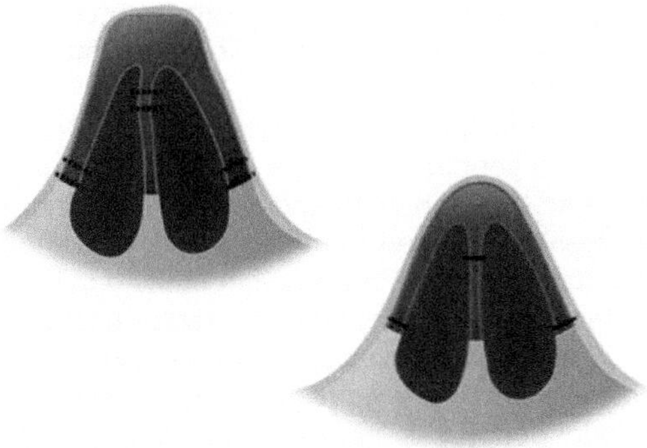

Fig. 2. Resected wedges of bone and the proportional part of the septum.

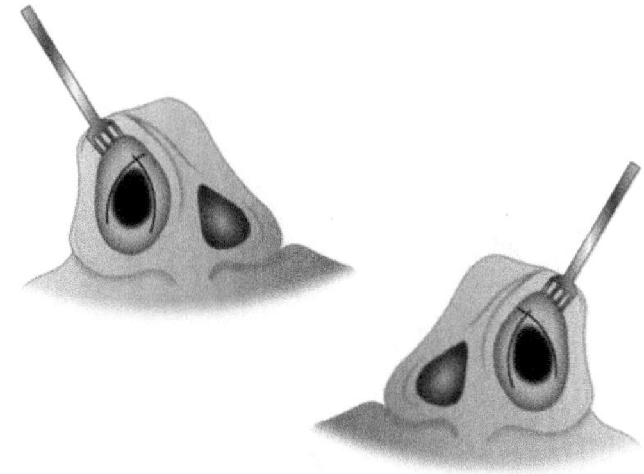

Fig. 3. Incisions made bilaterally to have good exposure of the dorsum and the septum through an endonasal approach.

The area is infiltrated with 3 to 5 mL of lidocaine 2% + epinephrine (1:100,000), in the conventional areas (nerves: external nasal, infraorbital, supratrochlear, supraorbital and nasopalatine) as well as the intercartilaginous (IC) area, cul-de-sac, and the transition from columellar skin to nasal mucosa. The caudal border of the upper lateral cartilage is identified and its scroll, with the help of a 4-prong retractor, and the application of digital pressure upon the lateral crus of the inferior lateral cartilage, to identify the cephalic border. A simple skin hook is placed in the cul-de-sac, applying medial traction to give the appropriate tension to the tissues, and perform its dissection. A left IC incision is made, followed by a hemitransfixion incision, and the incisions are replicated on the right side. The IC incision is situated on a horizontal plane, having first located the site where the caudal border of the upper lateral cartilage and the cephalic border of the inferior lateral cartilage where they meet. The IC incision of the skin is performed from a lateral to medial direction, beginning on the external border of the upper lateral cartilage, and upon reaching the cul-de-sac, the scalpel is inserted by applying pressure toward the nasal midline, with 2 objectives: deepening the incision so as to reach the dorsal cartilaginous plane and avoid the risk of continuing to cut and injuring the skin of the columella, maintaining absolute control of the length of the IC incision.

The hemitransfixion incision is performed from below upward, joining both incisions (hemitransfixion and IC) in a T-shaped incision (**Fig. 3**). The same procedure is performed on the right side.

Access to the septal tunnels is made, all the way to the keystone area, and any deflection or spur is corrected or resected. Removal of the perpendicular plate of the ethmoid along with the cartilage attached to it, all the way to the keystone area is performed to avoid resistance once the let-down maneuver is performed. The ventral border of the septum will be later resected according to the amount of bone that is resected to achieve the desired dorsal height. Therefore, repositioning, fixating and placing of transeptal sutures will be delayed until the bony pyramid reposition is achieved.

Once the approach is completed, one can proceed to make the osteotomies, as described for the Let-down technique.[7] The site of the intranasal incision is at the transition from nasal vestibular skin to mucosa just superior to the attachment of the head of the inferior turbinate. The incision is made perpendicularly to the skin, and dissection is carried on to identify the bone above the Webster triangle. The pyriform aperture is exposed on both the internal and external sides. A subperiosteal undermining is performed on both the internal and external surfaces of the frontal processes of the maxillary bone. The undermining proceeds first onto the deep aspect of the maxillary process. On the endonasal surface, the exposure continues upward to the lachrymal fossae and the head of the middle turbinate.

Then, bony wedges of the frontal process of the maxilla are resected using a small bone forceps or a Webster needle holder on both sides at the level of the facial plane, keeping Webster's triangle intact. The amount of bone resected will be assessed before the surgery and according to the height of the hump. Once the bony wedges are resected, the lateral osteotomies are continued following a high–low–high pattern toward the nasion (**Fig. 4**).

Next, a percutaneous perpendicular transection of the nasal spine is done according to Gola's technique.[12] A 2-mm osteotome is pushed through the skin at the nasion and a transverse

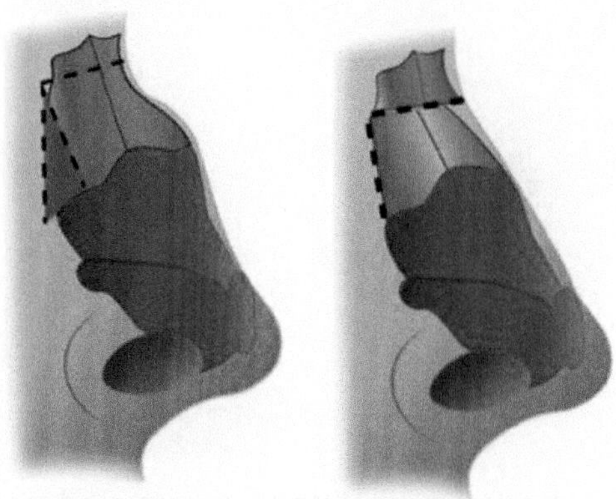

Fig. 4. Representation of the wedge resection and the lateral and transverse osteotomies to mobilize the dorsum en bloc.

root osteotomy of the nose is completed. This will allow an en bloc mobilization of the whole intact bony pyramid closing the gap created with the wedge resection (**Fig. 5**).

SEPTAL WORK

Once the bony dorsum is lowered, the cartilaginous dorsum should be addressed to match the new height without disrupting its attachment. There are several options described to adjust the height of the cartilaginous dorsum. Saban has proposed the resection of the cartilage in the middle portion from the anterior aspect to the perpendicular plate of the ethmoid, whereas Neves has described the split preservation technique more commonly known as the Tetris split technique, creating a measured gap below the junction of the upper lateral cartilages and the septum that is closed once the dorsum is lowered and suturing both portions to stabilize it.[1,13]

This author prefers the following maneuver to adjust the septum: Once the dorsum is lowered, the ventral portion of the septal cartilage should be carefully resected to match the new height of the bony dorsum, with the height of the cartilages and then fixated again to the nasal spine using a 3-0 PDS suture.[7] This maneuver favors also rotation and projection of the tip of the nose very similar to an extended septal graft or a tongue in groove (**Fig. 6**) Modifications of the dorsum must be the first step before any nasal tip surgery is done, because dorsal lowering can dramatically alter many of the extrinsic tip characteristics (**Fig. 7**).

A low radix can be found in many patients with kyphotic humps, and performing a transverse osteotomy can either increase a lower radix, or not solve it. Radix grafts are commonly used to deal with it in the small concavity that it is seen in these patients; augmenting the radix can soften an angry look; normal height in this area restores a high profile and separates or frames the eyes, creating a more aesthetically pleasing look. Augmentation of the radix by using an autologous cartilage graft with a precise pocket approach as described by Becker and Pastorek[14] can raise the apparent nasal starting point and thereby contribute to the illusion of nasal length (**Fig. 8**).

The use of crushed cartilage provides a more malleable material that adapts naturally to the radix,[12] providing a longstanding aesthetic effect; several studies have determined that cartilages lightly or moderately crushed maintain their viability and chondrocytic proliferation in remodeling of nasal contours, filling defects and/or camouflaging irregularities of the nasal dorsum.[15]

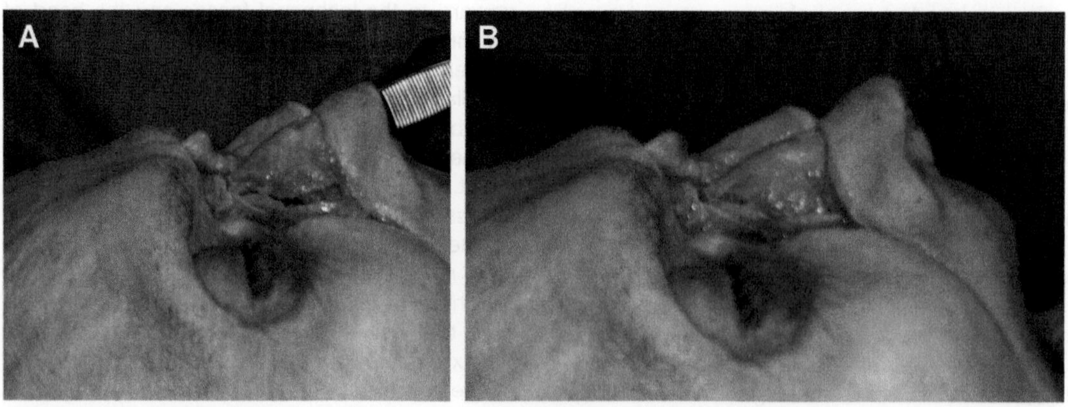

Fig. 5. (*A, B*) Cadaveric dissection showing the gap created by the wedge resection and its closure after lateral and transverse osteotomies.

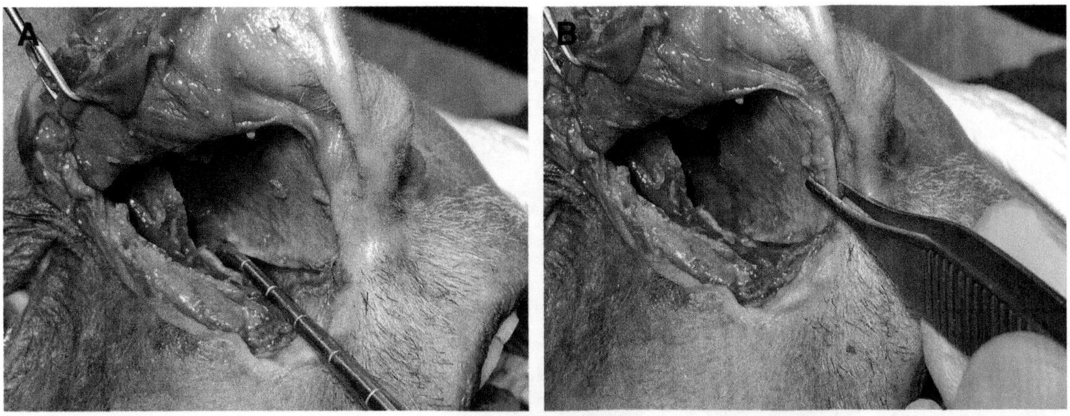

Fig. 6. (*A, B*) Cadaveric dissection showing the ventral part of the septal cartilage to be resected and the reposition at the nasal anterior spine, allowing for rotation of the tip of the nose.

There is a common finding in patients with tension noses: an altered facial volume or deficits in the midface, even more common in young patients that may be caused by nasal chronic obstructive diseases, these cases can benefit from a preservation rhinoplasty technique, which has the positive side effect as a midface filler, specifically in the malar region.

As described elsewhere by the author, the influence of the let-down technique on the midface allows a statistically significant increase in the malar contour by the mobilization of soft tissues adjacent to the nasal pyramid, and thus filling favorably and naturally this area, giving patients a better facial balance (**Fig. 9**). Finally, the skin and musculoaponeurotic system is separated from the dorsum, this will heal itself, again matching the new shape of the nose. This maneuver should always be performed at the end of the procedure because the musculoaponeurotic is the system that will provide certain stability while the surgeon is lowering the dorsum en bloc.[16]

SUMMARY

The goal of a dorsal preservation technique is to keep intact the K-area above the septum and the entire osseocartilaginous vault. The dorsal hump can be eliminated and no irregularities or discontinuity should be found either by the patient or the surgeon. It is imperative for the surgeon to recognize that every incision, reduction, and destabilizing step must be countered by a reinforcing supportive maneuver. An incision that is not reconstituted is left to unpredictable postoperative changes. Cartilage that is already weak before surgical manipulation is prone to postoperative deformity.

Over the years, a myriad of techniques and approaches for septorhinoplasty have been described, some based on minimally invasive surgery, which could complicate the task of the surgeon, her or his field of vision, and her or his action by working in a limited space. These factors argue that there is less trauma to the intranasal structures and the support mechanisms, and therefore, a lower number of complications.[17]

The approach that the author uses is based on basic surgical techniques, a knowledge of anatomy, and the surgeon's experience. The endonasal approach is a technique that combines various incisions, producing a complete, comprehensive, functional technique with enduring results that we have found to be useful for most of the primary patients.[18] Concerning the dorsum it is important to differentiate the push-down technique from the let-down technique. It basically involves the fact in the former, that the nasal bones are repositioned inside the nasal cavity, causing obstruction, whereas in the other, the nasal bones will rest at the maxillary plane, thus preserving the integrity of the bony pyramid, and improving function.[8] It will also maintain the tensegrity of the dorsum, a structural element present in the dorsum of the nose that require the understanding of the architecture of the nasal pyramid, and that preservation should be preferred over resection, and reposition over manipulation.[19]

Before working on the contour of the nasal tip lobule, the first step of tip modification is stabilization of the base or pedestal of the nose. This maneuver is critical to avoid postoperative loss of nasal tip projection. Some have advocated a preservation rhinoplasty method that preserves the caudal septal strut, to facilitate this.[20]

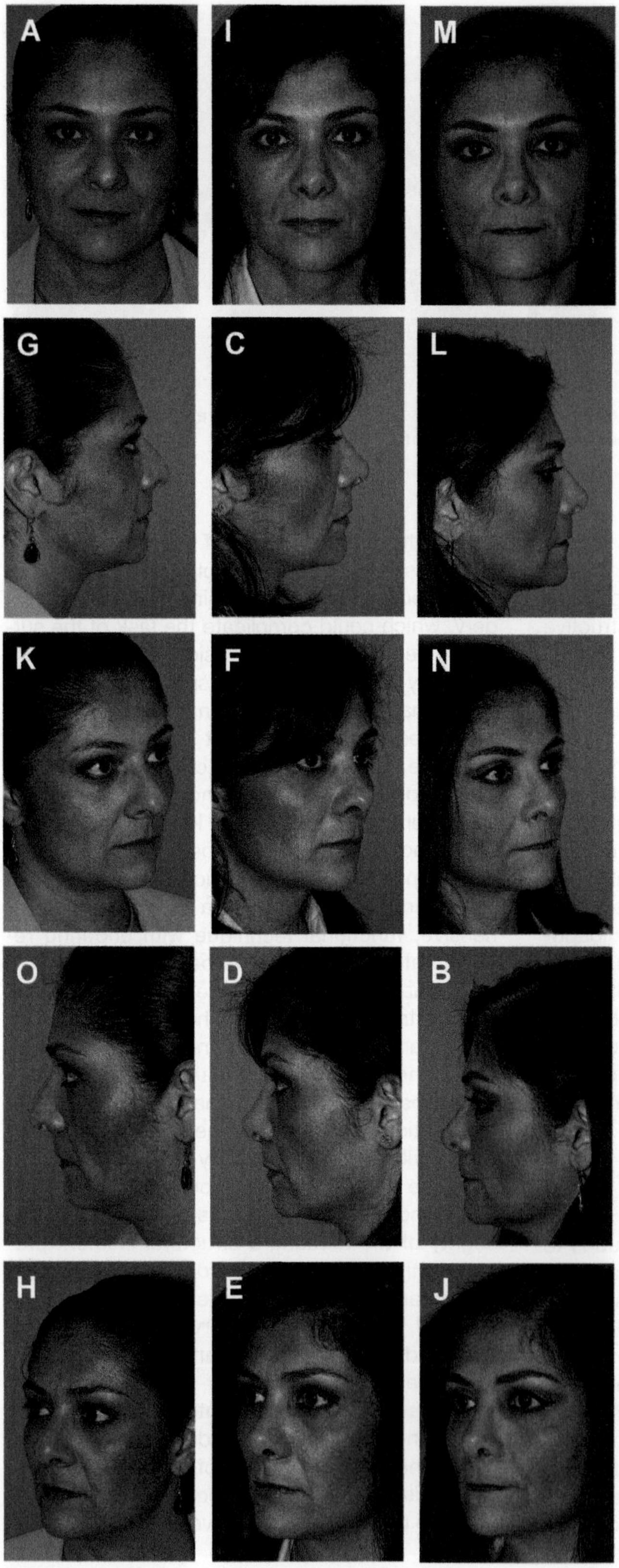

Fig. 7. (*A–O*) Patient who underwent a preservation rhinoplasty with no modification of the lower lateral cartilages. Results at 6 weeks and 10 years.

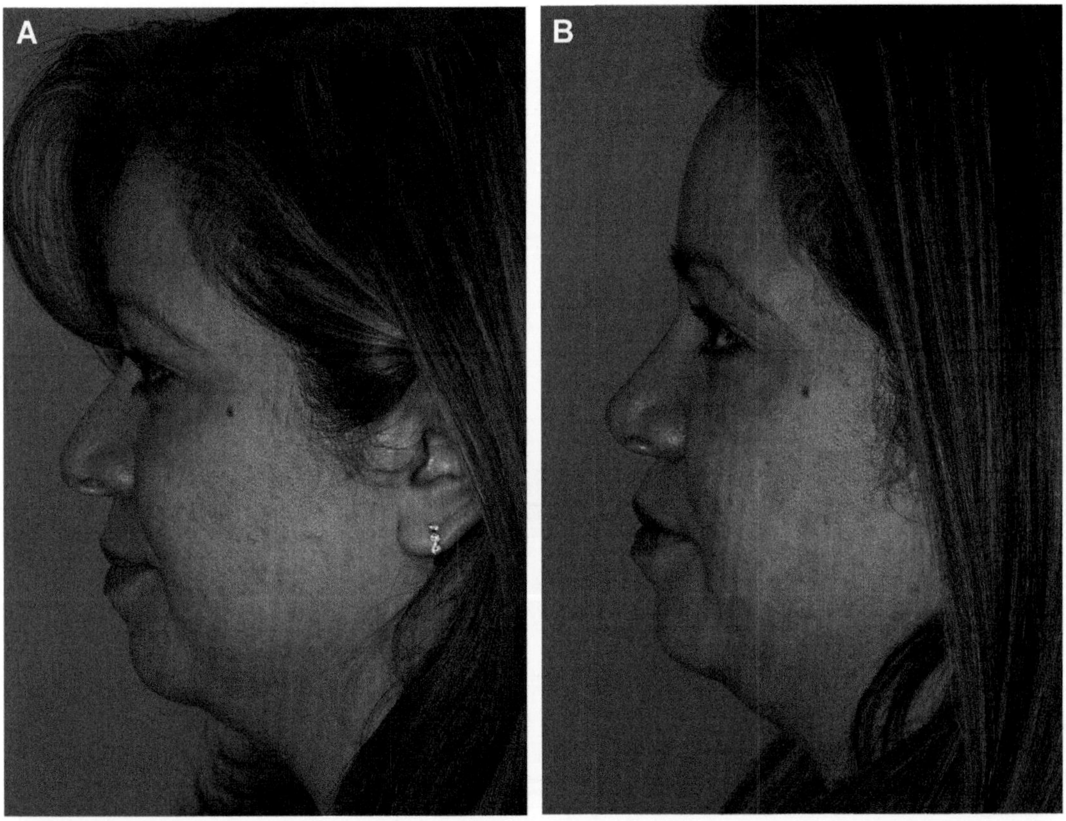

Fig. 8. (*A*, *B*) Patient with a moderate kyphotic hump and a deep radix. A preservation rhinoplasty was made with a small wedge resection and a crushed cartilage radix graft was placed to avoid shortening of the nose.

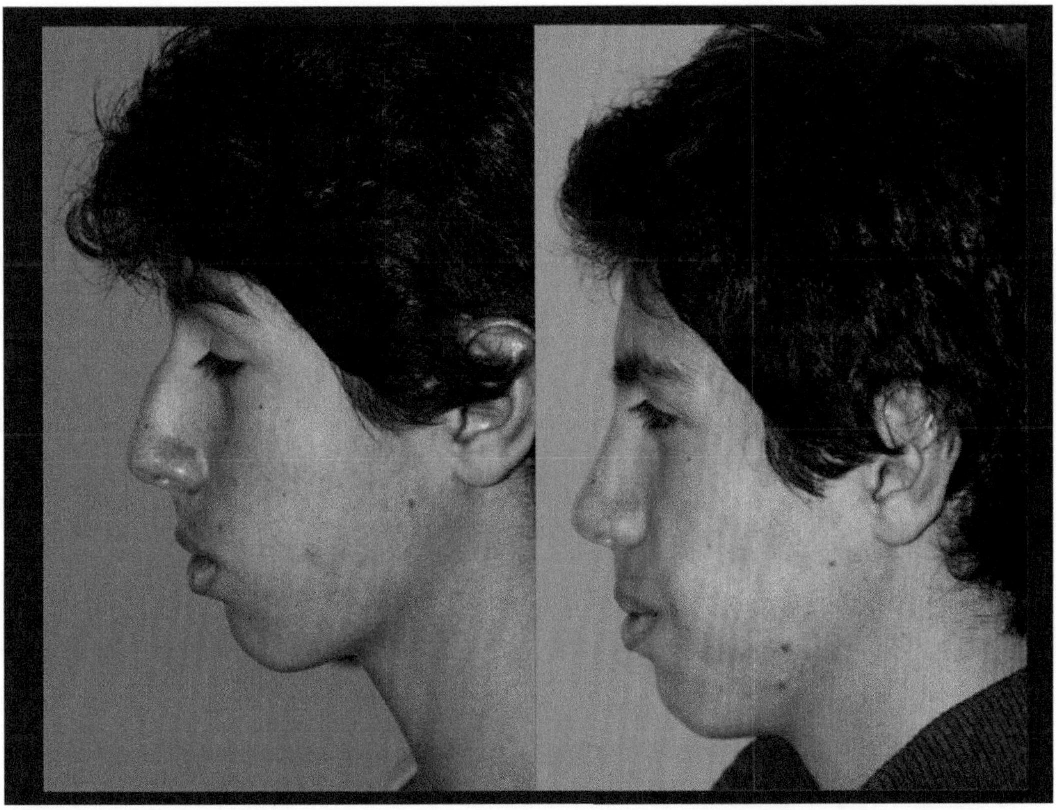

Fig. 9. Young patient with disproportion in the middle third of the face, and high dorsum. The let-down technique was used with improvement of the middle third by displacement of the soft tissues.

With all the techniques for septorhinoplasty available, it is extremely important to take into account the delicate balance between good and excellent results, as well as weighing the risk–benefit ratio, making it possible to achieve long-term predictable and reliable results, both functionally and cosmetically. A surgeon should realize that all techniques involve consequences; the more complicated the technique, the greater the consequences. This technique, like many others, is not the answer to every case, but will avoid those complications such as inverted V deformities, dorsal irregularities, and perhaps narrowing of the nasal valve.

CLINICS CARE POINTS

- Preservation technique.
- Difference between push down and let down techniques.
- Valve colapse prevention.

DISCLOSURE

No disclosures.

REFERENCES

1. Saban Y, Daniel RK, Polselli R, et al. Dorsal preservation: the push down technique reassessed. Aesthet Surg J 2018;38(2):117–31.
2. Yellin S. Aesthetics for the next millennium. Facial Plast Surg 1997;13:231–9.
3. Ricketts RM. Divine proportion in facial esthetics. Clin Plast Surg 1982;9:401–22.
4. Daniel RK. Mastering rhinoplasty. New York: Springer-Verlag; 2002.
5. Haight JSJ, Cole P. The site and function of the nasal valve. Laryngoscope 1983;93:49–55.
6. Kasperbauer JL, Kern EB. Nasal valve physiology. Otolaryngol Clin North Am 1987;20(4):699–719.
7. Montes-Bracchini JJ. Nasal profile hump reduction using the let-down technique. Facial Plast Surg 2019;35(5):486–91.
8. Abdelwahab MA, Neves CA, Priyesh NP, et al. Impact of dorsal preservation rhinoplasty versus dorsal hump resection on the internal nasal valve: a quantitative radiological study. Aesthetic Plast Surg 2020;44(3):879–87.
9. Ingber DE. The architecture of life. Sci Am 1998;1.
10. Dyer WK. Nasal tip support and its surgical modification. Facial Plast Surg Clin North Am 2004;12:1–13.
11. Tardy ME. Illusions in rhinoplasty. Facial Plast Surg 1995;11:117–38.
12. Gola R. Conservative rhinoplasty. Ann Chir Plast Esthet 1994;38(3):239–52.
13. Neves JC, Tagle A, Dewes D, et al. The split preservation rhinoplasty: "the Vitruvian Man split maneuver". Eur J Plast Surg 2020;43:323–33.
14. Becker DG, Pastorek NJ. The radix graft in cosmetic rhinoplasty. Arch Facial Plast Surg 2001;3(02):115–9.
15. Ozcan C, Fuat B, Zerrin Y, et al. Viability of cultivated nasal septum chondrocytes after crushing. Arch Facial Plast Surg 2005;7:407–9.
16. Saban Y. An anatomical study of the Nasal Superficial musculoaponeurotic system. Surgical applications in rhinoplasty. Arch Facial Plast Surg 2008;10(2):109–15.
17. Burke A, Cook T. Open versus closed rhinoplasty: what have we learned. Curr Opin Otolaryngol Head Neck Surg 2000;8:332–6.
18. Beaty MM, Dyer WK II, Shawl MW. The quantification of surgical changes in nasal tip support. Arch Facial Plast Surg 2002;4:82–91.
19. Daniel RK. The preservation rhinoplasty: a new rhinoplasty revolution. Aesthet Surg J 2018;38(2):228–9.
20. Patel PN, Abdelwahab M, Most SP. A review and modification of dorsal preservation rhinoplasty techniques. Facial Plast Surg Aesthet Med 2020;22(2):71–9.

Preservation Rhinoplasty
The Endonasal Cottle Push-Down/Let-Down Approach

Oren Friedman, MD[a,*], Fausto Lopez Ulloa, MD[b], Eugene B. Kern, MD, MS[c]

KEYWORDS

• Preservation rhinoplasty • Cottle rhinoplasty • Endonasal rhinoplasty • Rhinoplasty
• Dorsal preservation

KEY POINTS

- Endonasal Cottle rhinoplasty has been a preferred method of nasal surgery for more than 50 years.
- Preservation rhinoplasty is a new term for an established technique.
- The push-down/let-down technique is a tried-and-true method for dorsal reduction and has been used with great success as a conservative approach to the nasal dorsum.

INTRODUCTION

Rhinoplasty is a transformative operation aimed at enhancing an individual's quality of life through improved facial harmony and nasal breathing.[1] A myriad of techniques and approaches has been described in the past, each successful in allowing us to achieve the surgical goals, and each also with its own merits and shortcomings. The minimally invasive endonasal approach challenges the surgeon with a reduced field of view and limited access. The more extensive dissection as practiced with the external approach challenges the surgeon with a need for precise nasal restructuring, often with grafts and leaving an external scar. The endonasal "push-down" and "let-down" techniques, the subjects of this article, have been standard operations taught and practiced in the United States, Mexico, Brazil, Italy, Germany, the Netherlands, and France among many surgeons, with origins dating over a century by Lothrop and Goodale.[2,3] It should be clear that the techniques described herein are not part of a new surgical trend nor a new surgical technique, but rather a very well-established operation[4–6] that has been selectively used throughout the authors' careers and those of surgeons worldwide, including rhinoplasty giants, such as Cottle, Hinderer, Dewes, Sulsenti, Lopez-Infante, Huizing, Barelli, Saban, Drumheller, Goodale, Lothrop, Gray, and others. The long-term results have been very satisfying to both patient and surgeon alike.[7–9]

Recently, renewed interest in the endonasal approach for rhinoplasty has brought to light Dr Maurice Cottle's "Push-Down" operation[4,5] and Dr Egbert Huizing's wedge resection[8] called the "Let-Down" operation by Dr Vernon Gray of Los Angeles, California. Today's interest stems from the recent trends to preserve the nasal dorsum during rhinoplasty,[9] which has been newly branded "Preservation Rhinoplasty."[10] The rebranding of the operation through new terminology has popularized it and reopened possibilities for experienced surgeons to explore something "new" that is actually quite "old."

[a] Otorhinolaryngology, University of Pennsylvania School of Medicine, 800 Walnut Street, 18th Floor, Philadelphia, PA 19107, USA; [b] Otorhinolaryngology, Facial Plastic Surgery, ENT Department, Angeles Lomas Hospital, Mexico City, Mexico; [c] Otorhinolaryngology Head and Neck Surgery, State University of New York at Buffalo, 1237 Delaware Avenue, Buffalo, NY 14209, USA
* Corresponding author.
E-mail address: orenfriedman@hotmail.com

Facial Plast Surg Clin N Am 29 (2021) 67–75
https://doi.org/10.1016/j.fsc.2020.08.006

Surgeons approach rhinoplasty with options of performing the operation by either the endonasal or external structural approach. Currently, practicing surgeons seem to be embracing and adapting to a specific technique that best resolves a given pathologic condition. The "Push Down" or "Let Down" relies on reducing tension within the nose, whereas the classic external structural rhinoplasty relies on creating tension to insure the new nose can withstand the potentially deforming forces of wound-healing contracture. The reintroduction, popularization, and renaming/reclassifying of previously well-established but lesser-known and often even rejected techniques should not be confused with technical novelty or innovation and should therefore not be met with fear or concern regarding safety and efficacy.[4–9] Expert rhinoplasty surgeons who have enjoyed decades of outstanding results are trying something old for the first time, and they will contribute to innovations and improvements on the classic "Cottle operation."

History

In the early to middle twentieth century, the divergent rhinoplasty schools of Jacques Joseph and Maurice Cottle emerged based on differing surgical philosophies. Both the Joseph and the Cottle techniques were performed through the endonasal approach, but Joseph approached the dorsum directly with excision of the "hump," whereas Cottle reduced the "hump" by lowering the dorsum into the nose from below. Devout surgeons in each of the 2 schools continually worked to improve the basic techniques as they sought ways to optimize patient outcomes. Endonasal and external approaches evolved over time. The minimally invasive endonasal approach challenged the surgeon with reduced visualization compared with the extensive visualization attained by the external approach. The endonasal approach was also more demanding to teach because of limited visualization. The external approach and "hump" resection, although providing superior visualization, challenged the surgeon to construct the resected nasal structures with grafts and sutures. Outstanding techniques evolved out of a need to restructure the destabilized altered nasal dorsum and nasal middle third, in order to allow for excellent esthetic and functional breathing results.[11] External approaches also commonly detach or transect nasal ligaments, structures that have previously been identified as important structures to consider as early as 1965,[12–15] and to retain in more recent years.[16,17] Pitanguy and colleagues[12–14] described specific maneuvers to identify and transect the dermato-cartilaginous ligament: the ligament is bypassed and preserved in most endonasal surgeries, and Pitanguy himself described specific maneuvers useful to access, identify, and transect the ligament for situations he thought necessary.

Although it is more invasive, the external approach gained popularity for numerous reasons: excellent visualization permitting technical precision, visualization allowing anatomic comprehension, and straightforward student's understanding of the operational concepts. These factors, coupled with the abundance of talented teaching surgeons both training and producing outstanding results, contributed to the establishment of the external structural approach as the prevailing influence in North American and European rhinoplasty for the past 3 to 4 decades.[18,19] During the period of external approach structural rhinoplasty dominance, the results achieved were outstanding and exceeded the results obtained through earlier endonasal techniques. As a consequence, it appears that fewer surgeons were trained in the older endonasal rhinoplasty techniques. During these last decades, exceptional lessons were learned from the external structural approach. These lessons or pearls were adopted by endonasal surgeons to insure long-term outcomes and to help to avoid common sequelae of "old-fashioned" endonasal reduction rhinoplasty. The endonasal surgeons could also place columellar strut grafts, spreader grafts, spreader flaps, butterfly grafts, lateral crural strut grafts, batten grafts, and use other techniques used by external

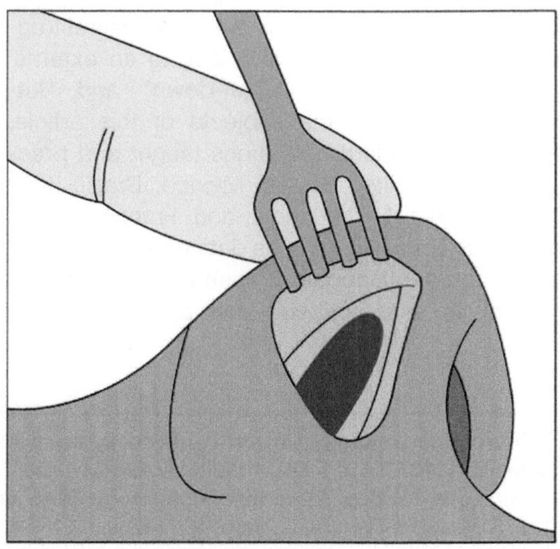

Fig. 1. The septum is scraped with a knife or scissor or sharp elevator until the subperichondrial plane is identified.

approach surgeons. Shaping the tip cartilages rather than resecting them, using spreader grafts and auto spreader grafts to straighten and stabilize the middle third, and using cartilage camouflage techniques helped secure strong long-term foundational nasal support by preserving and reinforcing native structures through an endonasal approach. It appears that the external rhinoplasty approaches still dominate the surgical landscape even today.

During the past few years, many surgeons have celebrated surgical success adopting concepts of dorsal preservation techniques. Many of these surgeons who follow the preservation rhinoplasty trend are performing the operation through the external approach. To make it an even more conservative and safe operation, the authors anticipate the future emergence toward endonasal preservation rhinoplasty. They present their long-standing endonasal Cottle surgical techniques and highlight some associated advantages over many of the other surgical techniques that they also use frequently. Through life-long learning and constant striving for improvement, the widespread renaissance or rebirth of the Cottle techniques among surgeons worldwide has added much excitement for the authors as they exchange ideas and explore new perspectives and variations on these traditional techniques. As new perspectives on an old technique emerge, the authors will all reexamine their rhinoplasty methods on the road to even better outcomes.

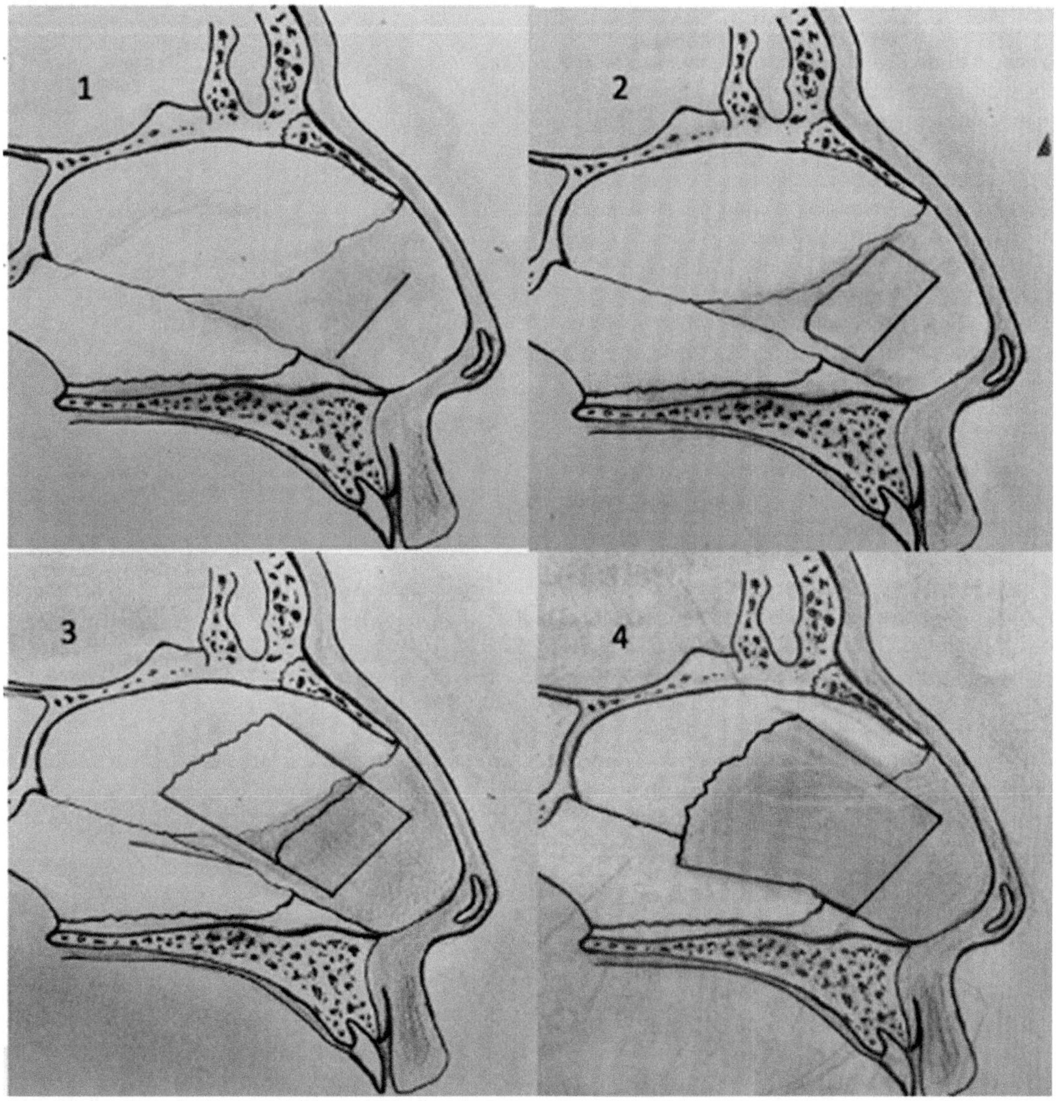

Fig. 2. Septoplasty approaches. 1. incision is made through the cartilage; 2. horizontal incisions through the cartilage and, 3. incisions extended to the bony septum, 4. window of septal cartilage and bone removed.

Technique

The endonasal Cottle technique forms the foundation of the authors' version of preservation rhinoplasty: a technique that combines various endonasal access incisions and produces comprehensive and enduring aesthetic and functional results. Standard endonasal Joseph access incisions, including a hemi-transfixion (HT) incision and an intercartilaginous (IC) incision, may be used. A Cottle retractor or a wide double skin hook may be used to access the intranasal cavity for these incisions. Alternatively, the Fausto Lopez Infante (FLI) "T" incision provided a nuanced modification of the incision to help prevent the often dysfunctional and potentially cosmetically deforming scar at the junction of the IC and HT incisions that were often found in patients who underwent reduction rhinoplasty through standard Joseph incisions. Using a 4-prong retractor along the rim of the nose for lateral and caudal traction and a single skin hook in the cul-de-sac at the internal valve angle applying medial traction, a left IC incision is made. The single hook is then repositioned toward the base of the columella for downward traction, and a HT incision is made. In the FLI approach, these 2 straight line incisions (HT and IC) come together as a "T" rather than an "inverted U," as in the standard Joseph approach, helping to minimize circumferential scarring at the valve angle in the "cul-de-sac." These incisions are replicated on the right side, thereby providing bilateral nasal access[20] (**Fig. 1**).

The caudal border of the septum is then exposed by elevating the perichondrial fibers that surround the septum. The septum is scraped with a knife or scissor or sharp elevator until the subperichondrial plane is identified. Bilateral anterior tunnels are elevated anteriorly. By grasping the columella with forceps, the authors are able to pull the columella caudally, separating it from the caudal septum in order to free the nasal tip complex by combining bilateral HT incisions into 1 complete transfixion through the thickness of the membranous septum just anterior to the caudal end of the septum. Using the FLI approach, the authors are able to access the entire osseocartilaginous structure, along with all aspects of the septum endonasally, thereby avoiding the complications of a rounded and narrowed scar at the internal nasal valve angle.

The nasal tip complex has now been freed, allowing visualization of the entire cartilaginous dorsum and the caudal edge of the septal cartilage. Next, the authors begin the subperichondrial septal dissection and complete the maxillary-premaxillary approach as described by Cottle.[21]

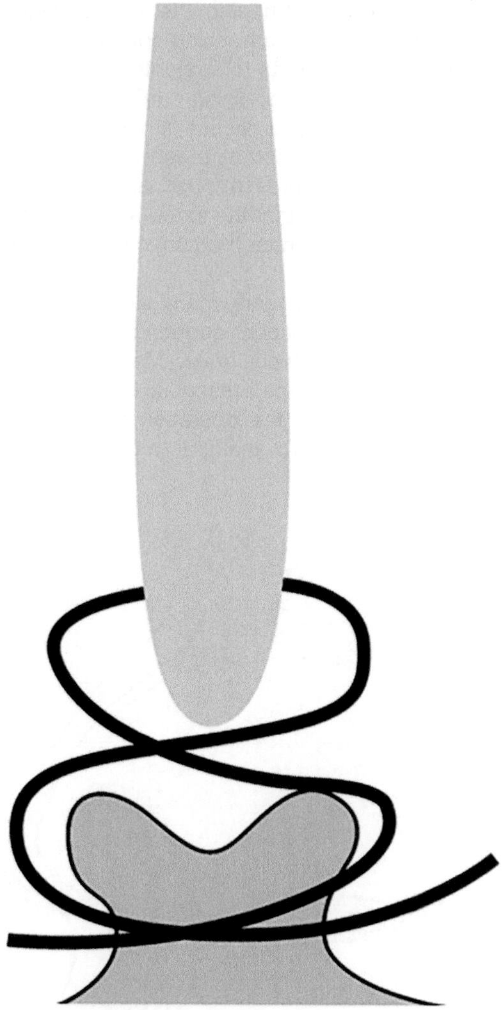

Fig. 3. Image-of-8 stitch.

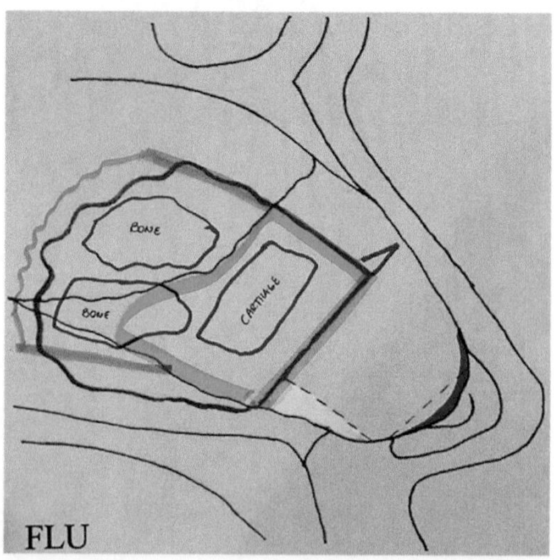

Fig. 4. Extensive septoplasty. Removal of all deviated cartilage and bone that is necessary to remove for airway improvement.

The Cottle method involves exposing 1 side of the septum from the anterior nasal spine, along the entire ventral border, extending dorsally to the upper lateral cartilages and posteriorly beyond the perpendicular plate of the ethmoid. The authors often prefer to elevate bilaterally to expose the entire septum, including cartilaginous and bony segments, and allow for better septal mobilization.

Various septoplasty techniques may be used. Commonly, the cartilage is incised with a Freer or Cottle elevator, a number 15 blade, an angled Beaver number 66 blade, or with an angled ophthalmologic crescent blade, perpendicular to the caudal edge of the septum, making sure to leave at least a 2.5-cm caudal strut and 1 cm of dorsal strut (**Fig. 2**).

Many surgeons use the Ballenger swivel knife to remove the window of cartilage beyond the remaining caudal and dorsal struts. Alternatively, the standard Cottle elevator or Freer elevator is used for the entire nasal septal dissection, including the incisions through the septal cartilage. The harvested cartilage is kept for ultimate replacement or for grafting as needed. The perpendicular plate of the ethmoid and vomer are then viewed and managed as needed to correct any bony airway pathologic conditions. This technique allows for effective septoplasty, opening the nasal airway while preserving or reestablishing solid structural support for long-term stability. Removal of large portions of the quadrangular cartilage and perpendicular plate of the ethmoid not only treats the nasal airway functionally but also provides space below the osseocartilaginous vault in order to displace downward the nasal pyramid. Once osteotomies are completed with either removal of a bony wedge from the pyriform aperture ("Let Down") or medializing the ascending (frontal) process of the maxilla after complete mobilization ("Push Down"), the dorsal height can be adjusted. The ventral border of the 2.5-cm caudal quadrangular cartilage remnant is freed from the maxillary crest and resected to control the final height of the cartilaginous dorsum. The ventral surface of the caudal septal cartilage is then fixed to the anterior nasal spine with a figure-of-8 stitch, pulling the caudal septum anteriorly and freeing dorsal septal attachments at the keystone (ie, 3-0 PDS, other suture) (**Fig. 3**).

The approach to the septum is as extensive as needed and can include removal and reconstruction of large portions of septal cartilage and bone

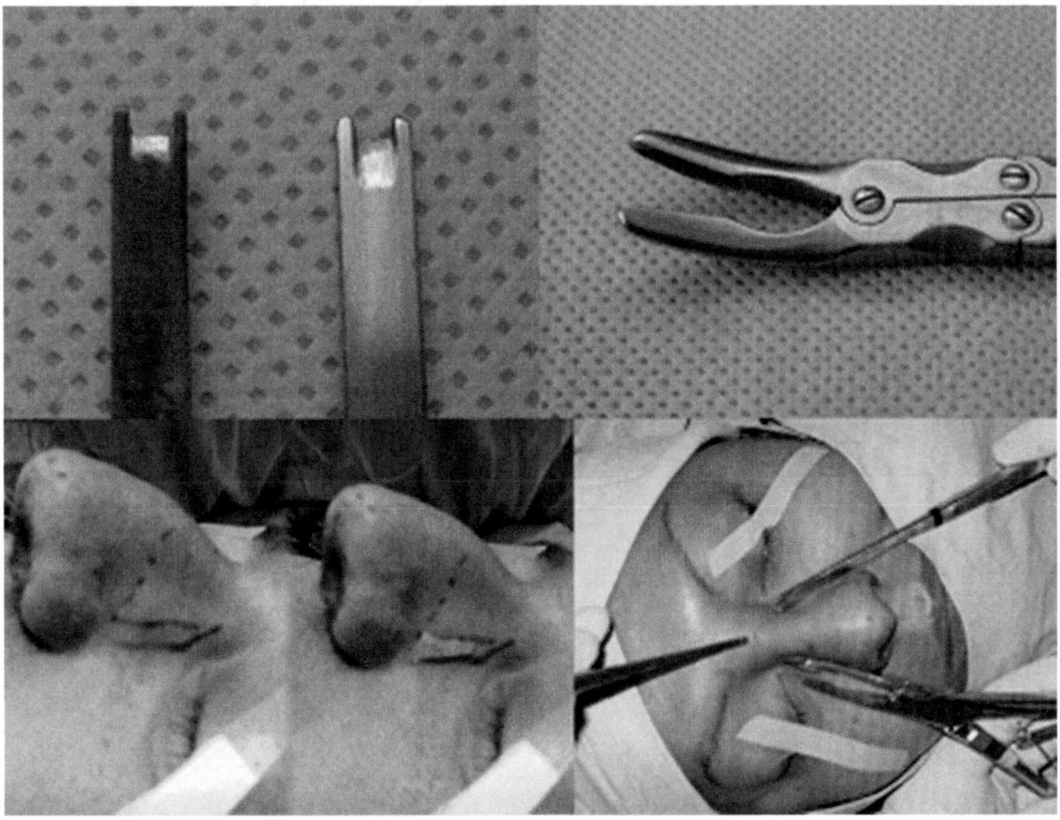

Fig. 5. Instruments for push down let down.

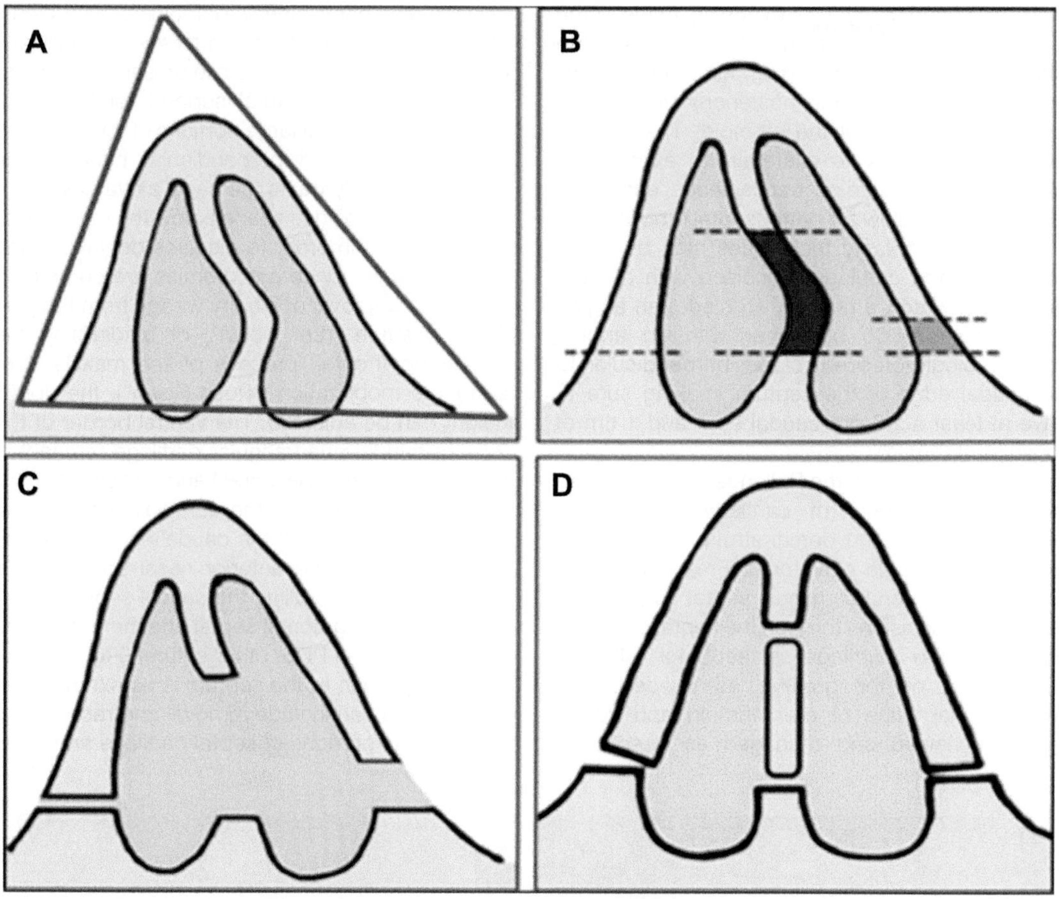

Fig. 6. Unilateral wedge resection with pyramidal alignment and septal work. Asymmetries of bone may be corrected with asymmetrical wedge of bone resection in the "let-down" approach.

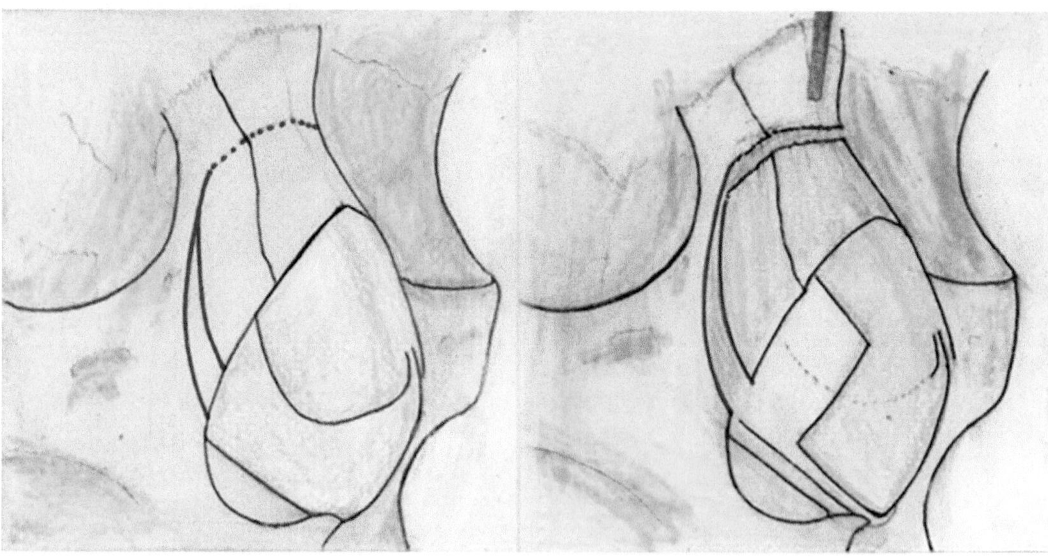

Fig. 7. Transvers root osteotomy.

in order to improve the nasal airway (**Fig. 4**). Other dorsal preservation techniques do not allow for the correction of septal pathologic conditions like this does, and it is therefore most suitable for functional rhinoplasty and combination functional and aesthetic rhinoplasty.

Let Down and Alignment of the Nasal Pyramid

A superficial incision is made just above the insertion of the inferior turbinate, allowing subperiosteal dissection along the pyriform aperture. Staying deep to the nasal muscles, sweeping them away with subperiosteal dissection, the authors avoid much of the bleeding that would be caused by cutting directly into the muscle, significantly decreasing postoperative edema and ecchymosis. The Cottle dissector is used to create subperiosteal tunnels medial and lateral to the ascending (frontal) process of the maxilla and nasal bones, along the length of the proposed lateral osteotomy sites. The width of the tunnel is determined by the size of the osteotome to be used and by the anticipated width of the wedge of bone that will need to be resected from the ascending (frontal) process of the maxilla for the "Let Down." A 2- to 3-mm Cook osteotome (single lateral guard and keel) or a 2-mm double-guarded curved osteotome (López-Infante) may be used to perform the lateral superior osteotomy first (parallel to the facial plane), which would correspond to the upper portion of the wedge, followed by the second lateral osteotomy for the lower portion of the wedge performed along the facial plane. The size of the wedge to be removed depends on the length amount of dorsal lowering desired. The bony wedge to be removed may also be excised with a bone rongeur in a single step once periosteal tunnels are elevated medially and laterally from the ascending (frontal) process of the maxilla bilaterally, or with an ultrasonic device. Once the wedge is removed, completion of the lateral osteotomies is performed from the apex of the excised wedge along the nasofacial groove of the ascending (frontal) process of the maxilla to meet the bony osteotomy cut of the transverse root osteotomy[4–9,22,23] (**Fig. 5**).

If the pyramid is symmetric and tall, then the traditional "Let Down" is performed symmetrically bilaterally. If the pyramid is deviated, for example, to the right, as in the illustration (**Fig. 6**), the authors would do a double osteotomy on the left side with resection of the osseous wedge fragment or a bigger wedge on the deviated side (longer left side). These maneuvers allow the nasal pyramid to fall toward the left, whereas on the right side a smaller wedge of bone or only a right lateral osteotomy would be required to be performed. Once the lateral osteotomies are completed, the authors release the nasal pyramid by means of a percutaneous transverse osteotomy with a 2-mm osteotome, in a greenstick fashion (which will work as a hinge, and height will not be lost in that area) or complete, which would allow mobilization of the osseous nasal pyramid as a single unit, toward the midline and downward (**Figs. 6** and **7**).

The combination of osteotomies and septal work allows repositioning of the entire nasal pyramid without instrumenting or directly modifying the nasal dorsum. The dorsal height is adjusted by changes made to the septum rather than adjustments made to the dorsum itself. In this way, the authors are able to preserve the anatomic relationships of the dorsum and avoid the complexities and complications of reconstructing the dorsum. The degree of downward displacement is directly related to the amount of osseous wedge resected

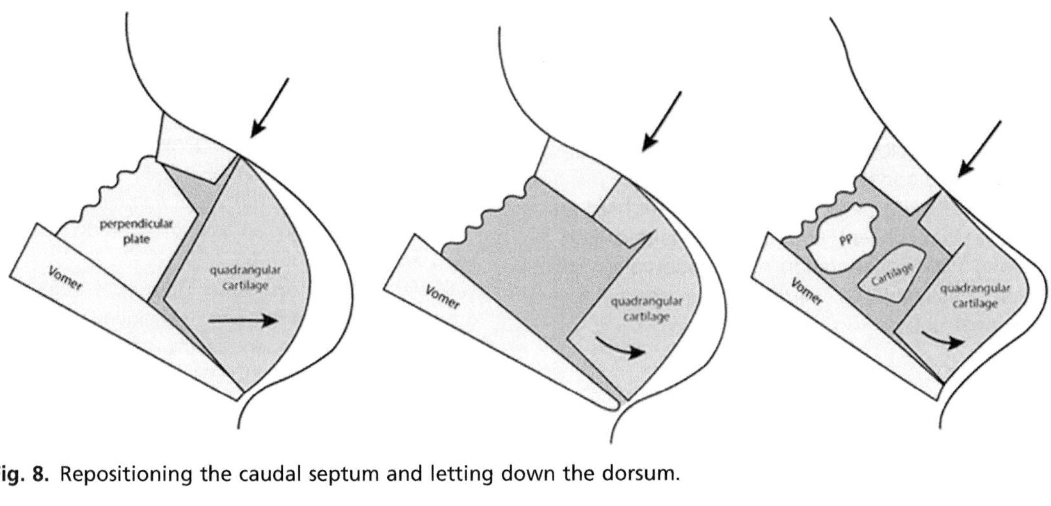

Fig. 8. Repositioning the caudal septum and letting down the dorsum.

and to the remnant height of septum that is anchored to the anterior nasal spine. The further anteriorly the caudal septal remnant is pulled, the lower the dorsum is lowered, and securing it in that position is a key step in insuring long-term dorsal height (**Fig. 8**).

SUMMARY

Preservation rhinoplasty and dorsal preservation rhinoplasty represent new terminology for old techniques. Regardless of which direction the rhinoplasty pendulum swings, conservative approaches and techniques will continuously provide predictable and secure aesthetic and functional breathing results. Cottle's endonasal approach to septorhinoplasty has provided us with a safe and effective means to satisfy patients' needs, both functionally and aesthetically. This operation is a tried-and-true operation that has enjoyed widespread use for generations of both contented surgeons and appreciative patients worldwide. Advances in structural rhinoplasty have enabled us to improve on the basic Cottle techniques by incorporating structural supports into the operation. Similarly, the authors expect the newfound popularity of "preservation rhinoplasty" among a much wider group of surgeons will lead to nuances and improvements to the basic conservative Cottle operation. As novel modifications are introduced and tested by innovative surgeons, there remains a reliance on the foundations of this established, consistent, stalwart operation always stressing and defending the consequence of nasal breathing function.

CLINICS CARE POINTS

- Endonasal rhinoplasty is a long established clinically proven approach to rhinoplasty.
- When considering preservation rhinoplasty, our goal is to conserve as much of the original structure and relationships between structures as possible. The endonasal approach allows us to conserve optimally.
- Cottle's endonasal preservation technique provides excellent access and visualization along with conservation and preservation of soft tissues to limit the need for reconstruction.

DISCLOSURE

The authors have nothing to disclose.

REFERENCES

1. Saleh A, Younes A, Friedman O. Cosmetics and function: quality of life changes following rhinoplasty surgery. Laryngoscope 2012;122(2):254–9.
2. Lothrop OA. An operation for correcting the aquiline nasal deformity; the use of new instrument; report of a case. Boston Med Surg J 1914;170:835–7.
3. Goodale JL. A new method for the operative correction of exaggerated Roman nose. Boston Med Surg J 1899;140:112.
4. Cottle MH, Loring RM. Corrective surgery of the external nasal pyramid and the nasal septum for restoration of normal physiology. Eye Ear Nose Throat Mon 1947;26(4):207–12.
5. Cottle MH. Nasal roof repair and hump removal. AMA Arch Otolaryngol 1954;60(4):408–14.
6. Kienstra M, Sherris DA, Kern EB. Osteotomy and pyramid modification in the Joseph and Cottle rhinoplasty. Facial Plast Surg Clin North Am 1999;7: 279–94.
7. Barelli PA. Long term evaluation of "push down" procedures. Rhinology 1975;13(2):25–32.
8. Huizing EH. Push-down of the external nasal pyramid by resection of wedges. Rhinology 1975;13(4): 185–90.
9. Saban Y, Daniel RK, Polselli R, et al. Dorsal preservation: the push down technique reassessed. Aesthet Surg J 2018;38:117–31.
10. Daniel R. The preservation rhinoplasty: a new rhinoplasty revolution. Aesthet Surg J 2018;38(2):228–9.
11. Kovacevic M, Riedel F, Goksel A, et al. Options for middle vault and dorsum restoration after hump removal in primary rhinoplasty. Facial Plast Surg 2016;32(4):374–83.
12. Pitanguy I, Salgado F, Radwanski H, et al. The surgical importance of the dermatocartilaginous ligament of the nose. Plast Reconstr Surg 1995;95(5): 790–4.
13. Pitanguy I. Surgical importance of a dermatocartilaginous ligament in bulbous noses. Plast Reconstr Surg 1965;36(2):247–53.
14. Pitanguy I. Revisiting the dermatocartilaginous ligament. Plast Reconstr Surg 2001;107(1):264–6.
15. Han SK, Jeong SH, Lee BI, et al. Updated anatomy of the dermocartilaginous ligaments of the nose. Ann Plast Surg 2007;59(4):393–7.
16. Daniel R, Palhazy P. The nasal ligaments and tip support in rhinoplasty: an anatomical study. Aesthet Surg J 2018;38(4):357–68.
17. Cakir B, Öreroglu AR, Doğan T, et al. A complete subperichondrial dissection technique for rhinoplasty with management of the nasal ligaments. Aesthet Surg J 2012;32(5):564–74.
18. Anderson JR, Johnson CM, Adamson P. Open rhinoplasty: an assessment. Otolaryngol Head Neck Surg 1982;90:272–4.

19. Johnson CM, Toriumi DM. Open structure rhinoplasty: featured technical points and long term follow up. Facial Plast Surg Clin North Am 1993;1: 1–22.

20. Schulte DL, Sherris DA, Kern EB. M-plasty correction of nasal valve obstruction. Facial Plast Surg Clin North Am 1999;7(3):405–9.

21. Cottle MH, Loring RM, Fischer GG, et al. The maxilla-premaxilla approach to extensive nasal septum surgery. AMA Arch Otolaryngol 1958;68(3): 301–13.

22. Atolini N Jr, Lunelli V, Pererira Lang G, et al. Septum pyramidal adjustment and repositioning - a conservative and effective rhinoplasty technique. Braz J Otorhinolaryngol 2019;85(2):176–82.

23. Ishida J, Ishida LC, Ishida LH, et al. Treatment of the nasal hump with preservation of the cartilaginous framework. Plast Reconstr Surg 1999;103(6): 1729–33.

Piezoelectric Osteotomies in Dorsal Preservation Rhinoplasty

Abdülkadir Göksel, MD[a,*], Priyesh N. Patel, MD[b], Sam P. Most, MD[c]

KEYWORDS

• Preservation rhinoplasty • Dorsal preservation • Piezotome • Piezo • Nasal bones
• Osseocartilaginous vault

KEY POINTS

- The primary methods of bony vault manipulation in preservation rhinoplasty are the let-down and push-down, with the former being preferred for airway preservation.
- The piezo device, with tips such as saws, rasps, and scrapers, allows for precise management of the osseocartilaginous vault.
- The drill tip allows for safe perforation of mobile nasal bones or the nasal spine.

INTRODUCTION

Piezoelectrical instruments (PEI) have been used for a long time in maxillofacial surgery and dentistry. These devices are useful in cutting through hard tissues such as bones and have the advantage of minimizing damage to soft tissues and reducing bleeding during the bone shaping process. Thanks to the new generation of the devices, procedures such as reshaping, cutting through and rasping of the nasal bones can be carried out much faster and easier. There are visibly less bruises on the skin in the postoperative period. Moreover, because this technique helps to avoid the unwanted fracture lines that may occur with traditional osteotomies carried out with osteotomes, it may help prevent typical complications during the reshaping of the bones. An excellent resource on this is Dr Gerbault's publication on piezo surgery.[1]

PIEZO-OSTEOTOMY AND PIEZO-OSTECTOMY

There are different ways to perform septal resections in dorsal preservation techniques.[2] High septal, mid septal, and low septal strip modifications all need precise cuts on the perpendicular plate of the ethmoid bone and removal of a piece of the cartilage and bone. The long saw insert of the piezo device is extremely useful to make a sharply defined cut on this thin layer of the bone without creating any additional fracture lines. We recommend making all excisions from the septum incrementally to decrease the risk of step-offs at the rhinion. If more lowering is required, we can incrementally excise small strips and recheck until the desired dorsal height is achieved. The piezo long saw insert allows us to make this step by step lowering safely (**Fig. 1**).

Especially in dorsal preservation techniques, the amount of lowering of the dorsum depends on the osteotomies and overlapping area of the low-to-low osteotomy sides (**Fig. 2**). As a result of this, precise osteotomies are more important and necessary in dorsal preservation.[3] To prevent a visible or palpable step deformity in the lateral osteotomy area, we perform our osteotomies as close as possible to the maxillary bone, right

[a] ENT Facial Plastic Surgery, Rino Istanbul, Bagdat Cad No:378/5 Saskinbakkal, Istanbul 34070, Turkey; [b] Division of Facial Plastic and Reconstructive Surgery, Department of Otolaryngology, Vanderbilt University Medical Center, 1215 21st Avenue, South Suite 7209 Medical Center East, South Tower, Nashville, TN 37232; [c] Division of Facial Plastic and Reconstructive Surgery, Stanford University School of Medicine, 801 Welch Road, Stanford, CA 94304, USA
* Corresponding author.
E-mail address: akgoksel@gmail.com

Facial Plast Surg Clin N Am 29 (2021) 77–84
https://doi.org/10.1016/j.fsc.2020.09.004

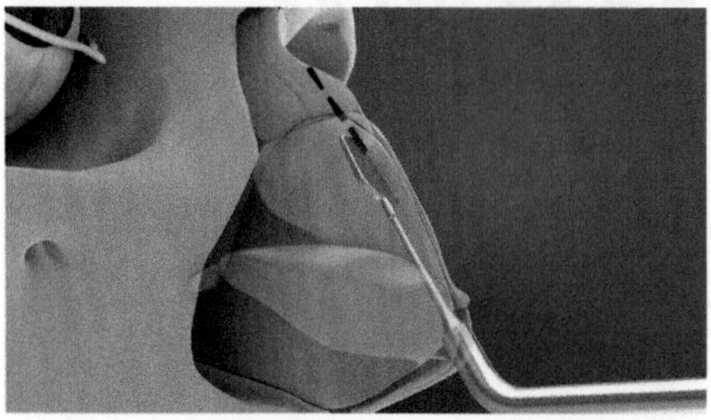

Fig. 1. High septal strip excision with piezo long saw.

above the nasofacial groove in a low-to-low approach.[4]

Depending on the ligament preservation technique used, different dissection approaches can be used for the osteotomies. If the skin attachments to the dorsum are to be preserved, we can create the tunnels on the frontal process of the maxillary bone posterior to the nasomaxillary suture line ligament. It is possible to use piezo instruments in a closed approach with this technique (**Fig. 3**).

Given the closed space when using endonasal methods and preserving the dorsal skin attachments, the heat generated from piezo instruments can be harmful to the skin and thus precludes their use in transverse osteotomies. Thus, we use the combination of hand saws and a 2-mm external osteotome for transverse and radix osteotomies in this group (**Fig. 4**). When we use an extended open approach, the piezo instruments can be used for all the osteotomies.

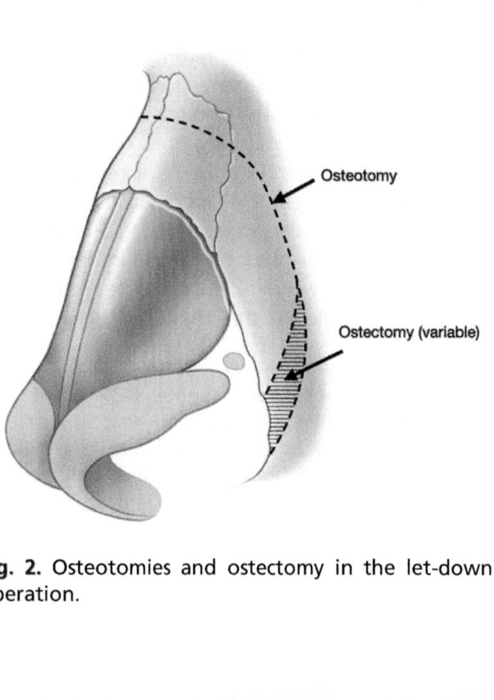

Fig. 2. Osteotomies and ostectomy in the let-down operation.

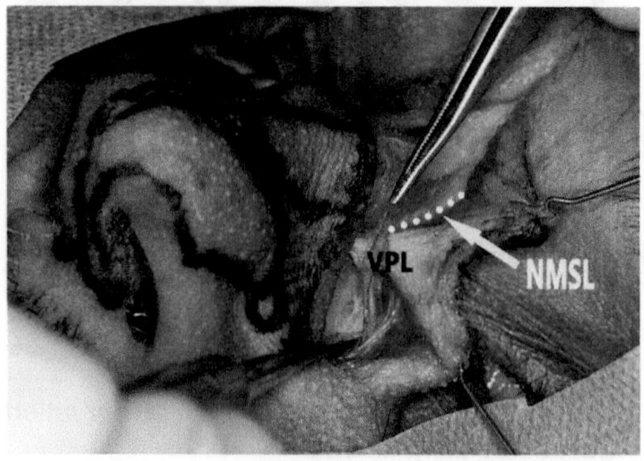

Fig. 3. Lateral ligaments of the nose. NMSL, nasomaxillary suture line ligament; VPL, vertical piriform ligament.

The most common complication of dorsal preservation rhinoplasty is a residual hump.[4] One of the most important reasons is resistance to movement of bone in the low-to-low osteotomy area. In traditional techniques, lateral osteotomies are needed for closing the open roof and narrowing the nasal pyramid's base. The direction of the osteotomes was horizontal to the maxillary bone to reduce posterior displacement of the nasal bones. As reviewed elsewhere, there are 2 different ways to handle the bony vault in dorsal preservation, the let down and the push down.[2] When we remove a strip of the bone on the facial groove, we call it let down. If we do osteotomies and overlap the bones, it is called a push down. Usually, we do the combination of these 2 procedures. In the cephalic portion of the bony pyramid, an osteotomy (without ostectomy) is performed, and is thus a push-down type of maneuver. In the caudal portion of the nasal bony pyramid (Webster triangle), an ostectomy is performed, thus creating a let down. In the push-down maneuver, the horizontal osteotomy creates resistance to posterior displacement, and thus the surgeon has to squeeze the nasal bony pyramid to force it to descend medial to the pyriform aperture. An

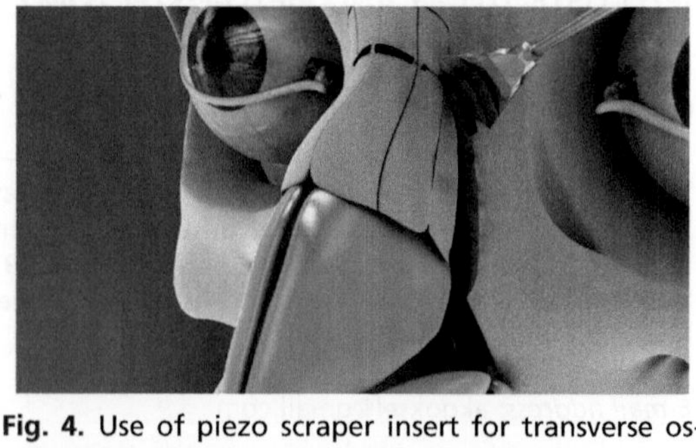

Fig. 4. Use of piezo scraper insert for transverse osteotomy in dorsal preservation rhinoplasty.

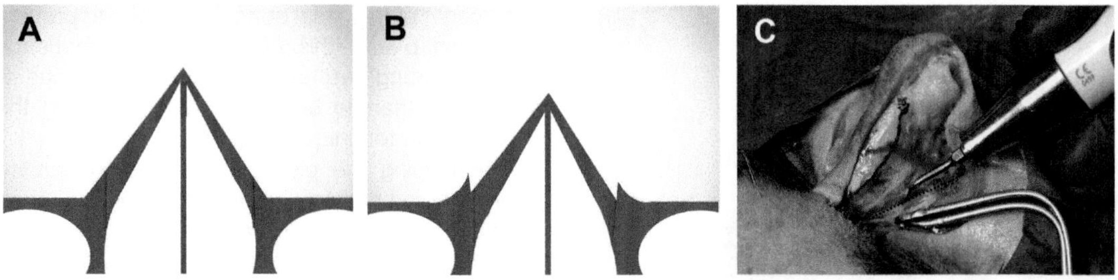

Fig. 5. Sagittal lateral osteotomies shown diagramtically (A and B) and in a cadaver specimen (C).

advantage of PEI is that it is possible to change the direction of the bony cuts from horizontal to sagittal, decreasing this resistance to posterior displacement.[5]

As the lateral osteotomy is performed in the sagittal plane, it is possible to easily push in the nasal dorsum, in both osteotomies and ostectomies, because the borders of the new bones are parallel to the sagittal plane (**Fig. 5**). It enables the dorsum to move lower and decreases the risk of a residual hump or recurrence of the hump in the late postoperative period.

Dorsal preservation is also a useful method to correct the crooked nose. The method chosen by the surgeon for correction of deviations depends on the pathology of the septum. For example, a low septal strip can be more useful for crooked nose correction. When it comes to designing osteotomies for correction of bony vault deviations, asymmetric osteotomies should be considered for correction of the unequal sides.

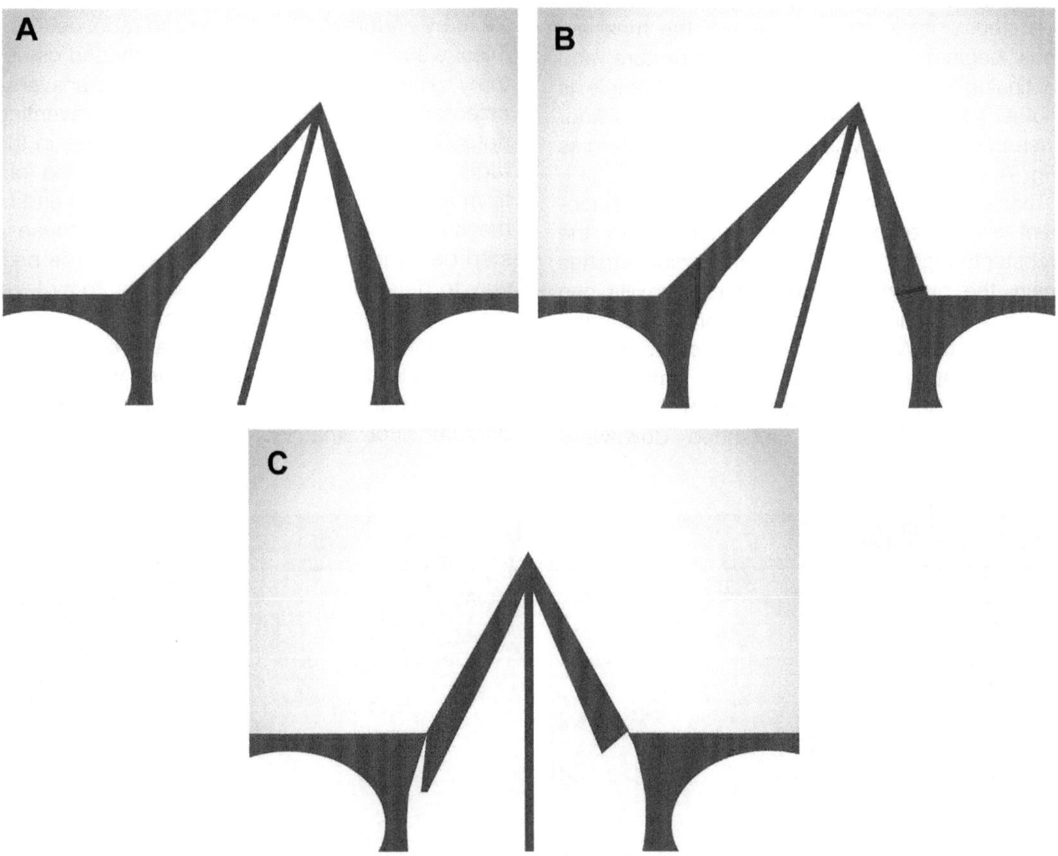

Fig. 6. Sagittal and horizontal osteotomies before (A) and after (C) crooked nose correction. The osteotomy on the short side of the pyramid is horizontal, to minimize posterior displacement (B). On the long side, a sagittal cut is used to allow posterior displacement and correction of the pyramid (B).

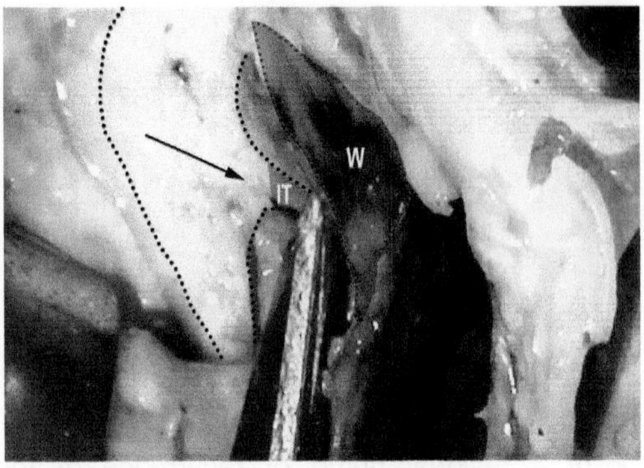

Fig. 7. Webster's triangle (*W, red dotted line*) and inferior turbinate (IT).

The direction of the osteotomies again becomes important: a horizontal lateral osteotomy is performed on the shorter side to decrease posterior movement and a sagittal osteotomy is performed on the longer nasal bone to allow posterior movement and correction of the crooked pyramid (**Fig. 6**).

After ostectomy and osteotomy, one can reduce any resistance to dorsal lowering by elevating the periosteum of the inner surface of the maxillary bone beginning at the pyriform aperture and continuing cephalically. The Webster triangle is another important anatomic landmark to consider when performing low-to-low sagittal osteotomies (**Fig. 7**).

The head of the inferior turbinate's bony attachment is located immediately posterior to the Webster triangle.[6] When the whole dorsum pushes down, the pyriform aperture of the maxilla can overlap with the inferior turbinate bony attachment exactly on the Webster triangle. This has the potential to cause unwanted residual hump recurrence because the bony fragment of the inferior turbinate can block the intended downward movement of the nasal bone. Therefore, to prevent this overlap and this undesirable consequence from occurring, we recommend that the bone of Webster's triangle be resected when using the preservation technique (**Fig. 8**).

When using the piezo, this resection can be easily and accurately performed. We feel that, because of the bone overlap providing bony support, resection of the Webster triangle does not result in breathing problems from lack of support of the internal nasal valve and subsequent collapse. A recent computed tomography study demonstrated improved patency of the nasal valve with resection of this area compared with push-down preservation rhinoplasty.[7]

In both let-down and the push-down cases, we conduct low-to-low lateral ostectomy on our patients. The scraper, straight, and angled piezo tips are the easiest, fastest, and most precise methods for achieving this goal. In the cephalic part of the bony pyramid, we conduct the osteotomy by thinning the bone and leaving a thin layer intact whereas in the caudal portion of the nasal bony pyramid, we use the scraper for thinning and then excising a bone strip as thin as needed. Next, by performing transverse and radix osteotomies, we merge the lateral osteotomy and ostectomy lines on both sides. The transverse osteotomy level is highly important for preventing potential step deformities and irregularities in the radix. If a transverse osteotomy is carried out from a level lower than the radix, from the end of the hump, the inferior radix part might cause a step deformity or a low projected radix. The best way to determine the transverse osteotomy level is to take the intercanthal area as a guide.

It is more difficult to reach the transverse osteotomy area and use piezo there when we preserve the ligaments and do not dissect the nasal dorsum. For that reason, in full ligament

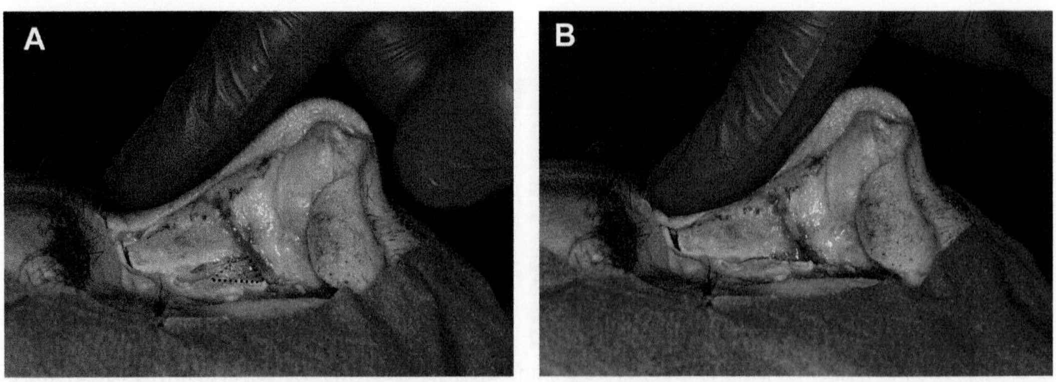

Fig. 8. Resection of Webster's triangle (dotted triangle, A) allowing bone to bone contact with the let-down method of dorsal preservation rhinoplasty (B).

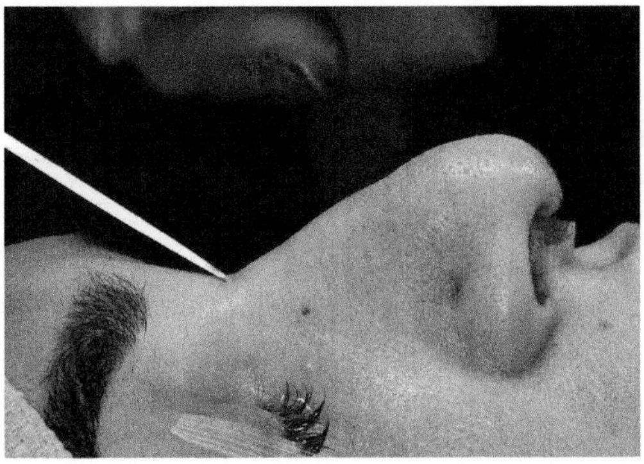

Fig. 9. Percutaneous transverse osteotomy.

preservation cases we conduct the lateral osteotomies sagittally using piezo, but transverse osteotomies are performed percutaneously, as noted elsewhere in this article. The transverse osteotomy is performed by making a 2-mm incision on the skin in radix area using a number 11 surgical blade followed by use of a 2-mm osteotome (**Fig. 9**).

In cases of an overprojected radix, after completing the transverse osteotomy and lowering the dorsum, there might be a step deformity caused by a high projection of the frontal process and nasal bones. In these cases, we can use the piezo scraper insert for equalizing the bone level. Also, for patients with an over projected radix, it should be remembered that the sub–superficial musculo-aponeurotic system layer in that area might be thicker and the procerus muscle prevents adequate redraping. In these cases, if the bone is rasped to lower the radix, excising the procerus muscle will help the skin to better conform to the bone and create a more defined nasal starting point.

OSTEOPLASTY WITH PIEZO

Anatomically and embryologically, the bony vault and cartilaginous vault are fused into a single entity—the osseocartilaginous vault.[7] Because PEI allows for precise bony cuts, it has led to greater precision in bony vault management.[3] The scraper or fine diamond insert of the PEI can easily remove the bony cap without damaging the upper lateral cartilage. When the bony cap is removed with piezo, there will be no open roof on the dorsum, because the piezo does not harm the underlying cartilage. If the patient has small bony hump, this osteoplasty can be enough without any other dorsal preservation or hump removing techniques. The cartilaginous hump can be trimmed if needed.

If the osteoplasty is not enough for reshaping the dorsum, dorsal preservation techniques can be used for flattening the dorsum. The main idea of dorsal preservation is to keep intact all the dorsal structures and not to destroy the dorsal key stone area. When a patient has V-shaped nasal bones, total preservation of the dorsum is easier, and the surgeon can create a straight flat profile. But most patients have an S-shaped bony dorsum.[8] Even if all the straitening maneuvers were done correctly, a residual hump can occur in patients with S shaped nasal bones. Rasping and reshaping the dorsum without disarticulating the dorsal Keystone area is necessary if the nasal bones are kyphotic. Piezoelectric instruments have different shaped rasps and scrapers, which allows us to reshape the bony dorsum without damaging the underlaying soft tissue. Comparing to conventional rasps, piezo rasps are slower but definitely safer and more precise. The most significant advantage of using piezo osteoplasty tools is that they give us an opportunity to reshape the bone even after full mobilization of the dorsum

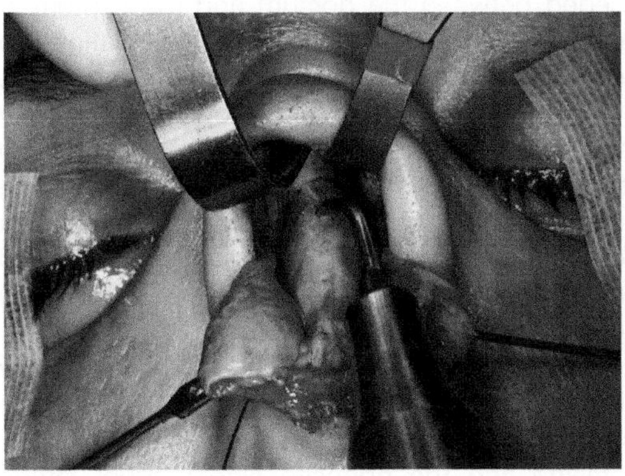

Fig. 10. The piezo scraper is used to remove the bony cap.

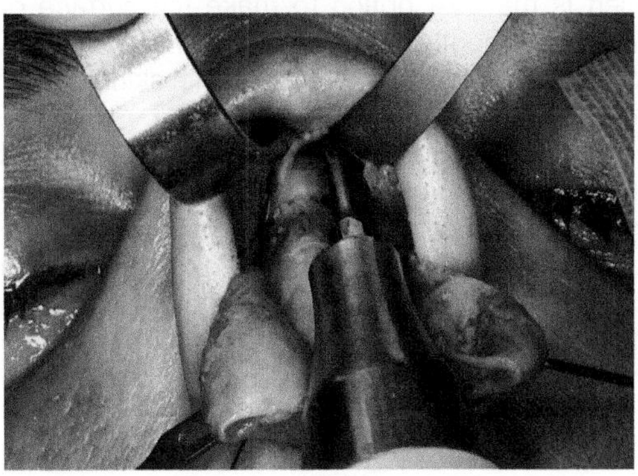

Fig. 11. Use of the piezo scraper to reduce a step-off at the transverse osteotomy site.

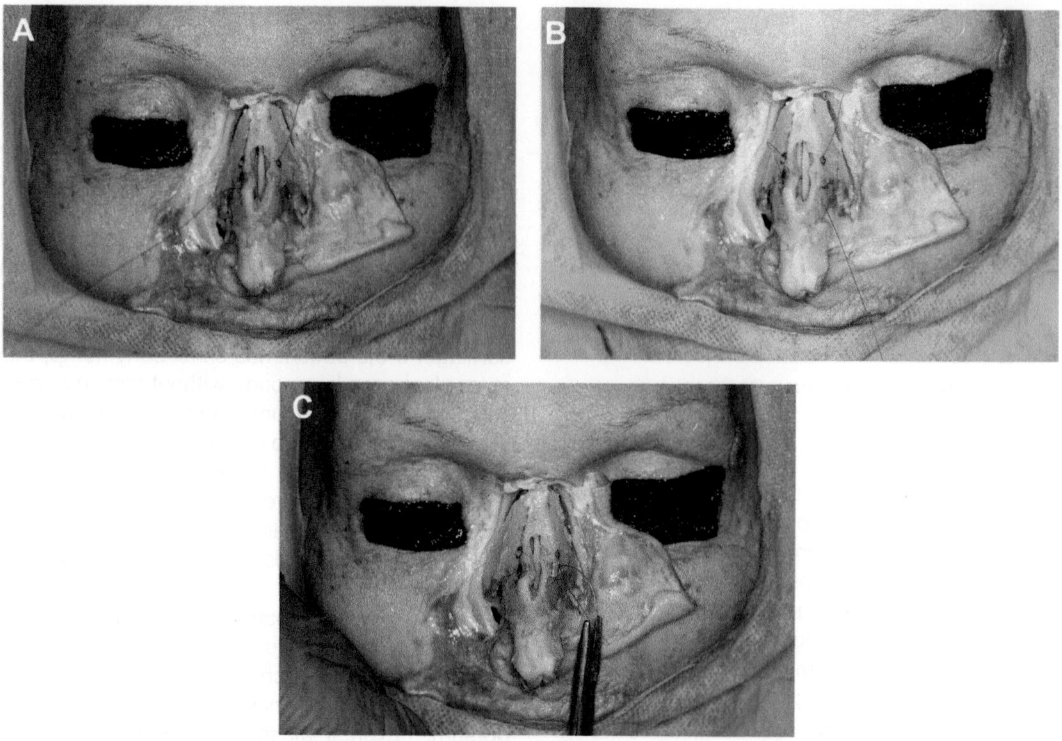

Fig. 12. The crisscross suture for dorsal stabilization. Drill holes are created in the nasal bones using the piezo. The suture is then passed through the bone and septum before exiting the opposite side upper lateral cartilage (A). Then the same procedure is performed on the other side and after passing through the septum, exiting on the starting side (B). When the stitch is completed, the nasal dorsum is stabilized to the septum (C). Note that the open roof is only for illustrative purposes, normally, the dorsum would be preserved.

because minimal pressure is required with this instrument (**Fig. 10**).

The scraper insert is the most powerful and the fastest tool to reshape the dorsum (see **Fig. 10**). Once we feel that the height of the dorsum has been reduced adequately, a fine rasp tip is used to polish the bone. Skin is very thin on the dorsal keystone area and even if we create small irregularities it can be easily visible. The fine piezo rasp insert is the best option to make the surface of the bone smooth. If reshaping of the dorsum is not required, we can preserve the skin attachments and avoid undermining the skin.

Having a palpable or sometimes visible step on the radix osteotomy area can be another common problem with dorsal preservation techniques. The scraper insert of the piezo is an extremely useful tool for fixing moderate step problems. When there is a step deformity on the radix osteotomy line, we can rasp the frontal portion of the step and make it smooth with the scraper tool (**Fig. 11**). If a severe step occurs, rasping may not be enough to solve the problem, and camouflage grafts will be required.

FIXING THE NEW POSITION OF THE DORSUM

Dorsal preservation techniques have the advantage of keeping intact the dorsal keystone and thus creating natural results. When preserving the dorsum, it is important to stably fix the dorsum in the new position. It is possible to perform this fixation with septal sutures in mid septal or low septal strip techniques. However, fixation is needed between the dorsum and the septum in high septal strip techniques. Once the relationship between the dorsum and the septum is separated, the entire dorsum becomes mobile without any resistance of a stabile unit. If it is not fixed to the stable part of the nose it can move and result in dorsal asymmetry. The crisscross suture is a good solution for fixating the dorsum. The piezo drill insert can be used for perforate the nasal bones, even when they are mobile.

A hole is made on the nasal bones using the piezo drill insert on both sides. A 5-0 PDS suture is passed through the dorsal area of the septal cartilage and the opposite side's upper lateral cartilage. Then, the suture is passed through the

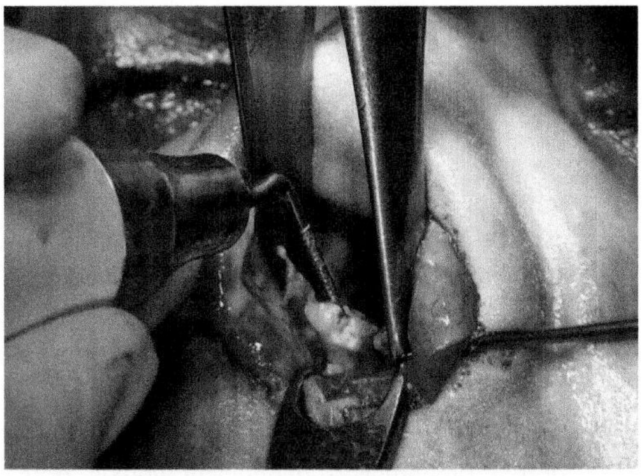

Fig. 13. Using the piezo drill tip to create precise holes in the nasal spine.

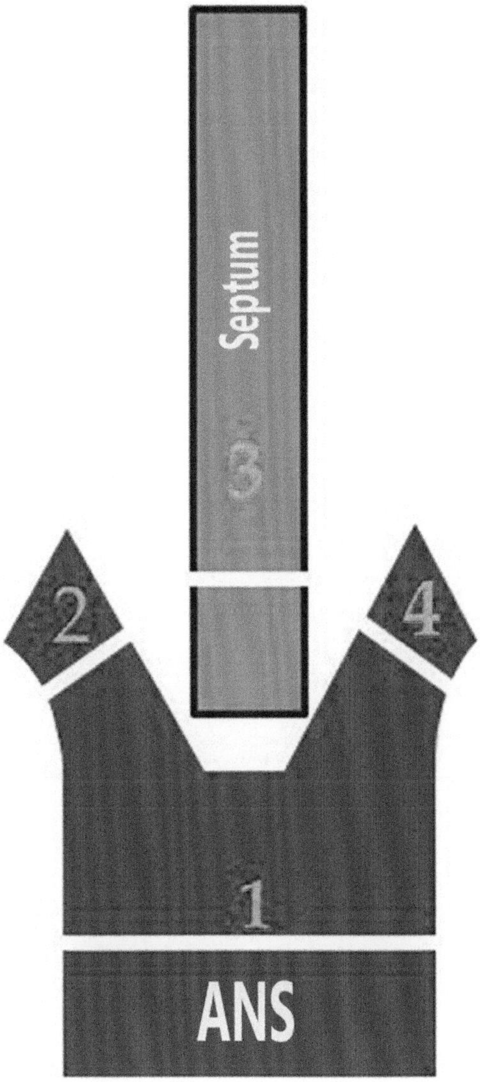

Fig. 14. Creating a notch on the ANS and the 3-hole method fixation of the caudal septum.

nasal bone hole on the other side. In **Fig. 12**, an open roof is created (for illustrative purposes) on a cadaver to demonstrate how the suture goes through the septum. At first, we pass through the bone and septum before exiting the opposite side upper lateral cartilage. Then, performing the same procedure on the other side and after passing through the septum we exit on the starting side upper lateral cartilage. When the sutures are completed, the nasal dorsum is fixed to the stable structure underneath the septal cartilage.

Also in low septal strip techniques (Cottle) it is important to attach the caudal portion of the released septum to the anterior nasal spine (ANS).[9,10] This connection will be the main fixation point for the new shape of the dorsum and is critical for the support of the septum. If the caudal portion of the septum is not strong enough, the suture material may tear through the cartilage, making fixation very difficult. There are different ways to fix the caudal septum to the ANS. This technique depends on the size and the shape of the ANS. Fixing directly through the ANS bone is the most stable method. After creating a notch with a 15 blade on the middle portion of the ANS, we drill a hole from one side to the other with the piezo drill insert (**Fig. 13**). As stated elsewhere in this article, the piezo tips, in this case the drill, does not harm soft tissue. Furthermore, as opposed to standard high-speed spinning drills, this device works with vibration so there is no risk of catching the soft tissue.

The second and third holes are also carefully created on the sides of the notch. A 4-0 PDS suture material can be used to fix the septum to the ANS, passing through the 3 holes created. In our experience, this ANS fixation is the strongest and most reliable method of single suture fixation (**Fig. 14**).

SUMMARY

Dorsal preservation rhinoplasty is a century-old method that has been seen renewed interest in the past decade. Although new approaches to exposure and septal resection have been described, the precise alteration of the osseocartilaginous vault while preserving the keystone remain as major tenets of the approach. The combination of newer approaches to dorsal preservation and ultrasonic piezo technology has allowed for more precise management of the osseocartilaginous vault.

CLINICS CARE POINTS

- The piezo device, with tips such as saws, rasps, and scrapers, allows for precise management of the osseocartilaginous vault and septum in preservation rhinoplasty.

- It is possible to use the piezo in a closed or open approach to rhinoplasty.
- An advantage of the piezo is that it is possible to change the direction of the bony cuts from horizontal to sagittal, decreasing the resistance to posterior displacement in push-down preservation rhinoplasty.
- The piezo allows for subtle reshaping of the dorsum even after osteotomies are performed and for drilling of holes needed for suture stabilization.

DISCLOSURE

Nothing to disclose.

REFERENCES

1. Gerbault O, Daniel RK, Kosins AM. The role of piezoelectric instrumentation in rhinoplasty surgery. Aesthet Surg J 2016;36(1):21–34.
2. Patel PN, Abdelwahab M, Most SP. A review and modification of dorsal preservation rhinoplasty techniques. Facial Plast Surg Aesthet Med 2020;22(2):71–9.
3. Goksel A. Piezo-assisted let down rhinoplasty. Instanbul: Bio Ofset; 2018.
4. Saban Y, Daniel RK, Polselli R, et al. Dorsal preservation: the push down technique reassessed. Aesthet Surg J 2018;38(2):117–31.
5. Goksel A, Saban Y. Open piezo preservation rhinoplasty: a case report of the new rhinoplasty approach. Facial Plast Surg 2019;35(1):113–8.
6. Saban Y, Polselli R. Atlas d'anatomie chirurgicale de la face et du Cou. Firenze (Italy): SEE Editrice; 2008.
7. Abdelwahab MA, Neves CA, Patel PN, et al. Impact of dorsal preservation rhinoplasty versus dorsal hump resection on the internal nasal valve: a quantitative radiological study. Aesthetic Plast Surg 2020;44(3):879–87.
8. Lazovic GD, Daniel RK, Janosevic LB, et al. Rhinoplasty: the nasal bones - anatomy and analysis. Aesthet Surg J 2015;35(3):255–63.
9. Cottle MH. Nasal roof repair and hump removal. AMA Arch Otolaryngol 1954;60(4):408–14.
10. Cottle MH, Loring RM. Corrective surgery of the external nasal pyramid and the nasal septum for restoration of normal physiology. Ill Med J 1946;90:119–35.

A Segmental Approach in Dorsal Preservation Rhinoplasty: The Tetris Concept

José Carlos Neves, MD, EBCFPRS[a], Diego Arancibia Tagle, MD, FEBORL[b,*], Wilson Dewes, MD[c], Mario Ferraz, MD, IBCFPRS[d]

KEYWORDS

• Preservation rhinoplasty • Intermediate split • Tetris concept • Segmental rhinoplasty

KEY POINTS

- Dorsal Preservation Rhinoplasty has seen considerable advances in the recent years since many doctors have improved and developed new ideas on the subject.
- The Split Preservation Rhinoplasty showed the real advantage of the intermediate resection in stabilizing the rhinion position by putting a suture from our free anterior dorsal septal cartilaginous flap to the basal posterior stabile septum.
- The Split Tetris is an evolution of the Intermediate Split Approach whose fundamental goal is the stabilization and predictability of the nasal dorsum final position. It was designed to avoid conceptual weakness, mainly regarding coronal axis deviations and causal septal border instabilities.

Video content accompanies this article at http://www.facialplastic.theclinics.com.

INTRODUCTION

Conservative dorsal rhinoplasty, until recently called the push-down rhinoplasty,[1–19] has been written about extensively. Since the end of the nineteenth century, some works have shown how to reduce a projected dorsum without impairing the surface anatomy of the nasal pyramid. By many, it was seen as an uninteresting and perhaps mistaken concept but by a few it was seen as the logical approach for preserving structures and avoiding massive complications. Recently, we have observed the rebirth of dorsal conservative concepts.[6] In some cases, the technique is incorrectly assumed to be new, and in others they are philosophies and details that really represent a step forward to achieving the best results in an accurate and predictable fashion.

DORSUM CONSERVATIVE TECHNIQUES

Even though the concept of dorsal preservation was already more than one-half of a century old, it was Cottle[2,3] who popularized the "push-down technique" in 1946, combining several steps described by other surgeons. The principle of the technique was to preserve the continuity of the nasal dorsum by impacting the bony and cartilaginous hump around the keystone point. His technique consisted of a basal strip resection of the septal cartilage, 1 or 2 paramedian osteotomies, the preservation of the keystone area, and lateral osteotomies allowing him to move the nasal pyramid downwards and inwards (or outwards) into the frontal process of the maxilla (**Fig. 1**, push down).

After the push down technique became popular, there were other surgeons such as Huffman and Lierle in 1954 and Huizing in 1975 who made

[a] MyFace, Clinics and Academy, Lisbon & Coimbra, Portugal; [b] Hospital Son Espases, Palma de Mallorca, Spain; [c] Facial Plastic Surgery Clinica Dewes, Lajeado, Brazil; [d] Facial Plastic and Reconstructive Surgery IBCFPRS, Campinas, Brazil
* Corresponding author.
E-mail address: arancibiadiego@gmail.com

Facial Plast Surg Clin N Am 29 (2021) 85–99
https://doi.org/10.1016/j.fsc.2020.09.010

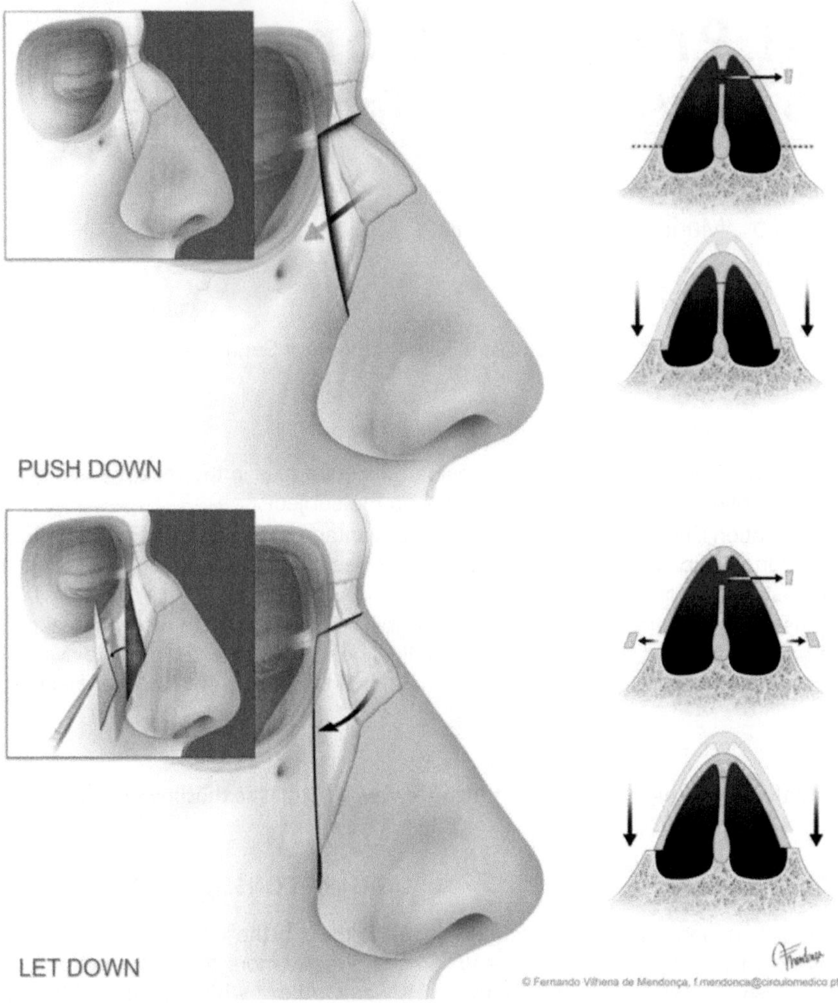

Fig. 1. Artist's sketch of push down technique and the let down technique.

variations of the technique as they argued that the amount of reduction that could be obtained in this way was limited.[11] The "let-down technique" was then popularized, even if authors like Lothrop in 1914 had already described the resection of a triangular bony wedge of the lateral nasal wall. This considerably facilitates the downward movement of the nasal bones and avoids the narrowing of the nasal cavity (see **Fig. 1**, let down).

In Lothrop's work, we can see that he already addressed the septum by removing cartilage and ethmoidal plate below the nasal vault.[8] In the 1980s Gola[12–14] and in the 1990s Saban and associates[6,7] refined the high strip approach. At the same time, Dewes[15–17] developed his concept, the septum and pyramid adjustment and reposition technique; his technique consisted in 2 possible conservative surgeries to reduce the septal height (type A, based on Gola's high septal strip concept, and B, based on low septal strip Cottle's concept, the approach more often performed) and one to augment the dorsum (type C). Later, many surgeons published modifications of these dorsal conservative techniques, such as Ishida and colleagues,[19] who in 1999 published an intermediated septal approach (see **Figs. 3–8**) that they have been performing for several years (**Fig. 2**).

The main author, a disciple of Dewes since 2008, gradually changed his preference from the low septal strip to the intermediate septal strip,[1] as explained elsewhere in this article, having taken into consideration the ideal indication of each case. Regarding the lateral wall, in the majority of cases the let-down technique is used.

THE SEGMENTAL PRESERVATION APPROACH

Whenever there are a considerable number of techniques describing how to achieve the same final surgical purpose, it means that the ideal

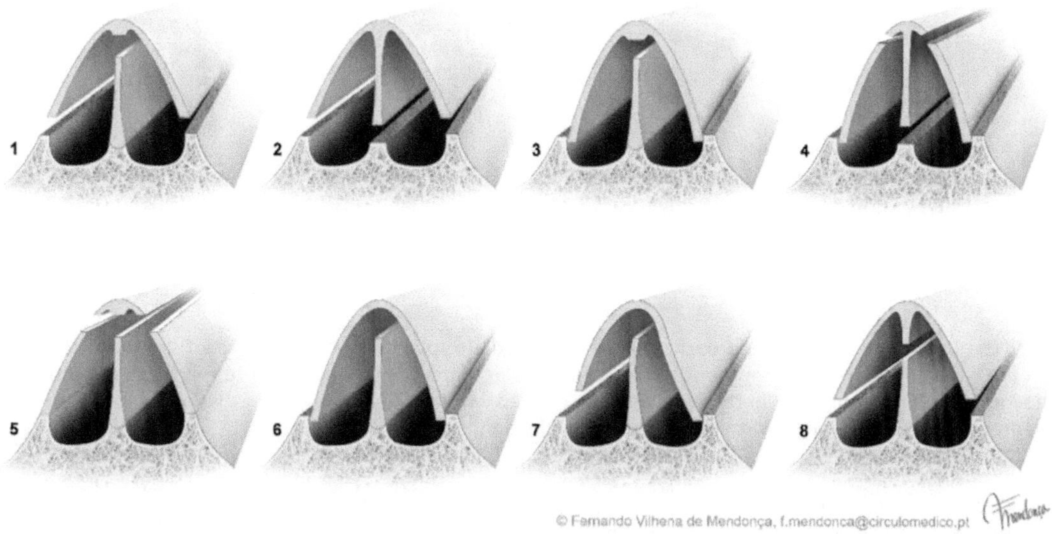

Fig. 2. Artist's sketch of different conservative techniques regarding lateral and medial walls. (1) Lothrop. (2) Sebileau and Dufourmentel. (3) Maurel. (4) Cottle. (5) Skoog (6, 7) Gola and Saban. (8) Ishida and Neves.

technique has not yet been found. We can also apply this rule to rhinoplasty techniques, and specifically to dorsal preservation concepts. Some disadvantages can be attributed to the push-down technique/let-down technique family. Bringing the nasal semirigid pyramidal unit down as a whole structure without addressing each segment for refinement can be the main disadvantage. The main disadvantages are a low radix and radix step, residual dorsal hump (being caused by a global hump relapse or by the inability to correct the residual bony hump), supra-tip saddle, wide dorsum, and eventual impairment of the nasal airway. Based on that factor, the pyramid must be addressed by segments and not as a single block. The Tetris concept in combination with the let-down technique aims to control each of them, regarding position and shape.

The main author has been doing preservation techniques for more than 10 years, with his preference being the intermediate approach. He has developed 1 modification of the let down technique with a septal intermediate resection, the split preservation rhinoplasty (**Fig. 3**A) that showed the real advantage of the intermediate resection in stabilizing the rhinion position by putting a suture from our free anterior dorsal septal cartilaginous flap to the basal posterior stabile septum. In fact, this is a critical stitch for predictably keeping the rhinion in the desired position with great accuracy.

The Tetris concept (**Fig. 3**B) is an evolution of the split preservation technique, with some advantages, which include suturing the free anterior septum (the Tetris block) in 2 vectors, craniocaudal and posteroanterior, conferring more stability to the pyramid in 2 axes and preserving a natural caudal septal strut, which allows us to control the supra-tip area and keep the caudal border and its relationship with the anterior nasal spine stable. As a general concept, these 2 techniques share the most relevant factor, the design of an intermediate fragment of cartilage below the rhinion to be anchored and consequently creating stability to the final dorsal profile.

For more details of the surgical technique we invite you to read the original articles "The Split Preservation Rhinoplasty, The Vitruvian Man Split Maneuver" and "The Segmental Preservation Rhinoplasty, The Split Tetris concept."

SURGICAL TECHNIQUE

Osteotomies and Pyramid Mobilization

The let-down technique is our preference for approaching the lateral nasal wall because it gives us better mobilization of the pyramid and avoids bone impaction into the nasal cavity (**Fig. 4**).

First, a transverse osteotomy is performed using a hand saw or an ultrasonic device under direct vision or alternatively a 2-mm osteotome that can be used percutaneously. The cut is made from the level of the medial canthal ligament up to the level of the lateral dorsum (**Fig. 5**A). The lateral osteotomy is part of the let down technique. It consists of 2 osteotomies followed by the removal of the intervening triangular bony wedge from the frontal process of the maxilla (**Fig. 5**B–D). The excision must be done very low laterally, in the nasofacial groove, to avoid any palpable or visible step (Video 1).

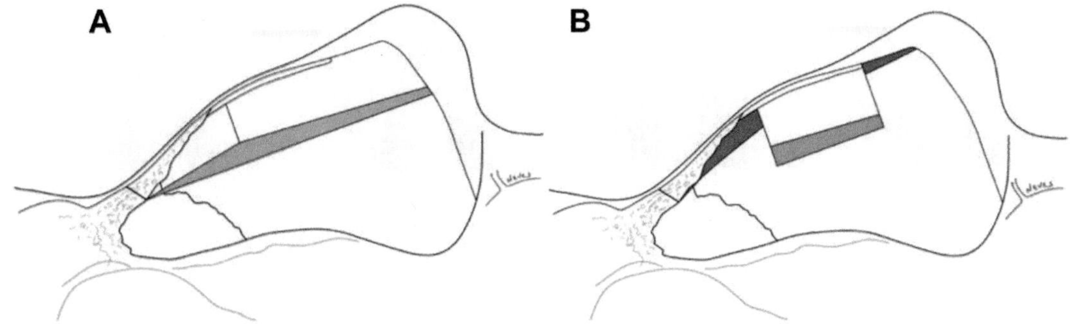

Fig. 3. The intermediate septal approach. (*A*) The intermediate split, where a fragment of septum is removed from the caudal border of the septum till the perpendicular plate at the level of the transverse osteotomy. (*B*) The segmental Tetris concept, where 3 segments are created with the key player being the Tetris block. The common gray area in both images is exactly at the same position.

The lateral wall split maneuver

To create the flattening of the dorsal profile, the lateral walls must show some plasticity. To achieve that goal, the lateral articulation between the upper lateral cartilage (ULC) and the nasal bones in its posterior cephalic border can be released so that the Lateral Wall Split Maneuver movement is facilitated. Recently, Goksel and Saban[20] also described this maneuver as the ballerina maneuver.

After the lateral bony wedge is removed, we dissect the inner surface of the lateral in a subperiosteal plane, to protect ULC and soft tissues. The pyriform ligaments are also liberated. This dissection will allow for an anterior and caudal sliding movement of the middle third of the lateral wall (see **Fig. 4**; **Fig. 6**, Video 2).

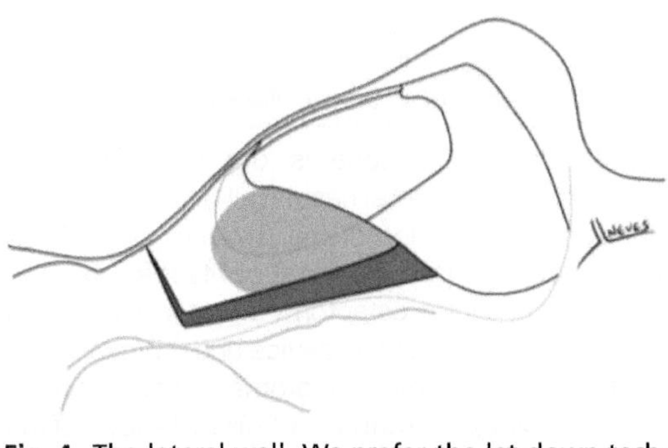

Fig. 4. The lateral wall. We prefer the let down technique. The blue segment represents the bone to be removed. Note that next to the medial canthal tendon we create some space where both osteotomies meet to facilitate the push down maneuver. The amount of bone removed will not influence the final dorsal profile position. The *gray shadow* represents the dissection area to perform the lateral splits movement.

Septal Resection

Conceptually, in preservation techniques the septum can be addressed lower in its base, by keeping the attachment with the cartilaginous vault intact and bringing all the structure down as a unit, and it can be addressed higher at the junction with the ULCs, exclusively pushing down the cartilaginous vault. It can also be addressed by splitting the septum in a strategic medial position, bringing the ULCs and the remaining attached septum down. Each one of these approaches has its pros and cons.

The intermediate split preservation rhinoplasty

The intermediate split preservation rhinoplasty consists of the following essential steps. (1) A tapered intermediate resection (that represents the amount of hump deprojection) begins at the caudal border of the septum and extending to the perpendicular plate of ethmoid, with its highest point in the most prominent aspect of the hump, at the rhinion level. (2) A vertical chondrotomy just toward this prominent point of the hump is performed, at the K-point or, most often, caudal to it. (3) A suture is placed for fixation from the free anterior dorsal septal cartilaginous flap to the basal posterior stabile septum (**Fig. 7**).

The medial wall split maneuver

A perpendicular chondrotomy below the most prominent point of the hump is performed to flatten the profile during the push down maneuver. Generally, this point is exclusively represented by cartilage, 1 to 3 mm caudally to the rhinion. This vertical section allows us to mobilize these 2 new septal segments, like the splits maneuver, allowing the surgeon to obtain the desired nasal dorsum esthetic line.

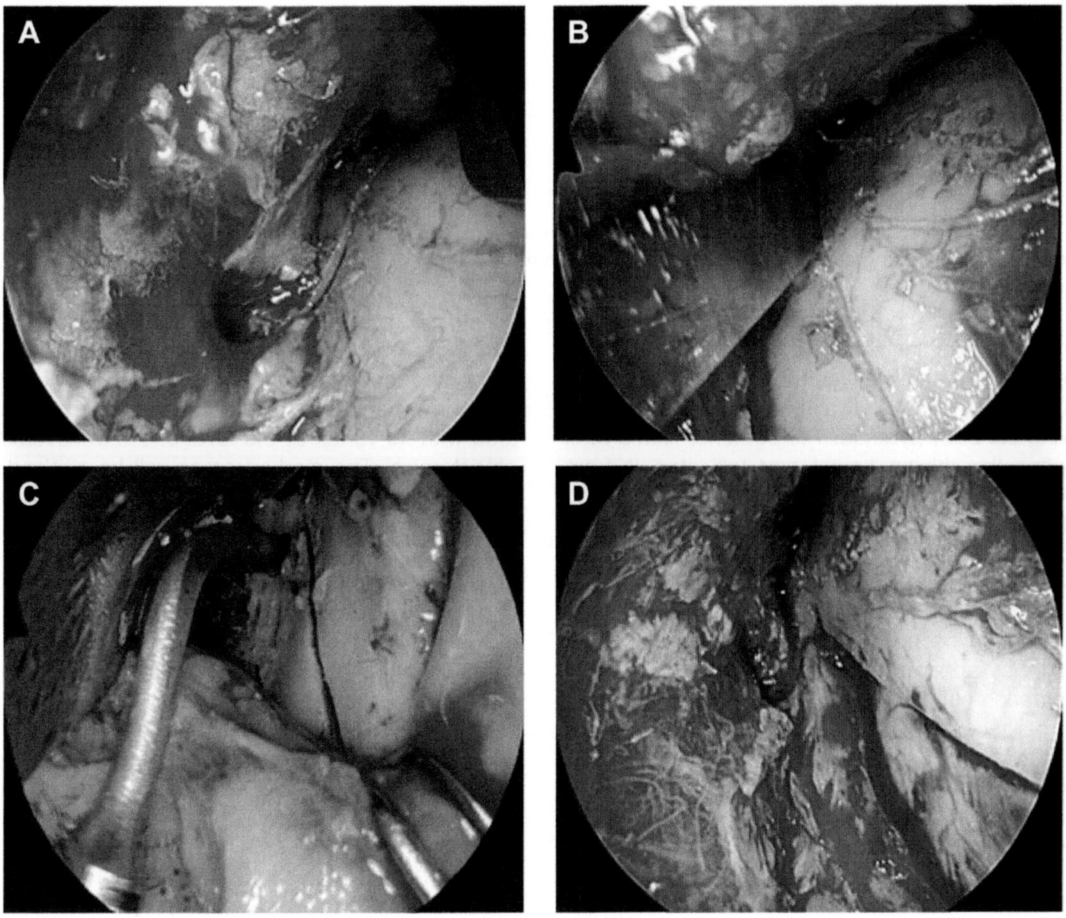

Fig. 5. The let down technique. Intraoperative pictures. (*A*) Upper left: A transverse osteotomy was performed with a Tastan-Çakir's saw, closed approach. (*B*) Upper right: The anterior osteotomy of the osseous wedge to be resected is being performed with a 3-mm osteotome, closed approach. (*C*) Lower left, the posterior osteotomy of the osseous wedge to be resected is being performed with an ultrasonic device, open approach. (*D*) Lower right, after the bony wedge resection with an osteotome in close approach; note the periosteum and its vessels were preserved.

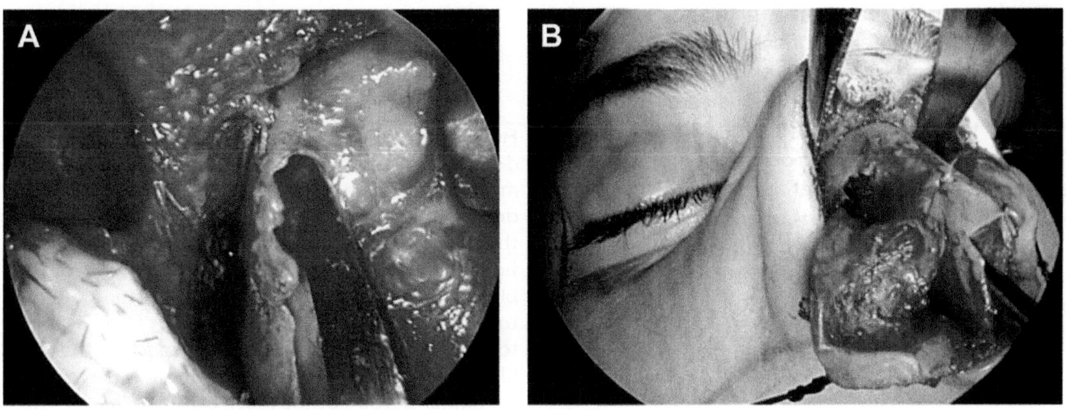

Fig. 6. The lateral wall split. Intraoperative pictures. (*A*) Left: Dissecting the ULC from the nasal bone with a delicate dissector. (*B*) Right: The triangular space created in between the ULC and the nasal bones after the anterior and caudal sliding movement.

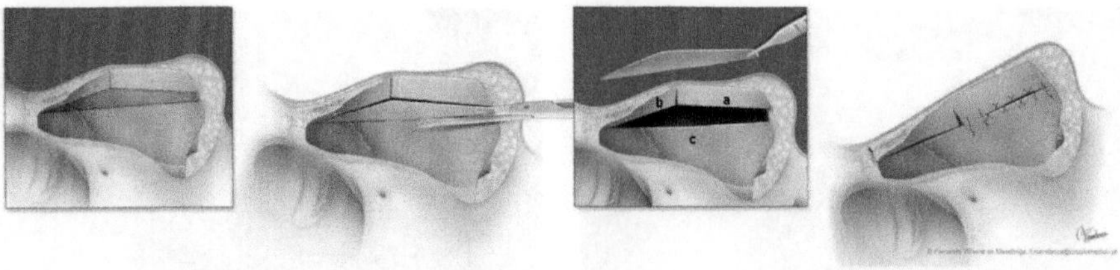

Fig. 7. Artist's sketch of the intermediate septal strip resection plus the perpendicular chondrotomy and the 8 figure sutures creating a very firm and stable cartilaginous septum.

We keep a 5- to 8-mm cartilage strip under the ULCs so we can suture it to the stable basal septum. A suture between these 2 septal pieces is mandatory and is always performed after mobilizing the bony pyramid. The posterior fixation will define the rhinion height and will stop it from popping up and creating a new hump, providing stabilization. This step is the main goal of this intermediate septal approach; that is, to create a stabilization point that guarantees the final position, and without any upward movement in the postoperative period because of relapsing forces, as seen in other approaches. In the last decade, this approach has been our workhorse, and attempts to be accurate with respect to the final position of the dorsum, by precisely stabilizing the point where more tension that leads to relapses is felt.

Additional sutures are placed until the caudal septal border, using figure of 8 stiches, 5-0 PDS. If more stability is needed, a strut side to side with the caudal septum can be used, which is sometimes useful as an extended septal graft.

The Segmental Preservation Rhinoplasty: The Split Tetris Concept

The Tetris concept is a modified intermediate septal resection consisting of the following steps (**Fig. 8**, Video 3). A 5- to 8-mm rectangular piece of septal cartilage will be designed below the cartilaginous hump in between the most prominent point of the hump (at or slightly caudal to the rhinion) and the caudal border of the ULC (the W point). The block is defined by 2 lines perpendicular and 1 horizontal to the dorsum (see **Fig. 6**; **Fig. 9**A). We prefer the block (quadrangular or rectangular) figure compared with a triangular shape, for instance. This is because it is designed to achieve a more stable structure, and once we have stabilized a vertical and a horizontal vector, we can avoid tilting of the free pyramid in the coronal and sagittal planes.

Two new shapes will be designed; one below the rectangular block and another below the bony hump. The shape below the block must have the height that we intend to decrease the dorsal projection. The shape of the excised area will usually be trapezoidal because the reduction will be bigger under the most projected point of the hump and less in the more caudal region. Below the bony hump, we draw a triangular excision area with its vertex at the level of the transverse osteotomies. The marked areas will be excised, which creates the space for the descending dorsum (**Fig. 9**B).

Using a 15 blade, the caudal, posterior, and cephalic borders of the rectangular block are cut. It is essential to free the cartilaginous hump. When pushed down, the block overlaps with the stable septal cartilage and we create a saddle nose below the UCL caudal border. Next, the triangular segment below the bony hump is removed using scissors. The cut always starts at a tangent to the undersurface of the bony vault to avoid an excess resection that can lead to a radix step. We initially remove a small triangular piece, and then perform the push down maneuver and analyze how much we have deprojected. If not

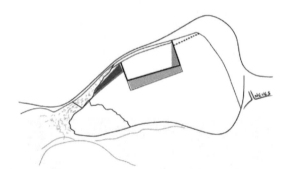

Fig. 8. The Tetris concept. A 5- to 8-mm height block is designed in between the WASA and the dorsal hump most prominent point (*red line*); a trapezoid figure is drawn bellow the block, it represents the amount of the hump to be reduced (*gray trapezoid*); a triangular figure is drawn below the bone pyramid, from the block till the lateral wall transverse osteotomy level to facilitate the push down movement (*blue triangle*); to avoid overlapping the caudal aspect of the Tetris block with the natural caudal septal strut we trim a triangular portion of the block cartilage (*purple triangle*); to adjust the new dorsal profile level a trimming of the anterior border of the caudal septal strut must be performed (*blue dots*).

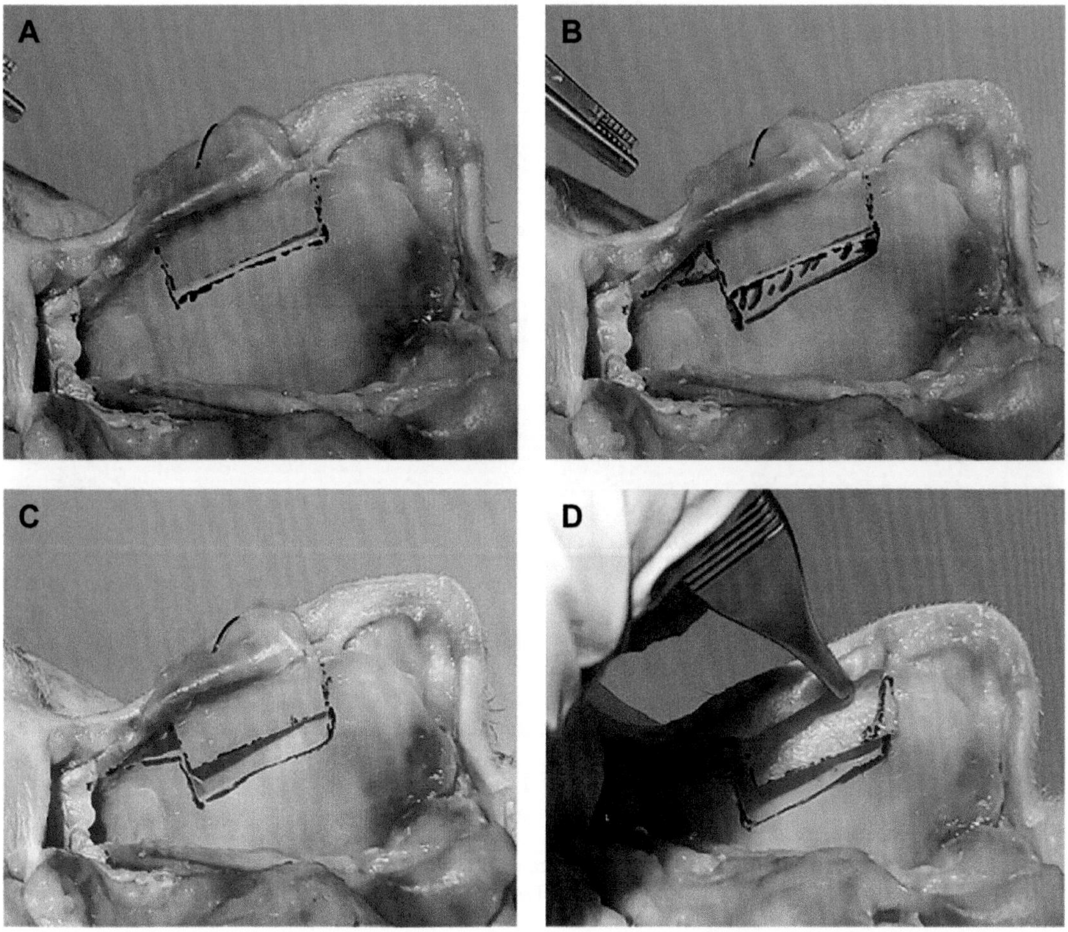

Fig. 9. The Tetris block designing (fresh specimen). (*A*) Designing the Tetris Block. (*B*) Designing the space slots. The trapezoid bellow the Tetris block, that determines the hump reduction, and the triangular below the bony pyramid. (*C*) The Tetris block and the pyramid are free and can be repositioned. (*D*) A triangle to be resected was marked in the caudal border of the Tetris block to avoid overlapping with the natural caudal strut.

enough, we go in again and remove another triangular slice until reaching the desired level. In some cases, we only remove cartilage, whereas in other cases we have to remove a small piece of bone, for which scissors are often necessary as well. Rarely, we use a baby rongeur, which we try to avoid, because it can create a bigger space than is needed and the radix step will appear as a consequence (**Fig. 9**C).

Now, the hump can be reduced and the cartilage block overlaps the stable basal septal cartilage; and because we have isolated the Tetris block we press it down, and by a rotational movement, posterior and caudal, we can create the side splits effect, thereby eliminating any residual dorsal hump. We are ready to remove the trapezoid slot, and thus create the space for our Tetris block.

The rotational movement of the block, downwards and caudal, creates an overlap of a small portion of cartilage of its caudal border with the caudal septum strut we have left intact. Thus, we trim the caudal border of the block so that it fits the slot created perfectly (**Fig. 9**D). This movement brings the pieces down into their spaces in a perfect match resembling the Tetris game, so we have called it the Tetris preservation concept. At this point in the operation, the surgeon decides how satisfied they are with the dorsal profile line. Sometimes, if the dorsum is too convex or a more concave shape is desired then a Tetris split is done at this time (as described elsewhere in this article).

The first suture of 5-0 PDS is placed between the posterior aspect of the caudal border of the Tetris block to the caudal septal strut, which stretches and helps to flatten the dorsum. This movement resembles what we performed in the Cottle push down technique,[2,3] and because of this here we can see a mini-Cottle, using an intermediate approach, with the advantage of

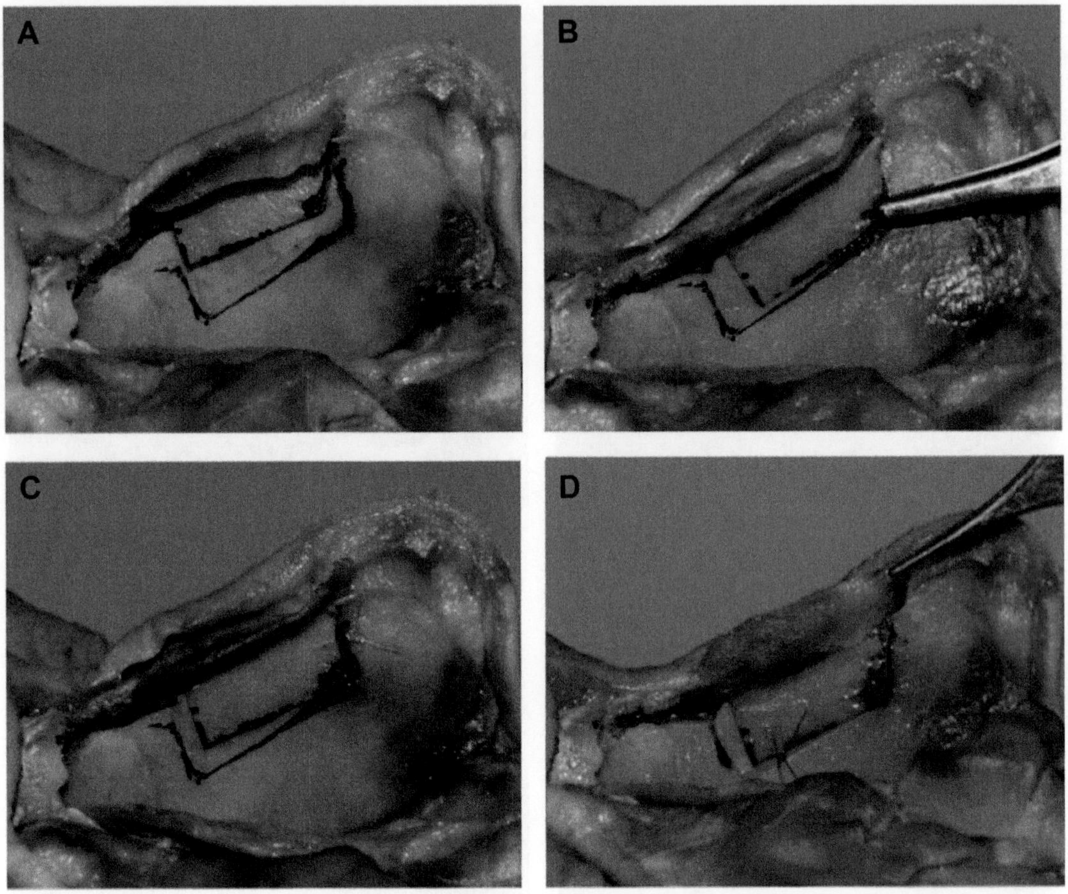

Fig. 10. The Tetris concept (fresh specimen). (*A*) The space slots are prepared to allow the push down movement. (*B*) Adjusting the Tetris block, the profile is checked. (*C*) Two PDS 5-0 sutures have stabilized the caudal border of the block; the stabilization of this border of the block is paramount to avoid pyramid lateralization. Note the spring effect bellow the rhinion, a gap is created in the cephalic aspect of the space slot below the rhinion. (*D*) The 5-0 PDS suture was placed below the rhinion. The stabilization of the dorsum in a predictable final nasal dorsum position is probably the greatest achievement of this technique.

preserving the stability of the rest of the septum. After performing this suture, the hump is reduced. Nevertheless, immediately we observe a small relapse of the hump that will slightly increase with time, the so-called spring effect (**Fig. 10**C). This phenomenon is responsible for the residual hump seen in a considerable number of cases, being a major problem of the dorsal preservation techniques. To prevent recurrent humps, we use a rhinion suture. At the level of the rhinion, we suture the cephalic border of the Tetris block to the underlying stable septal cartilage to guarantee precision and predictability (**Fig. 10**D). This suture can be performed as a simple interrupted one (**Fig. 11**) or as a figure-of-8 stitch, which is our preference. Additional sutures must be added between the caudal and the posterior borders of the Tetris block to the surrounding stable septal cartilage. To increase stability, we include the contralateral perichondrium and mucosa. With this

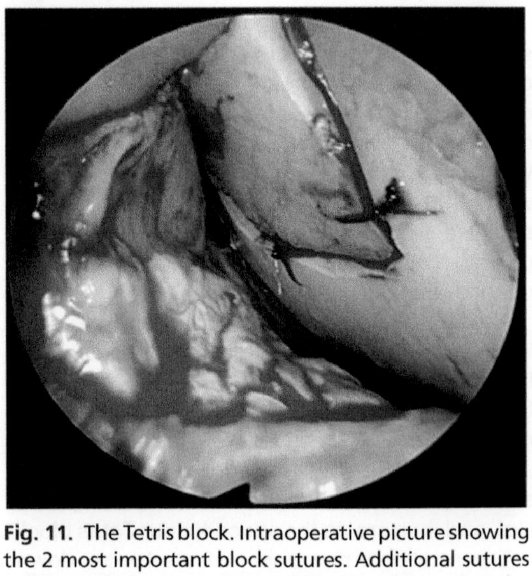

Fig. 11. The Tetris block. Intraoperative picture showing the 2 most important block sutures. Additional sutures will be added to complete stabilization. (Note that the stabilization of the 2 borders that are perpendicular promotes an affective stability to the pyramid, eventually like no other dorsal preservation technique.)

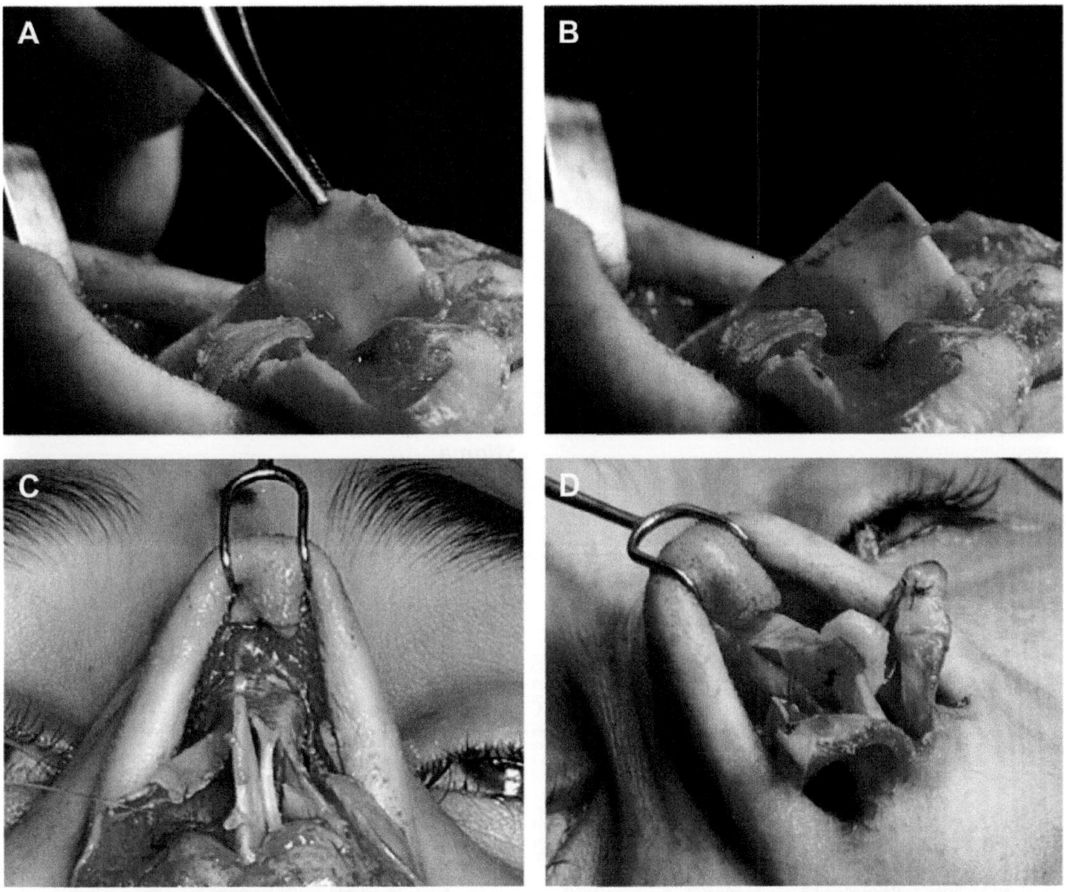

Fig. 12. The caudal septal strut. Intraoperative pictures showing the natural caudal septal strut. (*A*) The natural caudal septal strut before being addressed. (*B*) The septal profile after equalization of the caudal septal segment. Note the slight concave curve that the profile shows; it avoids the supra-tip saddling phenomena of some dorsal preservation techniques. (*C*) The caudal septal strut lateral to the Tetris back in a deviated pyramid. (*D*) The caudal septal strut supporting a septal extension graft (the anterior nasal septal angle banner).

approach, our incidence of recurrent cartilaginous humps has been negligible.

At this point, the dorsum has been brought down to its ideal position, except at the level of the caudal septal strut, which was previously preserved. In fact, one can often end up with a slight polybeak appearance. The anterior border of this natural strut must be addressed, and most often it is trimmed to achieve the desired dorsal height (**Fig. 12**B). Alternatively, it can be left partially at its maximum height to act like a strut to the tip or to support the stabilization of a septal extension graft (**Fig. 12**D).

In deviated noses, one can suture the overlapped cartilages side by side without resecting the trapezoid piece (gray trapezoid in **Fig. 6**). The rectangular block is sutured on the opposite side to the deviation so it can compensate (**Fig. 12**C, D, **13** and **14**).

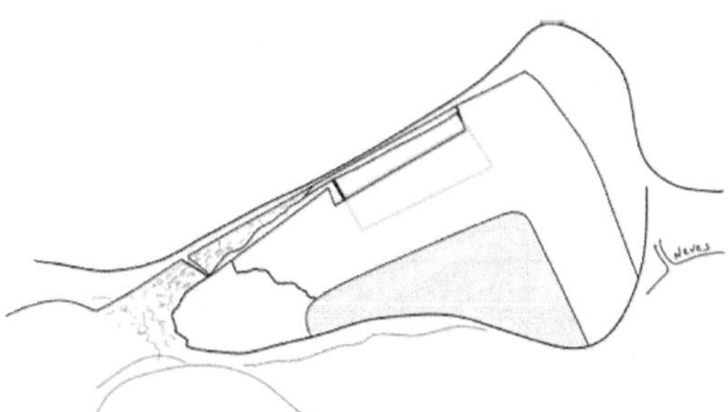

Fig. 13. The Tetris concept in deviated pyramids. When there is indication to perform the procedure in deviated pyramids there will be no slot creation below the Tetris block (*red line*) and consequently no trapezoid resection as seen in previous demonstrations; the block will suture to the stable septum in the opposite site of the deviation for compensation. The gray grid represents the septal harvesting leaving a stable L shape septum after suturing the Tetris block.

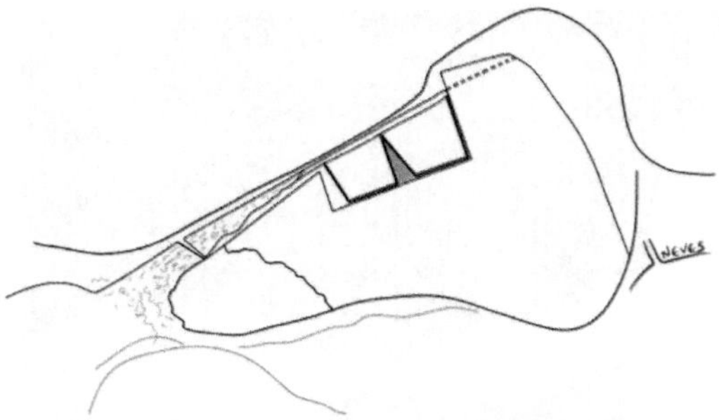

Fig. 14. The split Tetris concept. Splitting the Tetris block (*red lines*) allows the cartilaginous segment to flatten or eventually to become concave. The wider the gray triangle the more concave this segment will be.

In a nasal dorsal hump, the cartilaginous component tends to be convex. Even after hump reduction, a curved line can persist that creates a small hump in between the rhinion and the supra tip region; in some cases, it is essential to flatten this cartilaginous curve. One or 2 additional vertical cuts are made into the septal block converting it from a single entity into 2 or 3 new blocks that will be brought caudally into rotational movement (see **Fig. 14**; **Fig. 15**). The creation of multiple pieces allows the dorsum to flex, which resembles the spreading of fingers. This movement brings the pieces down into their spaces in a perfect match resembling the popular game and thus the name—the split Tetris preservation rhinoplasty. The more the block pieces are moved apart, the more concave the profile becomes.

Dorsal Segments and Strategies to Avoid Stigma

The split Tetris is an evolution of the intermediate split approach[1] whose fundamental goal is to stabilize and predict the nasal dorsum final position. It was designed to improve nasal pyramid stability,

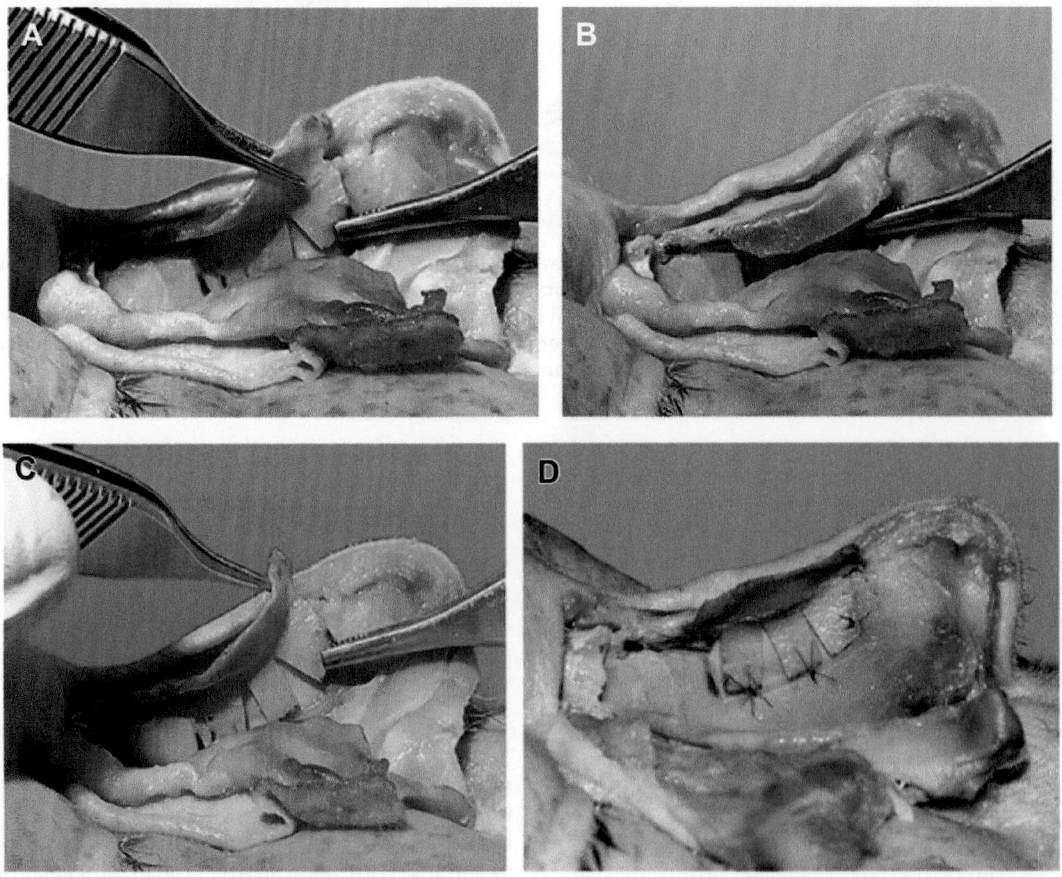

Fig. 15. The split Tetris concept (fresh specimen). (*A*) Upper left: one split of the block and defining the desired profile curvature. (*B*) Upper Right: one split of the block, we can see the eventual distortion of the caudal aspect of the UCL when bringing its caudal portion to a more anterior position. (*C*) Lower Left: 2 splits of the block; note the powerful effect of the craving effect. (*D*) Lower right: stabilization of the 3 small blocks to the underlying stable septum using 5-0 PDS.

regarding the coronal and sagittal axis, and to treat each segment of the dorsum more independently. At first, this technique may seem demanding, but once it has been learned it is relatively simple to perform. For many years the preservation techniques have been criticized for their lack of precision and the stigma of the outcome. With the segmental approach we aim to reduce its weaker aspects.

The bony pyramid segment

A lower transverse osteotomy must be avoided because it increases the probability of creating a radix step and a visible osteotomy. The thicker the soft tissue over the transverse osteotomy the better to work as camouflage. We must have perfect septal support below the nasion to avoid an excessive lowering of the bony dorsum, which would create a "radix step" or eventually a very low nasal radix. We prefer scissors to achieve a controlled septal removal. Eventually, in cases with thicker perpendicular ethmoidal plates a baby rongeur can be used but we definitely try to avoid it, because some undesirable bigger resections can be obtained. If, despite one's best effort, a radix step occurs then it can be minimized with a radix graft. Our choice is cartilage gel. Regarding the nasal bone shape, a final sculpture is performed to smoothen the profile line (especially in S-shaped bony dorsum[21,22]) and the transition in between bone and cartilage. Our preference is a 4- or 5-mm barrel burr, but an ultrasonic device or a rasp can be used. The burr can also gently reshape the dorsal cartilage. If the bony upper third is still wider than the goal, an osteotomy in both dorsal aesthetic lines is performed with an ultrasonic device and gently the lateral wall is medialized.

The rhinion and upper lateral cartilage segment

This segment is where the push down maneuvers show their fragility regarding accuracy and

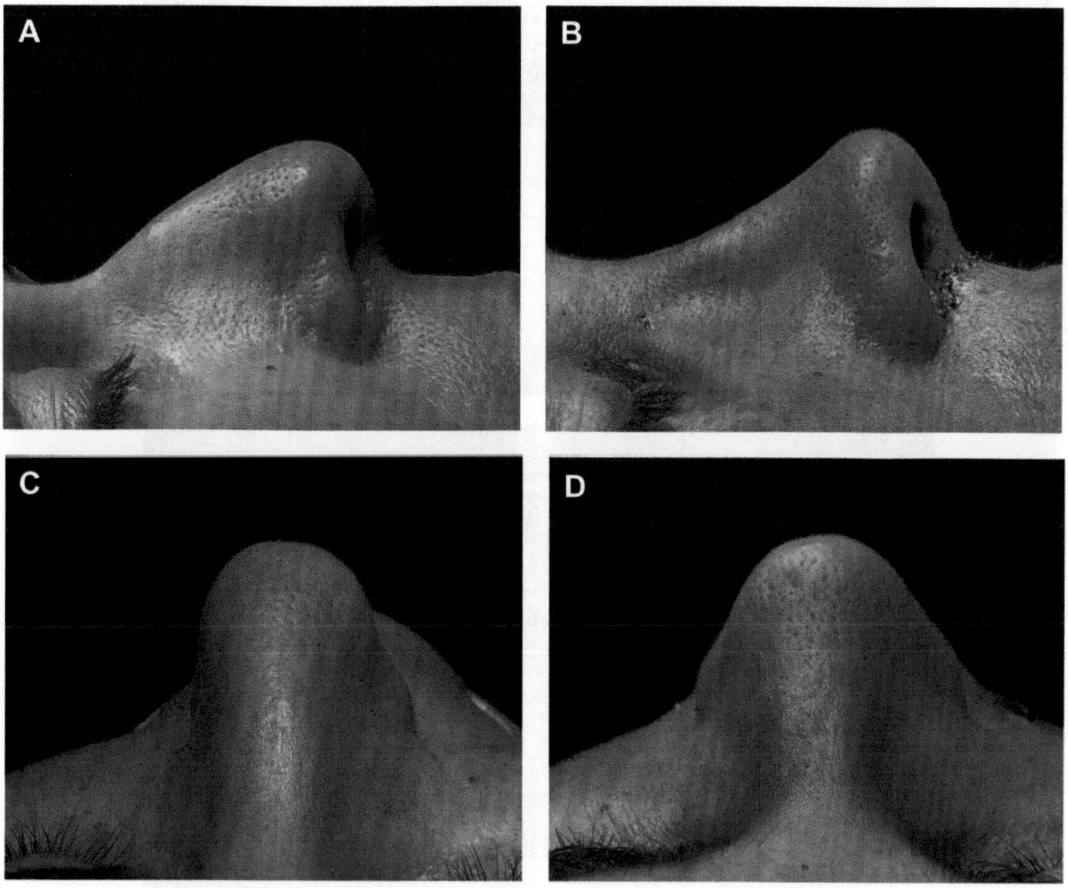

Fig. 16. Segmental dorsal preservation. A split Tetris approach to the septum was used plus an let-down technique in a close approach (a lip-lift was performed). The 2 split pieces of the Tetris block were suture to the right of the basal septum to compensate de deviated pyramid to the left (*C, D*). (*A*) Pre op lateral view. (*B*) Post op lateral view. (*C*) Pre op helicopter view. (*D*) Post op helicopter view.

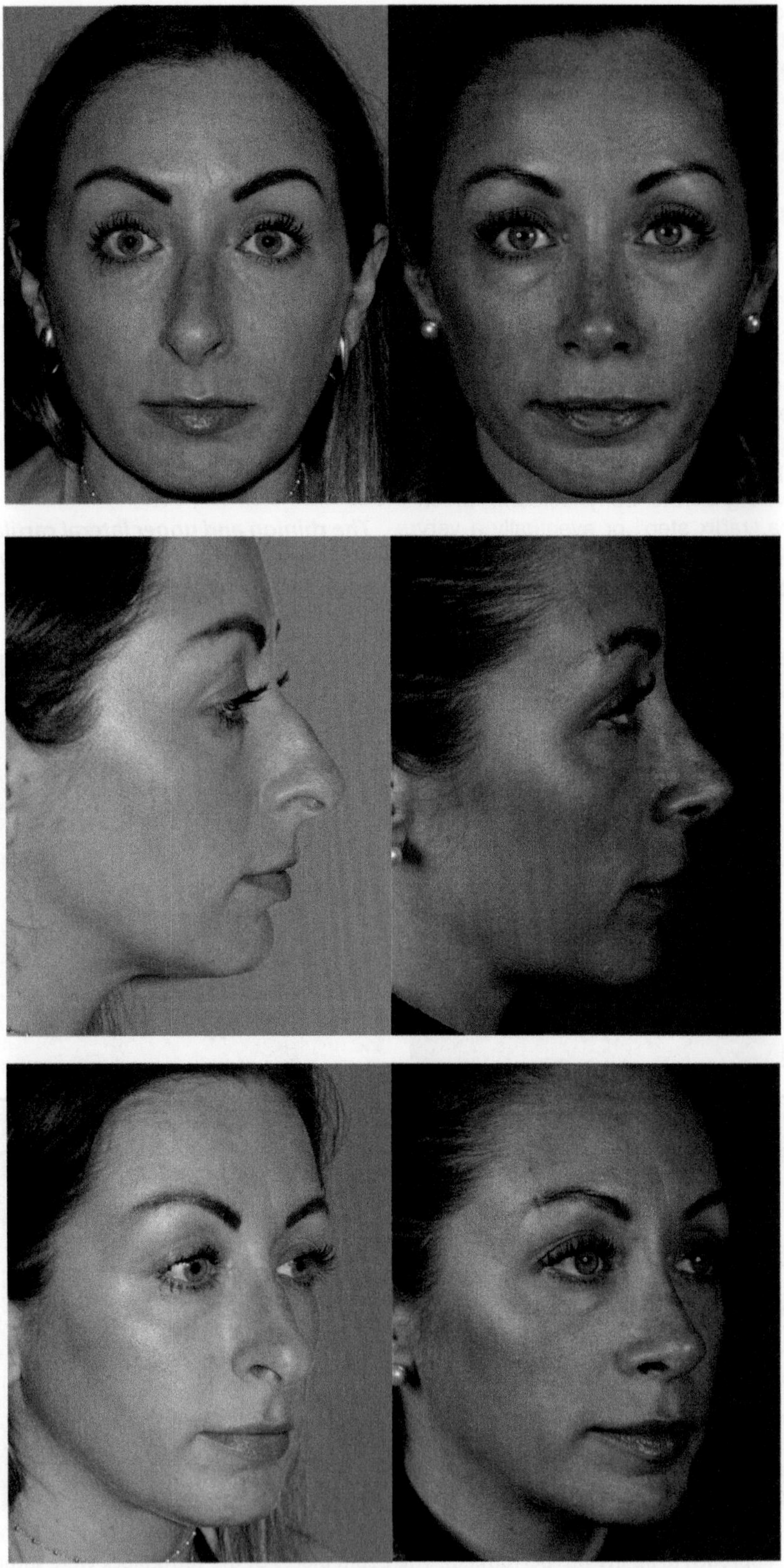

Fig. 17. Open approach; Segmental preservation approach, let-down technique with the Tetris Block being sutured to the left side of the septum to compensate pyramid deviation. Tip plasty was performed.

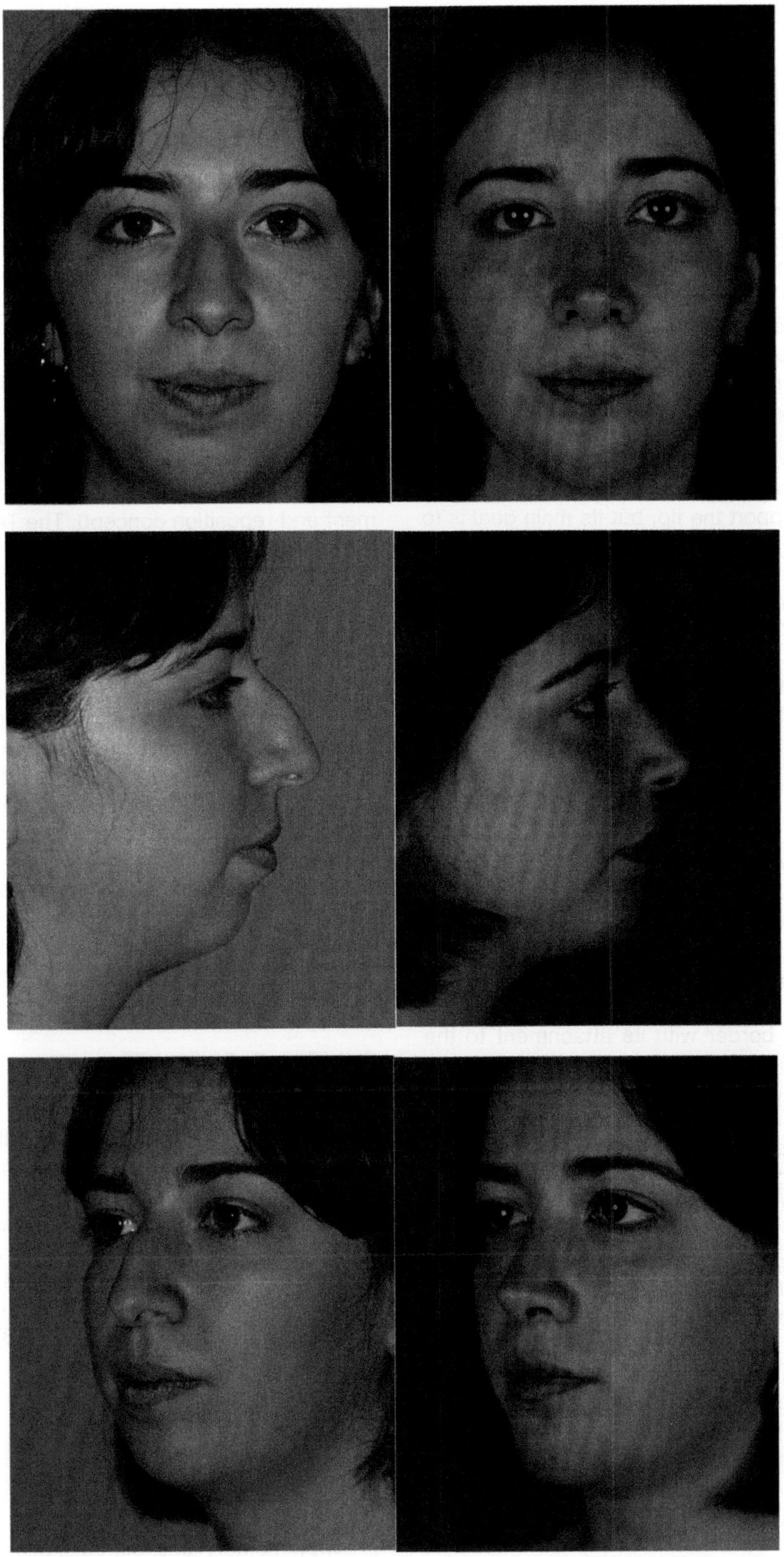

Fig. 18. Closed approach. Segmental preservation approach, let-down technique, and 7-mm Tetris Block stabilization. Tip plasty and alar base reduction were performed.

stability, and that is why we strongly believe the stabilization of the slice of septal cartilage below the UCL that was designed using an intermediate approach really helps to solve this problem. The suture below the rhinion gives precision and stability to the final dorsal height. In some cases, it is interesting to flatten the convex dorsal cartilaginous curvature; the Tetris block split is an elegant maneuver that can achieve this goal. It also helps if we want to achieve a concave profile. By performing the lateral wall split, decrease we reduce the elastic forces of ligaments and attachments, which are responsible for the spring effect and the consequent difficulty to achieving dorsal flatness and for relapses of the hump.

The supra tip segment

The natural caudal strut can be used as part of a strategy to support the tip, but its main goal is to design exactly the supra tip region. In fact, with this preservation we avoid supra tip saddling that is sometimes seen in push down maneuvers, mainly in Cottle's low strip ones. By keeping the caudal septal board and the septal/anterior nasal spine articulation intact, we do not promote an eventual instability of this region (**Fig. 16**).

DISCUSSION

In coronal straight noses, the segmental approach and other preservation approaches are indicated. In fact, the best candidate is the one with a straight narrow delicate nose with a dorsal hump. The greatest advantages of this approach are the stability of the rhinion area owing to the central suture, the rigidity of the caudal septal border with its attachment to the anterior nasal septum, the ability to achieve a flat or even concave profile of the cartilaginous segment, by splitting the Tetris block, and the avoidance of supra tip depressions.

The suturing of the 2 perpendicular borders of the block promotes a unique stabilization of the nasal pyramid in 2 axes. If the nose has a slight deviation, we can take advantage of the block overlap with the basal septum and suture it in an overlapping fashion with the block opposite to the deviation. If the septal deviation is mainly basal, we can perform a split Tetris preservation rhinoplasty and then the septoplasty. In fact, it works exactly as the L structure preservation in direct hump resection procedures. Because our Tetris block is around 5 to 7 mm high, if we stabilize it to a 5 bar of the stable septum it means that we end up with 10 to 12 mm of septum we cannot harvest. Below it we can proceed with a traditional septal harvesting (see **Fig. 7**).

The primary contraindications of this technique are crooked pyramids, severe septal trauma, and a wide cartilaginous dorsum. One prerequisite is that there must be sufficiently stable and relatively straight septum without major intrinsic high anterior septal deviations. In severe bigger deviations, we prefer a classical Cottle/septum and pyramid adjustment and reposition technique because it permits a more aggressive approach to the septal deviation or an open book technique.

SUMMARY

During recent years, and for more than a decade, the main author has been dedicated to achieving stable, accurate, and predictable results in preservation rhinoplasty, inspired by a modification of the Cottle operation (the septum and pyramid adjustment and reposition concept). The Tetris concept performed on indicated noses, is a technique that consistently achieves these goals.

At present, we recommend preservation rhinoplasty to around 30% of our patients. It means that the dorsal direct resection techniques[4,5] are still a part of our armamentarium in primary rhinoplasties. It is our belief that the more tools we have available, the better decision the surgeon is able to make, and the more accurate the choice of the technique will be in each individual case. Even though, whenever possible, we would rather use preservation rhinoplasty.

Achieving a natural and nonviolated dorsum in the proper position with the right shape is definitely the aim of any surgeon, and by performing the dorsal preservation techniques, we are definitely closer to this goal.

CLINICAL CARE POINTS

1. Open approach; segmental preservation approach, let-down technique with the Tetris block being sutured to the left side of the septum to compensate pyramid deviation. A tip plasty was performed (**Fig. 17**).
2. Closed approach; Segmental preservation approach, let-down technique and 7-mm Tetris block stabilization. Tip plasty and alar base reduction were performed (**Fig. 18**).

DISCLOSURE

No disclosures.

SUPPLEMENTARY DATA

Supplementary data related to this article can be found online at https://doi.org/10.1016/j.fsc.2020.09.010.

REFERENCES

1. Neves JC, Arancibia Tagle D, Dewes W, et al. The split preservation rhinoplasty: "the Vitruvian Man split maneuver". Eur J Plast Surg 2020. https://doi.org/10.1007/s00238-019-01600-3.
2. Cottle MH, Loring RM. Corrective surgery of the external nasal pyramid and the nasal septum for restoration of normal physiology. Ill Med J 1946;90: 119–35.
3. Cottle MH. Nasal roof repair and hump removal. AMA Arch Otolaryngol 1954;60(4):408–14.
4. Joseph J. The classic reprint: nasal reductions. Plast Reconstr Surg 1971;47(1):79–83.
5. Joseph J. Beiträge zur Rhinoplastik. Berl Klin Wochenschrift 1907;16:470–2.
6. Saban Y, Daniel RK, Polselli R, et al. Dorsal preservation: the push down technique reassessed. Aesthet Surg J 2018;38(2):117–31.
7. Saban Y, Braccini F, Polselli R. Morphodynamic anatomy of the nose. In: Saban Y, Braccini F, Polselli R, et al; The monographs of CCA group n°32. Paris; Rev Laryngol Otol Rhinol 2006;127(1):15-22.
8. Lothrop OA. An operation for correcting the aquiline nasal deformity; the use of new instrument; report of a case. Boston Med Surg J 1914;170:835–7.
9. Sebileau P, Dufourmentel L. Correction chirurgicale des difformités congénitales et acquises de la pyramide nasale. Paris: Arnette; 1926. p. 104–5.
10. Maurel G. Chirurgie maxilla-faciale. Paris: Le François; 1940. p. 1127–33.
11. Huizing EH. Push-down of the external nasal pyramid by resection of wedges. Rhinology 1975;13(4): 185–90.
12. Gola R. Conservative rhinoplasty. Ann Chir Plast Esthet 1994;38(3):239–52.
13. Gola R. La Rhinoplastie Fonctionnelle et Esthétique. Paris: Springer-Verlag; 2000. p. 360.
14. Gola R. Functional and esthetic rhinoplasty. Aesthetic Plast Surg 2003;27(5):390–6.
15. Ferraz MBJ, Zappelini CEM, Carvalho GM, et al. Cirurgia conservadora do dorso nasal – A filosofia do reposicionamento e ajuste do septo piramidal (SPAR). Rev Bras Cir Cabeça Pescoço 2013;42: 124–30.
16. Dewes W. Rinoplastia conservadora: Septo Piramidal, Ajuste e Reposicionamento De A. Tratado de Otorrinolaringologia e Cirurgia Cervicofacial Da ABORL-CCF. Philadelphia: Elsevier; 2017. p. 149.
17. Atolini N Jr, Lunelli V, Lang GP, et al. Ajuste e reposicionamento da pirâmide e septo nasal - uma técnica conservadora e eficaz em rinoplastia. Braz J Otorhinolaryngol 2019;85(2):176–82.
18. Ulloa FL. Let down technique. Rhinoplasty Archive (free online surgical textbook). 2011. Available at: http://www.rhinoplastyarchive.com/articles/let-down-technique. Accessed January 11, 2017.
19. Ishida J, Ishida LC, Ishida LH, et al. Treatment of the nasal hump with preservation of the cartilaginous framework. Plast Reconstr Surg 1999;103(6): 1729–33 [discussion: 1734].
20. Goksel A, Saban Y. Open Piezo preservation rhinoplasty: a case report of the new rhinoplasty approach. Facial Plast Surg 2019;35(01):113–8.
21. Lazovic GD, Daniel RK, Janosevic LB, et al. Rhinoplasty: the nasal bones – anatomy and analysis. Aesthet Surg J 2015;35(3):255–63. https://doi.org/10.1093/asj/sju050.
22. AM Kosins. Expanding Indications for Dorsal Preservation Rhinoplasty with Cartilage Conversion Techniques. Aesthet Surg J 2020. https://doi.org/10.1093/asj/sjaa071.

Incorporating Dorsal Preservation Rhinoplasty into Your Practice

Aaron M. Kosins, MD

KEYWORDS

- Dorsal preservation • Preservation rhinoplasty • Keystone area • Pushdown • Let down
- Osteotomy

KEY POINTS

- Dorsal preservation represents a new frontier in surgery of the nasal dorsum.
- Multiple new techniques are evolving allowing for increased applicability of dorsal preservation.
- An algorithm is presented for the different forms of dorsal preservation and how to incorporate them into your practice.

INTRODUCTION

For rhinoplasty surgeons, surgery of the dorsum is increasingly dynamic and exciting. An expanding repertoire of reproducible techniques offers excellent results that can be difficult to attain in certain patients using conventional methods.[1] Once surgeons understand dorsal preservation (DP), they will look for every opportunity to preserve the dorsum. An enlarging body of techniques is evolving as the most creative and innovative rhinoplasty surgeons push the limits of the philosophy. For beginners, easier techniques should be chosen initially on patients with the most appropriate indications. As the learning curve progresses, it makes sense to advance to the next phase of the preservation journey and to learn the more complicated operations. Each DP operation builds on the others, and, over time, these philosophies make clinicians not only better surgeons of the nasal dorsum but also better surgeons of the septum and the nose in general. To understand DP, surgeons needs to gain a new appreciation of the septum, the perpendicular plate of ethmoid, osteotomies, and anatomy of the nose where they rarely operate with traditional L-strut philosophy.[2] Through this journey, I have evolved as a surgeon, and now I approach rhinoplasty in ways that I did not before. The result is more natural and beautiful noses where the anatomy has been preserved.

Dorsal Preservation

Control of the bony vault, especially the keystone area, is enhanced with the popularity of the full open approach and piezoelectric surgery. However, keystone irregularities, bony spicules, callus formation, asymmetric osteotomies, asymmetries of the middle vault, and long-term contraction can affect dorsal aesthetic lines years after the operation was performed. However, dorsal irregularities (especially in the middle vault) continue to be an issue for rhinoplasty surgeons over the long term. This situation is where DP takes the lead in the rhinoplasty revolution.

PERSONAL EXPERIENCE WITH DORSAL PRESERVATION

My introduction to DP came in 2016. The concept was intriguing: preserve the dorsum by lowering the osseocartilaginous vault into the pyriform aperture. Because the keystone would remain intact and the middle vault would not be opened, irregularities/asymmetries/contraction could potentially be avoided. In addition, the prospect of a narrow but stable middle vault was exciting. Up to that point in my career, I learned the hard

Plastic Surgery, UC Irvine School of Medicine, 1441 Avocado Avenue, Suite 203, Newport Beach, CA 92660, USA
E-mail address: aaronkosins@gmail.com

Facial Plast Surg Clin N Am 29 (2021) 101–111
https://doi.org/10.1016/j.fsc.2020.09.001

way that the only way to maintain stability was restructuring, which sometimes widened the middle vault and/or deteriorated over time. After dozens of hours of discussion with Drs Yves Saban and Rollin Daniel, I did my first DP at the end of 2016. Over the next year, other surgeons, including Drs Baris Cakir, Milos Kovacevic, Olivier Gerbault, Charles East, Peter Palhazi, and Abdulkadir Goksel, also began in parallel performing high septal strip DP as advocated by Saban and colleagues.[3] Through hundreds of hours of casual conversations, emails, roundtable discussions, presentations, and meetings, we learned the technical details and were able to understand how to perform the high septal strip push/letdown technique and to achieve stable and predictable results. With 2 years of experience performing the high septal strip DP operation, I found that one-third of my primary rhinoplasty patients were good candidates.[4] What came next was astounding:- the resurgence, development, and modification of techniques that expanded my indications for DP.[5] Throughout 2018 to 2019, several techniques came to the forefront of rhinoplasty surgery, including Valerio Finnochi's modification of the Cottle technique, as well as the cartilage pushdown techniques championed by Ferreira and colleagues[6] and Ishida and colleagues.[7] More than half of my patients can now successfully undergo DP with excellent results using a variety of techniques, each with its own best indications.

THE SPECTRUM OF DORSAL PRESERVATION (TYPES 1–4)

Preservation rhinoplasty is not just DP, and DP is not just a pushdown or letdown impaction procedure.[8] DP is a spectrum of techniques whereby the surgeon preserves all or part of the osseocartilaginous dorsum. More simply, DP can be divided into both impaction techniques as well as surface dorsal modification (DM) techniques. Impaction techniques lower the entire osseocartilaginous vault by (1) first separating the nose from the septum, followed by (2) separating the nose from the face. In contrast, surface or DM techniques lower only the central cartilaginous vault (with or without the bony cap), and the bones are treated separately as in component reduction. Technically, surface techniques are easier to learn and to execute for surgeons beginning DP. In addition, surface techniques widen the applications of the preservation philosophy (**Fig. 1**).

As surgeons become more experienced with DP, it is preferable to preserve the dorsum and to avoid midvault reconstruction in select patients.

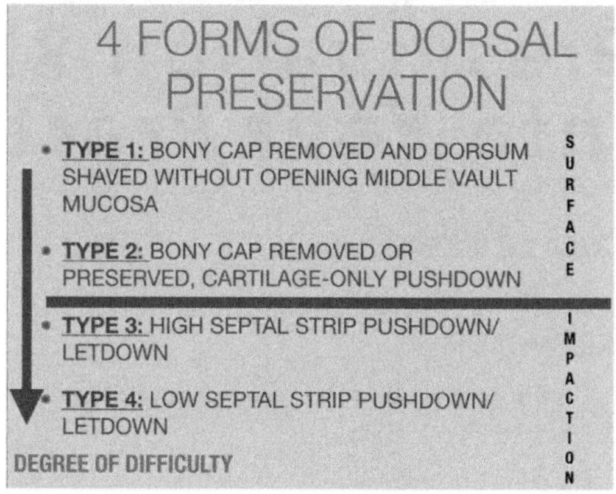

Fig. 1. The different DP procedures in order of increasing complexity. Types 1 and 2 are surface techniques whereby the cartilage is lowered, and the bones are treated separately without impaction of the osseocartilaginous vault. Types 3 and 4 are foundational techniques. A septal strip is removed either directly under the septum (type 3) or from the floor of the septum (type 4) and the nose is then impacted into the pyriform aperture.

Although some surgeons prefer a specific technique for all patients, I prefer to apply the optimal technique for each patient. A summary of my indications for each DP procedure follows, in order of increasing complexity. I have not invented any of these techniques, nor do I prefer 1 technique. I have used all these techniques in hundreds of cases over a 3.5-year period and have become aware of each technique's inherent advantages and disadvantages in different patients. Each surgeon selects which technique to use based on personal experience and the patient population. The step-by-step technical details of these procedures are summarized elsewhere in this issue, so this article focuses on indications and thought processes.

Type 1 Surface Technique: Dorsal Modification/Cartilage Vault Modification

Cartilage vault modification (CVM) is the simplest technique for DP and an easy entry for beginner surgeons.

CVM modification is a hybrid DP technique that consists of 4 parts:

1. Incremental modification and ostectomy of the bony cap to convert the bony dorsum to cartilage
2. Shaving excess upper lateral cartilage shoulders and/or dorsal septum without opening the mucosa
3. Piezoelectric rhinosculpture and/or osteotomies to narrow and to sculpt the bony pyramid

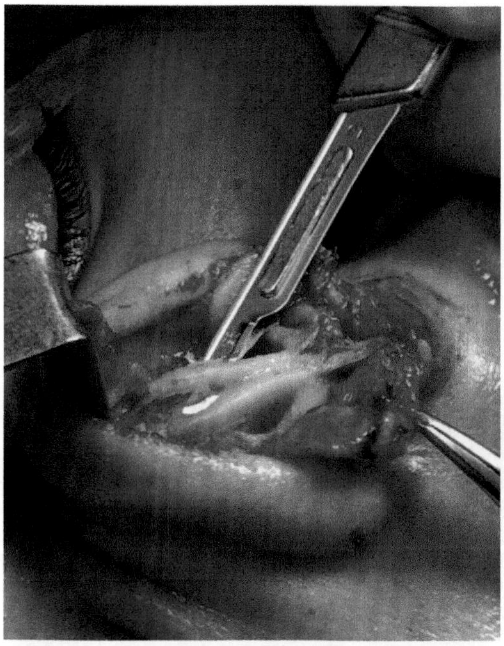

Fig. 2. Piezoelectric removal of the bony cap followed by shaving of the shoulders of the upper lateral cartilage without opening the middle vault. This is DM/CVM.

4. Closing any cartilage defect over the underlying mucosa and shaping the upper lateral cartilages (**Fig. 2**)

Thus, CVM is a surface technique whereby only the bony cap is removed, and the cartilaginous vault is modified/lowered. The bones are dealt with separately (as in a component reduction) and no impaction of the osseocartilaginous vault into the pyriform aperture is performed.

My indications are as follows (**Fig. 3**):

- Small hump/convexity less than 2 mm
- Small hump with need for tip projection
- Small hump with wide bones and/or need for osteotomies

The main advantage of the CVM technique is simplicity, particularly in an open approach. With a small osseocartilaginous hump, the osseous part is removed up to the desired profile line, and any excess cartilage is shaved. The cartilaginous vault is kept mostly intact, as is the internal valve mucosa. Because the upper lateral cartilages have not been separated from the dorsal septum, there is no need for midvault reconstruction. In addition, endonasal spreader grafts can easily be placed in submucosal pockets to treat asymmetries. The bones are modified as needed with standard osteotomies for narrowing dorsal or base bony width. Of note, the septum remains available for septoplasty and harvesting of graft material, and, if the surgeon gets in trouble, conversion to a standard component reduction is simple.

Type 2 Surface Technique: Dorsal Modification/Cartilage Vault Preservation

Cartilage vault preservation (CVP) is a critical category of techniques in my rhinoplasty practice. It is widely applicable, easy to learn, fast, and has a very low complication rate. CVP can be done using a high or low septal strip.

CVP is a hybrid technique that consists of 4 parts:

1. Preservation or ostectomy of the bony cap to convert the bony dorsum, thereby permitting a cartilage-only pushdown
2. Septal strip resection under the dorsum by removing a high or low septal strip
3. Precise downward fixation of the cartilaginous vault
4. Piezoelectric rhinosculpture and/or osteotomies to narrow and to sculpt the bony pyramid (**Fig. 4**)

Thus, this technique is also a surface technique whereby only the cartilaginous vault is lowered with or without the bony cap. The bones are dealt with separately (as in a component reduction) and no impaction of the osseocartilaginous vault into the pyriform aperture is performed. If the bony cap is flat, it can be preserved and lowered along with the cartilage vault. If the bony cap is curved (convex) or irregular, it is better to remove it or to modify.

My indications are as follows (**Fig. 5**):

- Small hump/convexity 2 to 3.5 mm
- Small hump with S-shaped nasal bones where bony cap and high septal strip removal break the convexity of the dorsum
- Small hump with underprojected tip and/or low radix
- Small hump with need for osteotomies

If a patient has a hump greater than 2 mm, it is better to lower the entire cartilage vault rather than to modify it by shaving the upper lateral cartilages (type 1). Aggressive shaving eventually opens the middle vault mucosa and further violates the preservation philosophy. If the hump is bigger than 2 mm and the nasal bones have an S shape, it is better to remove the bony cap and to lower the whole cartilage vault. Like the type 1 cartilage modification (CVM), the main advantage of this technique is simplicity. The bony cap can either be released from the nasal bones with osteotomies or removed, and the cartilage vault is lowered

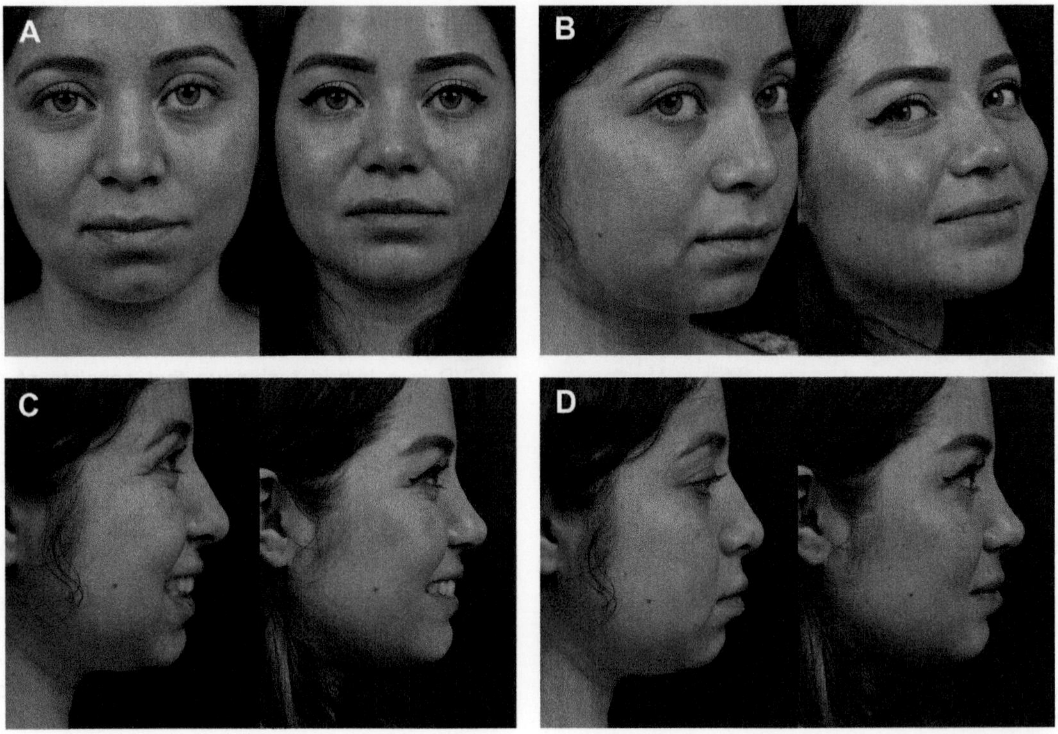

Fig. 3. DM/CVM. A 20-year-old woman presents with a 2-mm dorsal hump, a bulbous tip, wide nasal bones, and plunging tip on smiling. She has an underprojected nasal tip. The patient is shown preoperatively (*left*) and postoperatively (*right*) after removal of the bony cap with piezoelectric surgery and modification of the cartilaginous vault. The upper lateral cartilages and a small amount of the dorsum are shaved with a 15-blade without opening the middle vault mucosa. Medial oblique, low-to-low, and transverse osteotomies were performed with piezoelectric instruments. A septal extension graft was used to support the nasal tip. Her tip was dissected sub–superficial musculoaponeurotic system (SMAS) and her dorsum in a subperichondrial plane. Her ligaments were preserved, and no cartilage was removed from her alars (only tip suturing). Therefore, she underwent a complete preservation rhinoplasty. Postoperatively, she shows improved dorsal aesthetic lines, relief of the dorsal hump, and excellent tip contour.

independent of the nasal bones by removing a septal strip.

My preference is to perform type 2 CVP by removing a high septal strip for 4 reasons:

1. Removing 2 to 3 mm of subdorsal cartilage allows for incremental lowering of the cartilaginous vault
2. Minimal release is needed at the lateral keystone area to allow lowering of the cartilage
3. The cartilage vault can be precisely sewn down to the underlying septum, and sutures are used to modify width and asymmetries
4. The technique is easily converted to component reduction if necessary. Number 3 is what makes this technique so valuable: the dorsum is preserved in continuity, but sutures can be used to modify the postoperative width, symmetry, and shape of the cartilage vault.

When a low septal strip is used, the cartilage must be completely released from the bone to allow lowering, and this in my mind is destabilizing. Also, any of the low strip procedures cannot be converted to component reduction. Nevertheless, select patients present with a small hump and cartilaginous axis deviation. These patients are optimal for a low septal strip cartilage preservation.

Type 3 Impaction Technique: Dorsal Preservation (High Septal Strip)

High septal strip DP as advocated by Saban and colleagues[3] consists of 4 parts:

1. Septal strip resection (directly underneath the dorsum) to flatten the dorsal hump and to separate the dorsum from the septum
2. Mobilization of the bony pyramid with osteotomies to separate the dorsum from the face
3. Lowering of the dorsal profile via impaction into the pyriform aperture
4. Fixation of the osseocartilaginous vault to the underlying septum

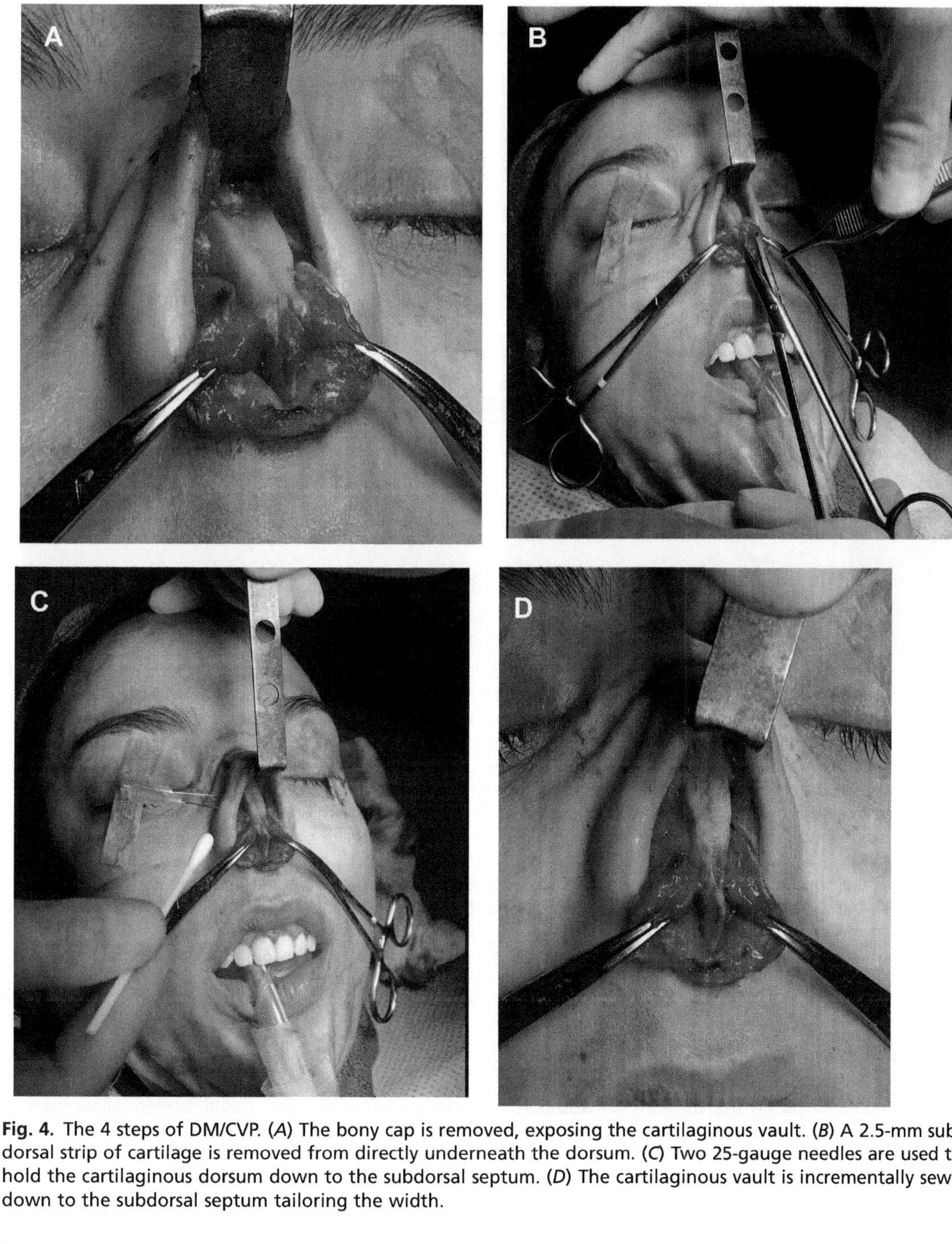

Fig. 4. The 4 steps of DM/CVP. (*A*) The bony cap is removed, exposing the cartilaginous vault. (*B*) A 2.5-mm subdorsal strip of cartilage is removed from directly underneath the dorsum. (*C*) Two 25-gauge needles are used to hold the cartilaginous dorsum down to the subdorsal septum. (*D*) The cartilaginous vault is incrementally sewn down to the subdorsal septum tailoring the width.

Thus, this is an impaction technique whereby the entire osseocartilaginous vault is lowered.

My indications are as follow (**Fig. 6**):

- Over projected or slightly convex dorsum
- Cephalic hump
- V-shaped nasal bones
- Normal or high radix
- Cartilaginous nose (tension nose)
- Large amount of septal cartilage needed for grafting (Hispanic noses)

Of all the techniques, the high septal strip DP is the most widely applied to almost any patient population. The technique can be used in humps of any size, is easy to conceptualize, only has 1

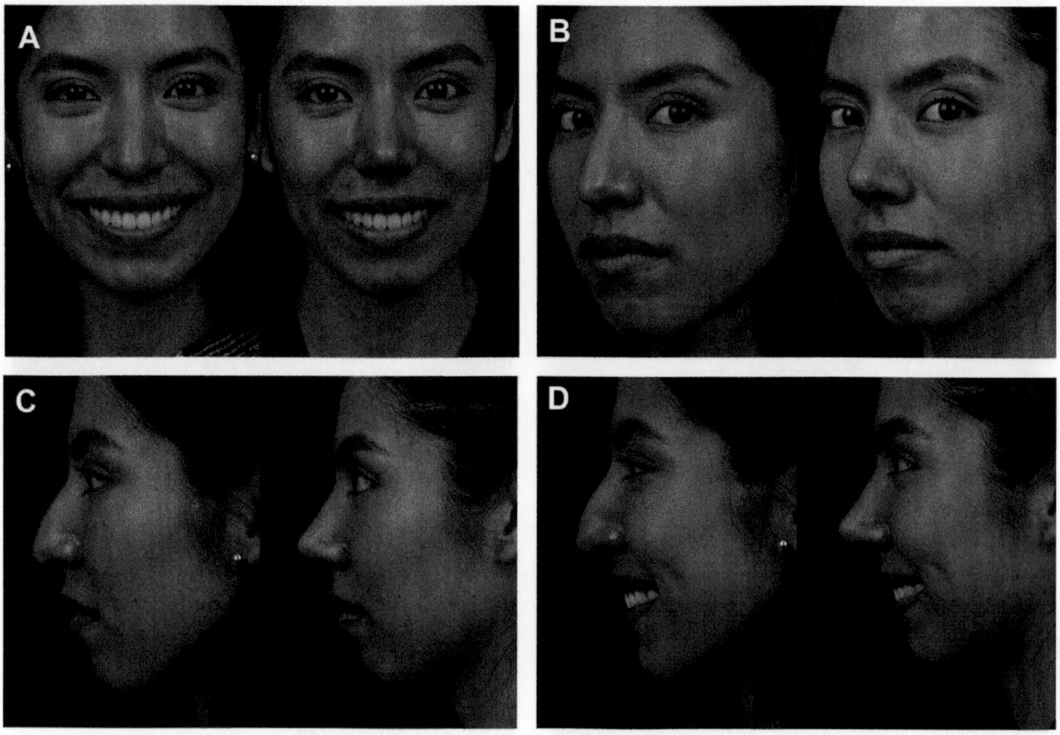

Fig. 5. DM/CVP. A 22-year-old woman presents with a 3-mm dorsal hump, a wide and asymmetric bony vault, and a plunging tip on smiling. The patient is shown preoperatively (*left*) and postoperatively (*right*) after she underwent a cartilage pushdown after bony cap modification. The patient has an ideal cartilaginous vault with wide and asymmetric nasal bones and a hump of approximately 3 mm. After removal of the bony cap with piezoelectric surgery, a 3-mm strip of subdorsal septum is removed. The cartilage vault is conservatively disarticulated at the lateral keystone area from the nasal bones. Once mobilization has occurred, 5-0 PDS sutures are used at multiple points to sew the preserved cartilaginous vault down to the underlying septum. Piezoelectric medial oblique, transverse, and low-to-low osteotomies were performed to narrow the bony dorsum and bone base after piezoelectric rhinosculpture of the lateral keystone areas was performed. In this way, the cartilage vault is preserved, and the bones are narrowed. Her tip and dorsum were dissected in a subdermal plane with en bloc SMASectomy. The tip was supported with a septal extension graft and all ligaments were preserved. No cartilage was removed from her alars (only tip suturing). Therefore, she underwent a complete PR other than a subdermal dissection of her nasal tip. Postoperatively she has improved dorsal aesthetic lines and a narrow and symmetric bony vault. The profile line is improved without opening the middle vault.

degree of movement (down), and is easily converted to a component reduction if the surgeon is having trouble lowering the dorsum. In addition, large amounts of septum can be harvested (very important in underprojected tips), midvault width can be tailored with sutures, and dorsal hump flattening is easily achievable if patients are chosen properly.

An important factor that must be evaluated when selecting patients for a high septal strip DP procedure is the shape of the osseocartilaginous hump. Based on our previous work on the nasal bones, there exists 2 types of bony humps with either a V or S shape.[9] V-shaped nasal bones have a straight-line configuration from nasion to kyphion to rhinion, with 1 locus of angulation. In contrast, S-shaped nasal bones have a curved configuration that starts at nasion and rises abruptly to the kyphion, giving a second locus of angulation. V-shaped nasal bones allow easier flattening of the osseocartilaginous joint.

When doing a high septal DP procedure, 2 concurrent factors allow flattening of the hump: lowering the dorsum and a flexion of the osseocartilaginous joint. Assuming all blocking points are released, flexion of the KA joint is easier when more cartilage is present than bone. Bone can never be flattened, so convex bone must be modified or removed.

If the surgeon has difficult flattening the hump, it becomes easier with 3 steps:

1. Removing bone
2. Doing a limited lateral keystone release

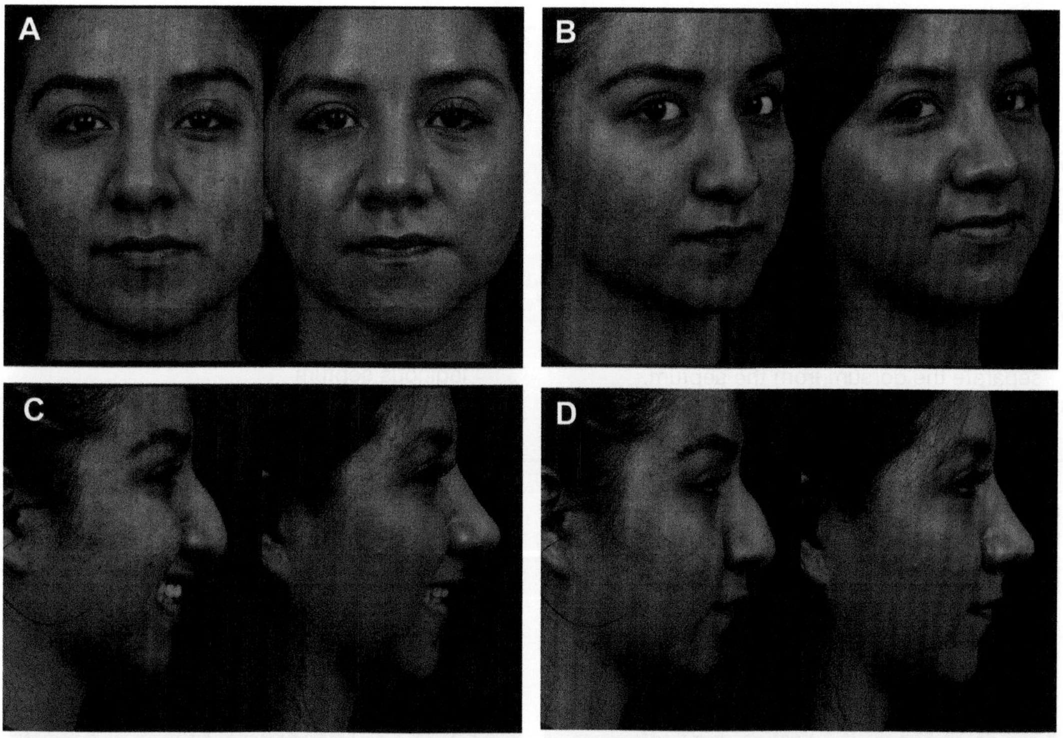

Fig. 6. A DP/high septal strip. A 26-year-old woman presents with a 4.5-mm dorsal hump, an ideal osseocartilaginous vault, and a plunging tip on smiling. The patient has very thick skin. The patient is shown preoperatively (*left*) and postoperatively (*right*) after she underwent a high septal strip pushdown. The patient has an ideal osseocartilaginous vault and a hump of approximately 4.5 mm. A 5.5-mm strip of subdorsal septum is removed and piezoelectric osteotomies are performed to release the bony vault from the face. The tip was supported with a septal extension graft to stabilize the nasal base and no cartilage was removed from the alars (only suturing). Therefore, she underwent a complete PR. Postoperatively the profile line is improved without opening the middle vault.

3. Fixating the cartilage vault down to the underlying septum

With good 3-point fixation, none of my patients have needed revision surgery for a recurrent dorsal hump in 3 years of high septal strip DP.

It is important to understand aesthetically that, with high septal stirp DP, flaring of the middle vault and widening of the internal valve occurs. In addition, widening of the dorsal aesthetic lines becomes evident. These changes in the dorsal aesthetic lines must be kept in mind when doing a DP procedure. The advantage of an open approach is that the dorsum can be fixed to the underlying septum with 2 25-gauge needles and middle vault width can be adjusted with sutures just as in the high septal strip cartilage-only DP. This advantage is key because it allows surgeons to tailor dorsal width and modify any asymmetries.

In addition, controlling the radix osteotomy is critical in any impaction technique. With the radix osteotomy, the nose is released from the face and, if there is a gap below the osteotomy site (from removal of septal cartilage or perpendicular plate of ethmoid [PPE]), the radix can lower. Two points are important to consider. First, in most cases only cartilage needs to be removed under the dorsum. Ethmoid bone (PPE) is only removed if it is impeding the impaction of the dorsum. Second, accurate osteotomies can be done with piezosurgery or osteotomies to achieve an incomplete (greenstick) fracture at the radix. In an open approach, the transverse osteotomies are brought anteriorly with a piezoelectric saw up to the radix bilaterally. The radix bone is left intact for approximately 2 to 3 mm and then a partial cut is made. Gentle pressure is applied to the dorsum, which clicks down as the greenstick fracture occurs. I have found this method to be the best way to control radix movement in an open approach. In a closed approach, it is best to leave the periosteum attached to the bone at the radix and to do the osteotomy in an oblique fashion with the osteotome pointing toward the chin (as opposed to a perpendicular cut).

Type 4 Impaction Technique: Dorsal Preservation (Low Septal Strip)

Low septal strip DP consists of 4 parts:

1. A vertical cut in the quadrangular cartilage at the highest point of the nasal hump.
2. Septal strip resection (along the maxilla and vomer) to lower/flatten the dorsal hump and to separate the dorsum from the septum.
3. Osteotomies to mobilize the bony pyramid, to separate the dorsum from the face, and to lower the dorsal profile via impaction into the pyriform aperture.
4. Precise fixation of the quadrangular cartilage flap to the anterior nasal spine. Thus, this is an impaction technique whereby the entire osseocartilaginous vault is lowered.

My indications are as follows (**Fig. 7**):

- Asymmetric developmental deviation of the nose (axis deviation)
- High and/or complicated septal deviations that do not involve the caudal half of the cartilaginous septum
- Small amount of cartilage needed from the septum for structural tip grafting

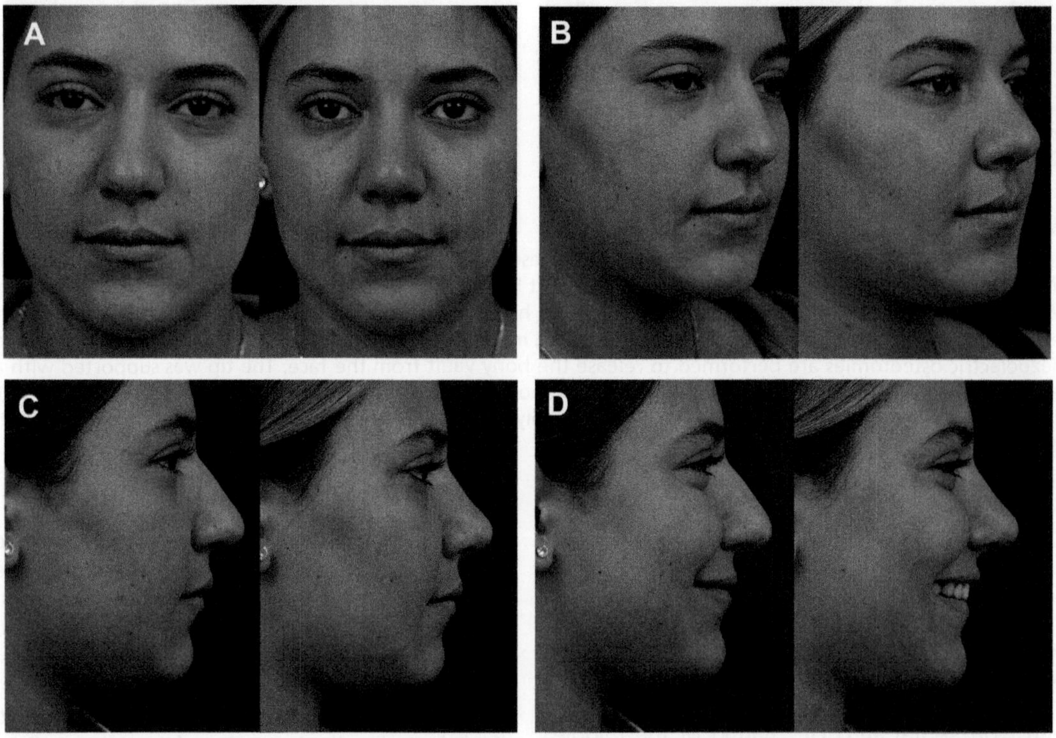

Fig. 7. A DP/low septal strip. A 24-year-old woman presents with asymmetric developmental deviation of the nose. This patient has an ideal osseocartilaginous vault with a small hump and straight-line deviation to the right. She also has a bulbous tip. The patient is shown preoperatively (*left*) and postoperatively (*right*) after undergoing a low septal strip, asymmetric letdown. The quadrangular cartilage was disarticulated from the anterior nasal spine, vomer, and PPE creating a so-called swinging door. A pushover of the osseocartilaginous vault was performed and profile line lowered by removing a 2.5-mm low septal strip and performing low-to-low and transverse osteotomies bilaterally as well as a radix osteotomy. On the long (left) side, a 3-mm strip of lateral nasal bone was removed at the face of the maxilla. On the short side, a low osteotomy was performed without bone removal. Once the osseocartilaginous vault was mobilized, the nose was pushed over and impacted on the long side. The caudal septum was then reattached to the anterior nasal spine via a drill hole. The tip was supported with a columellar strut and only tip suturing was performed. No cartilage was removed from the alars. A total subperichondrial dissection was done of the tip and dorsum with preservation of ligaments. Postoperatively, the dorsal aesthetic lines remain ideal and the osseocartilaginous vault has been centralized on the face. In effect, the nose was straightened without opening the middle vault or performing multiple open-book and closed-book osteotomies. Interestingly, the nasal tip deviation is fixed once the septum is placed in the midline. The patient underwent a complete PR.

Of all the DP techniques, the low septal strip is the most powerful, but it is the most difficult to learn and to understand. Unlike the high septal strip DP, there are 3 degrees of movement: posterior, lateral, and rotation/advancement, which allows the correction of very complex deformities. However, once the vertical cut is made in the septum, the technique cannot be converted to component reduction. In addition, smaller amounts of septum are available to harvest, and midvault width cannot be tailored with sutures compared with the high strip techniques.

When doing a low septal strip DP procedure, 2 concurrent factors allow the flattening of the hump. First, the entire osseocartilaginous hump lowers during a letdown or pushdown procedure. The second factor is rotation and advancement of the quadrangular cartilage flap that allows the osseocartilaginous joint to flex. As the bone moves down, the flap swings caudally and anteriorly. Flattening of the joint becomes easier when more cartilage is present than bone along the dorsum. Cartilage flexion becomes easier by removing bone and by doing a limited lateral keystone release. Using this technique, it is paramount that all tension is taken off the osseocartilaginous joint and that the neocaudal septum is securely fixed to the anterior nasal spine. Unlike the high strip DP, there is only 1 point of fixation.

Perhaps the best indication for this technique is axis deviation of the nose: a straight nose that is deviated off the midline axis in both its bony and cartilage components. A low strip technique combined with an asymmetric letdown of the bony vault results in impaction into the midline. The cartilage flap follows because the vertical cut releases the dorsum from the deviated PPE. In traditional component reduction rhinoplasty with an L strut, the PPE translates tension onto the cartilaginous portion of the septum. With a low strip DP, total release of the dorsum from the PPE is achieved and the bone and cartilage can swing into the midline without tension. These procedures have been the most exciting DP techniques for me. Very difficult, asymmetric noses can be corrected without the necessity of a total or subtotal septoplasty. However, if the flap of cartilage is deformed or curved, it is better to do an extracorporeal septoplasty.

DECISION MAKING

It is my opinion that no 1 operation is useful in 100% of patients. When I see or read about a new technique, my primary goal is to understand which of my patients would benefit and how. I began DP with the high strip Saban technique and expanded my skill set from there. Being in southern California, my rhinoplasty practice has a large percentage of Middle Eastern, Hispanic, and Asian patients. Initially, DP seemed to be a good option in approximately 15% to 20% of primary rhinoplasty patients. However, with better understanding of DP/high septal strip, I was able to apply the technique to 33% of my patients. Now, with the addition of cartilage conversion techniques and low septal strip DP, I choose to preserve the dorsum in more than 50% of patients. Thus, my rule is: if I can, I preserve.

The initial decision is made based on the anterior view of the patient. During physical examination, I decide whether the natural dorsum is ideal in terms of width and shape of the cartilaginous dorsal aesthetic lines. In selected cases, cartilage modification or cartilaginous preservation can be done while treating the bones separately. Once a surgeon has examined the anterior view and decided to preserve the dorsum, the next step is to examine the profile. Based on my ultrasonography studies and hundreds of postoperative results with each technique, the following key points must be assessed:

1. Position of radix. As described earlier, the radix lengthens in the vertical plane with DP techniques and the starting point of the nose (nasion) moves caudally if the radix drops. Ideal patients for impaction techniques have a normally positioned radix or slightly high radix. In these cases, a movement in radix position is not detrimental to the final result. In contrast, patients with a low radix must be approached much more carefully and a radix graft considered. Because the radix does not drop with surface techniques, radix issues can be dealt with separately and do not affect decision making. Performing a DP in the wrong patients or unintentionally dropping the radix can result in infantilization of the nose
2. Type of hump. The easiest patients for DP have a straight dorsum that is too high or overprojected. In these cases, the whole dorsum can be lowered or only the cartilaginous dorsum because there is no true hump.

   However, most patients have a hump, and understanding the difference between a V-shaped and S-shaped hump is critical to choosing initial patients for DP. It is much easier to flatten the osseocartilaginous vault in patients with a V-shaped hump because they have only 1 locus of angulation. S-shaped humps are much more difficult. It has been my experience that these noses are more difficult to flatten and any convexity in the bone must be removed.

3. Length of bony vault. The length of the bony vault is a critical determinant of how easy it will be to flatten a hump. Longer nasal bones are harder to flatten because cartilage is easier to flex than bone. Initial DP patients should be chosen who have primarily cartilaginous noses.
4. Position of anterior septal angle (ASA). The position of the ASA must be inspected carefully preoperatively. Early on, surgeons would take out a strip of septum to find that they had caused what appeared to be a saddle. With any DP technique, it is important to modify the caudal septum last. Using the high septal strip techniques, the W-ASA segment should be modified last. Using the low septal strip techniques, the posterior portion of the caudal septum should be modified last.

TECHNICAL DETAILS AND LESSONS LEARNED

Patient selection is the number 1 determinant of success with any rhinoplasty technique, including DP. As discussed earlier, surgeons should begin with patients who have ideal dorsal aesthetic lines with minimal deviation, asymmetries, and width discrepancies. Looking at the profile, ideal patients have a well-positioned or high radix, a V-shaped dorsal hump or no hump (only overprojection), and shorter nasal bones. The septum should be without major deviations. Overall, avoid patients with a prominent glabella or premaxilla as well as radix hypoplasia. Keeping these things in mind, patients typically look good immediately after surgery. It is also important to note that, because the middle vault is not be opened, the patients have minimal bleeding under the skin and photograph well even at 10 days postoperatively.

How to Learn Dorsal Preservation Surgery

If I were to start my journey over again, I would take a slightly different route to minimize my own stress. The best technique to start with is the type 1 cartilage modification (DM/CVM). Surgeons can become adept at removing the bony cap and preserving the underlying cartilaginous vault. This procedure is done in patients with small humps, and surgeons can easily convert to component reduction if they become uncomfortable. Next, the surgeon progresses to type 2 high septal strip, cartilage-only DP (DM/CVP). Now that the surgeon has become familiar with bony cap removal, a subdorsal strip of cartilage only can be removed. This step is the scariest part of learning the operation for surgeons who perform and understand the standard L-strut philosophy. The type 2 operation is also done in patients with small humps, and surgeons can convert to component reduction while doing traditional osteotomies. Once the surgeon is comfortable removing a subdorsal strip, it is time to progress to traditional DP procedures with impaction of the osseocartilaginous vault. The surgeon must have proper instrumentation: a small rongeur to remove PPE incrementally, as well as precise osteotomes. The first few type 3 high septal strip DP procedures are very stressful. However, over time, surgeons begin to feel comfortable. Even with this technique, it is easy to transition to component reduction at any point if things are not going smoothly. In addition, the low septal strip DP procedure can be learned. This technique has the steepest learning curve by far and is the hardest to control. Low strip techniques cannot be converted to a component reduction. To learn these procedures, it is imperative to visit a surgeon who performs them in order to see it being done and to have the opportunity to ask questions.

SUMMARY

All new techniques come with a learning curve. Because I am a younger surgeon in this group of physicians, I have built my rhinoplasty practice on the shoulders of giants and have had hundreds of opportunities to discuss and to develop these techniques with the help of spectacular surgeons. As a group, we worked hard and thought a lot about these techniques to make them safe and predictable. Pick your first patients correctly, and you will be successful. Visiting surgeons who do DP regularly is a must. For me, this technique only applies to a subset of patients in my practice. However, it is the best technique for these patients. No dorsum looks as good as a natural dorsum, and long-term issues with the middle vault and keystone area can be avoided.

DISCLOSURE

The author has no conflict of interest. Dr A.M. Kosins is a designer of instruments for Micrins and the Kosins Preservation Rhinoplasty Set. He is also a shareholder and consultant for ZO Skin Health. No outside funding was received.

REFERENCES

1. Daniel RK, Kosins AM. Current trends in preservation rhinoplasty. Aesthet Surg J Open Forum 2020;1–8.

2. Palhazi P, Daniel RK, Kosins AM. The osseocartilaginous vault of the nose: anatomy and surgical observations. Aesthet Surg J 2015;35:242–51.
3. Saban Y, Daniel RK, Polselli R, et al. Dorsal preservation: the push down technique reassessed. Aesthet Surg J 2018;38(2):117–31.
4. Kosins AM, Daniel RK. Decision making in preservation rhinoplasty: A 100 case-series with 1-year follow-up. Aesthet Surg J 2020;40(1):34–48.
5. Kosins AM. Expanding indications for dorsal preservation rhinoplasty with cartilage conversion techniques. Aesthet Surg J 2020;sjaa071 [online ahead of print].
6. Ferreira MG, Monteiro D, Reis C, et al. Spare roof technique: A middle third new technique. Facial Plast Surg 2016;32(1):111–6.
7. Ishida LC, Ishida J, Ishida LH, et al. Nasal hump treatment with cartilaginous push-down and preservation of the bony cap. Aesthet Surg J 2020;sjaa061 [online ahead of print].
8. Daniel RK. What is preservation rhinoplasty: rationale and overview?. In: Cakir B, Saban Y, Daniel RK, et al, editors. Preservation rhinoplasty. Septum Publications; 2018. p. 17–29.
9. Lazovic GD, Daniel RK, Janosevic LB, et al. Rhinoplasty: the nasal bones – anatomy and analysis. Aesthet Surg J 2015;35(3):255–63.

Combined Functional and Preservation Rhinoplasty

Priyesh N. Patel, MD[a], Mohamed Abdelwahab, MD, MS[b,c], Sam P. Most, MD[b,*]

KEYWORDS

- Dorsal preservation rhinoplasty • Septoplasty • Nasal obstruction
- Patient-reported outcome measures

KEY POINTS

- In dorsal preservation surgery, the nasal vault is treated en bloc without disarticulation of the upper lateral cartilages from the septum.
- Cadaveric studies imply that the let-down dorsal preservation procedure may be superior to the push-down; however, clinical correlation is necessary.
- The techniques used to treat the septum in dorsal preservation surgery differ in location of septal cartilage resection.
- Dorsal preservation limits damage to nasal mucosa and nasal ligaments with resulting functional implications.
- Robust patient-reported outcomes are needed to elucidate the functional implications of dorsal preservation surgery and compare breathing outcomes between conventional and preservation hump reduction techniques.

INTRODUCTION

Dorsal hump reduction with the classic technique of removing dorsal nasal bone and cartilage as championed by Joseph has become a hallmark of rhinoplasty.[1] Variations in techniques for tissue removal (eg, composite vs component hump reduction), for osteotomies to close subsequent open roof deformities, and for midvault reconstruction exist in literature.[2] More recently, there has been renewed interest in techniques that prevent resection of the dorsal hump and rather preserve the overall architecture of the nasal pyramid.[3–7] Much of the interest in dorsal preservation (DP) is due to the avoidance of the potential negative implications of excisional techniques. The maintenance of the structural integrity at the nasal keystone, dorsal aesthetic lines, and the patency of the internal nasal valve are points of DP.[8,9] The anatomic and technical considerations of preservation rhinoplasty have been comprehensively reviewed in a book entitled *Preservation Rhinoplasty*, written by rhinoplasty experts Daniel, Saban, Palhazi, and Cakir.[10] Several experienced surgeons have also reported exceptional aesthetic results with DP techniques.[4–7,11–14] However, despite the often stated theoretic benefits of DP on nasal airflow, few studies have explored the effect of these techniques on functional outcomes.[4,5,15] This article provides a review of the functional considerations in DP surgery and available literature on functional outcomes.

THE INTERNAL NASAL VALVE

The internal nasal valve contributes to the narrowest portion of the nasal airway and is bounded by the caudal edge of the upper lateral cartilage (ULC)

[a] Division of Facial Plastic and Reconstructive Surgery, Department of Otolaryngology, Vanderbilt University Medical Center, 1215 21st Avenue, South Suite 7209 Medical Center East, South Tower, Nashville, TN 37232, USA; [b] Division of Facial Plastic and Reconstructive Surgery, Stanford University School of Medicine, 801 Welch Road, Stanford, CA 94304, USA; [c] Department of Otolaryngology–Head & Neck Surgery, Division of Facial Plastic and Reconstructive Surgery, Mansoura University, Faculty of Medicine, 25 El Gomhouria St, Dakahlia Governorate 35516, Egypt
* Corresponding author.
E-mail address: smost@stanford.edu

Facial Plast Surg Clin N Am 29 (2021) 113–121
https://doi.org/10.1016/j.fsc.2020.09.005

laterally and the nasal septum medially.[16,17] This angle of articulation is generally 10° to 15°.[18] Inferiorly it is bounded by the nasal bony floor and posteriorly by the anterior head of the inferior turbinate. The degree of collapsibility of the internal nasal valve wall depends in part on the intrinsic stability of the ULCs, and minor changes in the internal nasal valve size result in large changes in resistance of nasal airflow. Given the attachment of the ULCs to the nasal bones, changes in position of the nasal bones are translated to the upper lateral cartilage and thereby may impact the internal nasal valve.

In the standard Joseph hump takedown, the upper lateral cartilages are disarticulated from the septum and the cartilaginous and bony pyramid are reduced in height. The resection of the cartilaginous middle vault disrupts the important relationship between the upper lateral cartilage and the dorsal septum. The upper lateral cartilage is more prone to medial collapse and careful midvault reconstruction is, therefore required.[19] Moreso, it may decrease the cross-sectional area of the internal nasal valve.[20] Overall, this procedure can result in impaired nasal ventilation.[12] In DP surgery, the nasal vault is treated en bloc without disarticulation of the upper lateral cartilages from the septum. This precludes the disruption of the internal nasal valve angle or the need for midvault reconstruction.[21] Overmobilization and mediatization of the nasal sidewalls can occur with standard lateral and medial osteotomies used to close an open roof deformity. This can lead to a narrower nasal vault and nasal obstruction. Because DP techniques treat the entire nasal pyramid en bloc, there is a decreased risk of overmedialization of the nasal sidewall.

The bony pyramid in DP surgery can be managed using one of two strategies: the push-down (PD) or let-down (LD) operation.[4,7,13,22–25] In the PD technique, lateral and transverse osteotomies are performed to allow for mobilization of the entire bony vault. In the LD operation, similar osteotomies are performed, but a wedge of bone at the frontal process of the maxilla is also removed. After osteotomies in the PD technique, the lateral aspect of the bony pyramid is advanced into the nasal cavity medial to the frontal process of the maxilla (**Fig. 1**). Theoretically, although the internal nasal valve angle is not directly disrupted with this technique, the medial movement of the bony vault could narrow the angle. In addition, when combined with the inferior descent of the pyramid into the nose, there may be a reduction in the cross-sectional area of the nose at this site. Alternatively, with the LD technique, because the nasal pyramid is not impacted within the nose and rather lowered to rest on the maxilla, there is a theoretically lower risk of narrowing the area of the internal nasal valve (see **Fig. 1**).

A recent cadaveric radiologic study from our group has examined the impact of DP (both LD and PD) and standard hump take down with autospreader reconstruction of the midvault on internal nasal valve dimensions.[15] In the cadavers with conventional joseph hump take downs, the internal nasal valve angle decreased from a mean of 10.72 preoperatively to 9.98 postoperatively, although this difference only approached significance (P = .068). The cross-sectional area at the level of the internal nasal valve did not significantly change (1.92–1.87; P = .156). In cadavers undergoing the PD procedure, both the internal nasal valve angle and cross-sectional area decreased (11.36–9.3 [P = .016] and 1.89–1.59 [P<.001], respectively). The LD group did not show significant reduction in the internal nasal valve angle or in cross-sectional area (P = .437 and P = .331, respectively). As such, the LD procedure may be superior to the PD with regard to narrowing of the nasal passage. Whether this difference has clinical relevance for patients is an area of ongoing research and may have implications for the selective use of the LD over the PD technique. Moreover, it remains unclear if there are dynamic differences in narrowing of the internal nasal valve in addition to the static differences between dorsal hump reduction procedures elucidated in this study.

The placement of spreader grafts to widen a narrow internal nasal valve has not been described with DP techniques, although it is theoretically possible to place spreader grafts endonasally without release of the ULCs. Certain methods of DP, including the modified subdorsal strip method described elsewhere in this article, allow access to and release of the caudal upper lateral cartilage attachments. Therefore, the placement of spreader grafts is facilitated. This method allows for unilateral or bilateral widening of the internal nasal valve for functional or aesthetic purposes.

A cartilaginous DP surgery (termed spare roof technique by the authors), has also been described to impart benefits on the internal nasal valve.[26] In this technique, the cartilaginous midvault is preserved with subdorsal resection of septal cartilage. However, an ostectomy of the caudal edge of the nasal bones is performed with subsequent need for lateral osteotomies to close an open roof. As such, this technique differs from DP techniques in which the entirety of the dorsum is preserved. However, in preserving the upper lateral cartilage attachments to the nasal septum, the internal nasal valve is importantly

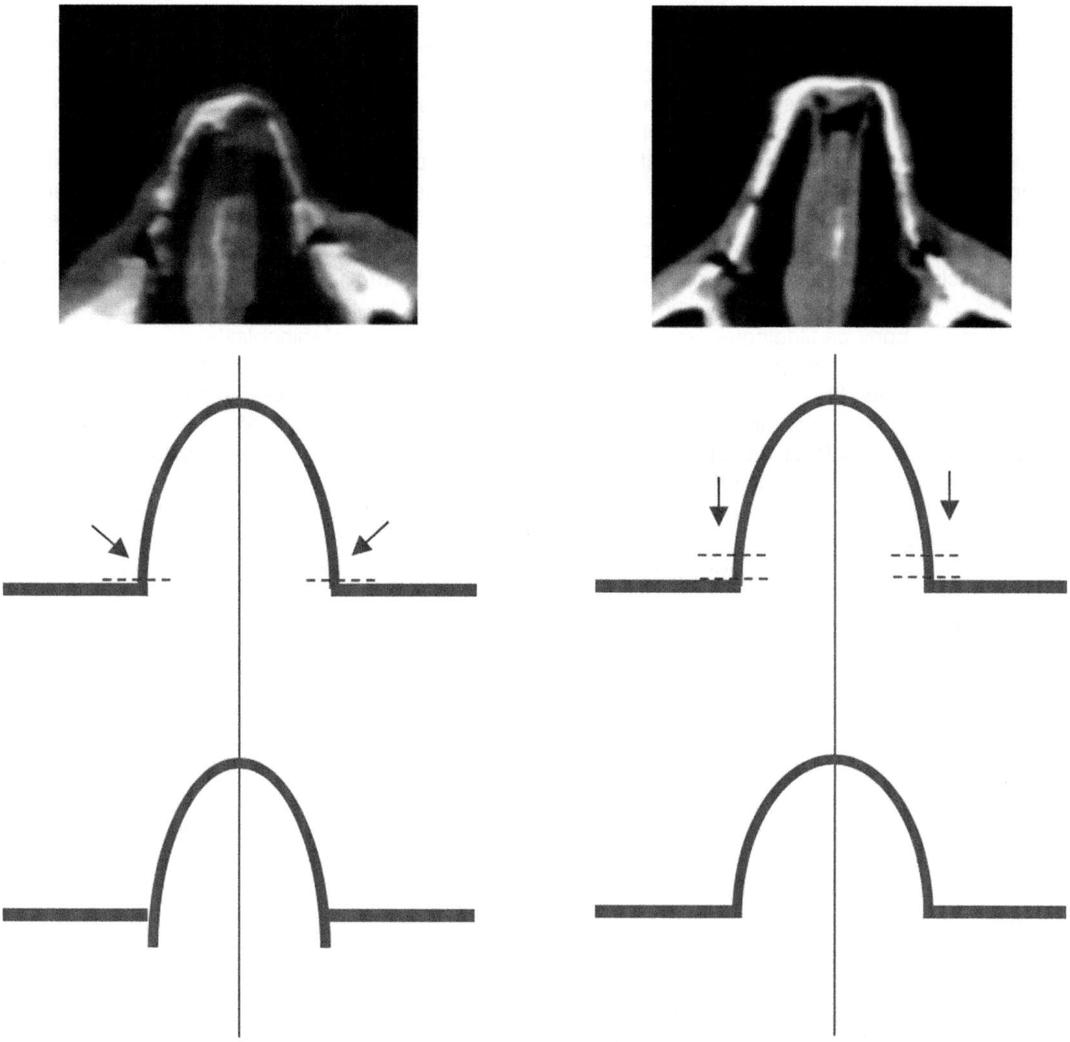

Fig. 1. (*Left*) In a PD technique, lateral osteotomies (*red dotted line*) are performed and the nasal vault is impacted into the nasal cavity as is seen on computed tomography imaging. The posterior and medial displacement (*blue arrows*) of the bony pyramid can result in narrowing of the internal nasal valve. (*Right*) In a LD technique, lateral osteotomies combined with an additional wedge resection of bone (*red dotted line*) are performed and the nasal vault is lowered onto the frontal process of the maxilla. The posterior displacement (*blue arrows*) of the bony pyramid is not combined with medialization into the nasal cavity, thereby preventing narrowing of the internal nasal valve.

preserved. The authors suggest that this technique has functional benefits secondary to the widening effect on the midvault and internal nasal valve as the dorsum descends.

NASAL SEPTUM

In patients who present with a dorsal hump, the presence of a septal deviation may contribute to concomitant obstructive complaints. In addition, the septum provides support to the overlying nasal bone and upper lateral cartilages. Therefore, regardless of whether the LD or PD technique is used, descent of the dorsum requires excision of a portion of the septum. Several techniques to manage the septum have been described in DP surgery, each primarily differentiated by the location of septal cartilage excision. Although these techniques have been described in detail elsewhere, several differences that contribute to functional outcomes are briefly summarized here.[4,5]

A subdorsal resection of cartilage originally described by Goodale and championed by Saban and associates, involves a strip of cartilage removed immediately under the dorsum.[4,27,28] The resection extends to the anterior septal angle.[4,12,14] A recently described modified subdorsal strip method performed by the senior author involves resection of a strip of cartilage high on the septum with the preservation of a 3- to 5-mm subdorsal strip of cartilage.[5] Unlike other techniques, the resection terminates posterior to the anterior septal angle, and a 1.0 to 1.5 cm caudal strut of septal cartilage is maintained. A third method, described by Cottle, involves inferior cartilage excision along the maxillary crest. This is combined with a resection of a vertical 4 mm segment at the bony cartilaginous junction (from the keystone to the vomer) and a resection of the ethmoid bone under the nasal bone.[29] Another method, described by Ishida and colleagues,[9] involves excision of a strip of cartilage at the mid aspect of the cartilaginous septum.

Both the subdorsal technique and modified subdorsal strip method would allow for removal of any septal deviation in the mid or posterior aspects of the cartilaginous septum. This is because the excision of cartilage performed for descent of the nasal pyramid is higher up on the septum. As long as a strut of cartilage is maintained superiorly, portions of deviated septum inferiorly can be resected without disrupting nasal support. Alternatively, the Cottle and Loring method relies on resection of inferior cartilage and manipulation of cartilage along the entire bony–cartilaginous junction. This precludes the removal of any further cartilage. Similarly, midseptal resection of cartilage for the purposes of dorsal hump descent limits the amount of cartilage that can be removed inferiorly for the purposes of septal deviations without the risk of loss of nasal support. For these reasons, cartilage grafts for the purposes of providing lower lateral cartilage support can be harvested more easily in the subdorsal and modified subdorsal technique.

Although posterior septal deviations can be managed with standard endonasal septoplasty approaches, deviations of the anterocaudal septum pose unique structural challenges.[30–32] A variety of repair techniques have been described to address deformities of the caudal septum in nonpreservation rhinoplasty cases, including swinging door, cartilage scoring, septal extension grafts, and septal batten grafts.[30,32,33] These techniques are aimed at stabilizing or recontouring native cartilage and may be applied to DP rhinoplasty. This technique, however, must be undertaken with caution because the caudal aspect of the septum is already violated during excision of the cartilaginous strip needed for dorsal descent in the majority of techniques, and there is a risk of overweakening of the cartilage to occur (ie, if it is scored). In the Cottle technique, the anterior septum is disarticulated from the maxillary crest and excised inferiorly. As such, this method incorporates elements of the swinging door technique for correcting caudal deviations. The anterior septum can theoretically be positioned into the correct position in both the anterior–posterior and transverse dimensions. The caudal septum is tensioned to the anterior nasal spine and is critical to success of the dorsal reduction. If the caudal septum is severely deviated, weakening and scoring methods will weaken the critical structure of this type of rhinoplasty.

Even in cases of nonpreservation rhinoplasty, these techniques addressing septal caudal deviations can be variably effective because most depend on an inherently misshapen cartilage structure.[30] Conventional extracorporeal septoplasty techniques that are used for extensive caudal septal deviations are difficult to perform with DP techniques given both the septal excisions performed for dorsal lowering and the need to maintain the keystone and the stability of septum to support the overlying nasal vault.

Subtotal septal reconstruction and the anterior septal reconstruction (ASR) techniques, both modifications of extracorporeal septoplasty, preserve the dorsal septum and thereby maintain the integrity of the keystone area.[34–37] In the ASR method, the anterocaudal septal deviation is removed and a new caudal strut is reconstructed from either rib or septal cartilage. This strut is anchored to the remaining dorsal strut and placed into a groove in the nasal spine. The modified subdorsal strip method, by maintaining a strut of subdorsal cartilage, allows for the use of ASR in this particular DP method (**Fig. 2**). In this technique, the ASR graft can be directly sutured to the dorsal strut in a side-to-side configuration (see **Fig. 2**A) or it can be sutured in an end-to-end configuration (see **Fig. 2**B). In the latter configuration, bilateral extended spreader grafts are used to stabilize the ASR graft. Notably, these spreader grafts differ from traditional spreader grafts because they do not sit between the native dorsal septum and the upper lateral cartilages (as the upper lateral cartilage attachment to the dorsal septum is preserved), but instead sit high along the remaining dorsal strut, just beneath the upper lateral cartilage. **Fig. 3** demonstrates representative photographs of a patient undergoing an LD procedure with the modified subdorsal strip method technique combined with an ASR.

INFERIOR TURBINATES

Inferior turbinate hypertrophy may represent a cause of nasal obstruction in patients presenting

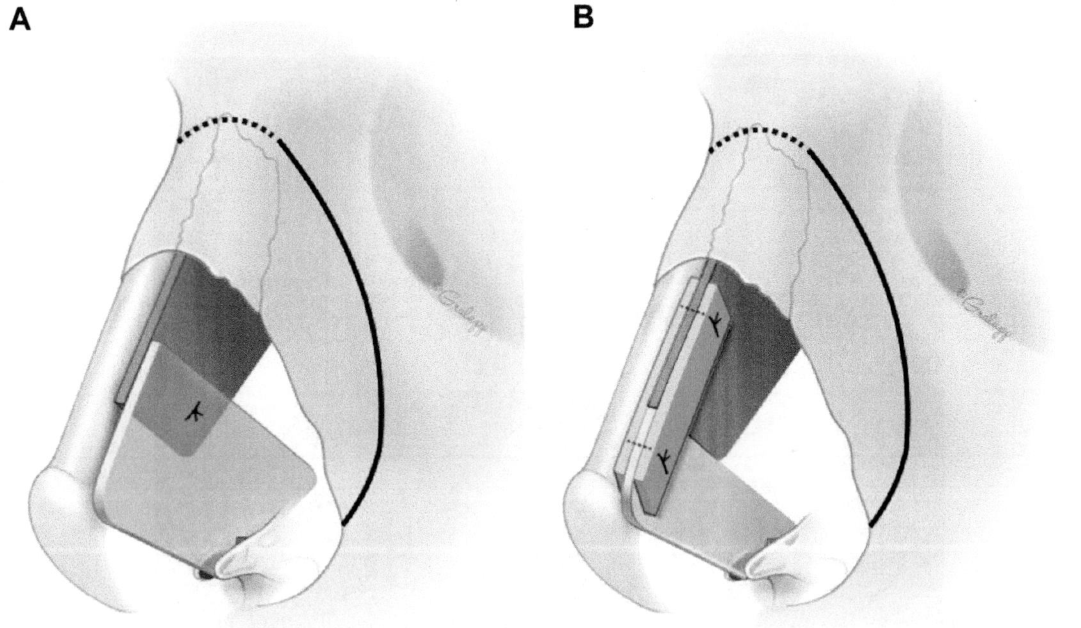

Fig. 2. In a structural preservation rhinoplasty approach using the modified subdorsal strip method, modified extracorporeal septoplasty techniques such as the ASR can be used. Osteotomies are performed to allow for either a LD or PD maneuver, followed by techniques to lower the dorsum. Note that in this figure, the LD has already been performed. In the modified subdorsal strip method a dorsal strip of cartilage (*purple*) is maintained. The remaining underlying septum, including anterior deviations, can be resected and either septal cartilage (or autologous rib cartilage) is then fashioned into an ASR graft (*blue*). This is positioned to sit in a groove created in the maxillary spine. The ASR graft is secured to the dorsal strip of cartilage either in a side-to-side orientation (*A*) or in an end-to-end configuration (*B*). In the latter configuration, extended spreader grafts attached to the subdorsal strip are used to stabilize the ASR graft.

for aesthetic rhinoplasty. Turbinate reduction can be safely performed in DP procedures with several important considerations. In general, turbinate reduction should be performed before any delicate work with the septum or osteotomies. A variety of techniques exist and although the best strategy remains controversial, submucosal resection combined with lateral displacement has been suggested to be the most effective at decreasing nasal obstruction.[38] Submucosal reduction can be performed with cautery, radiofrequency ablation, or a microdebrider with or without additional removal of anterior turbinate bone. Importantly, poorly placed lateral nasal osteotomies can lead to medialization of the inferior turbinate with resulting nasal obstruction. It can be avoided if the lateral osteotomy is performed in a high–low–high fashion with preservation of a triangular area of the caudal aspect of the frontal process of the maxilla near the internal valve (Webster's triangle).[39]

NASAL MUCOSA

Candidates for DP rhinoplasty with concomitant nasal obstruction may have underlying nasal mucosal disease including allergic rhinitis or chronic sinusitis. Patients with nasal obstruction should have a thorough examination of the nasal mucosa to assess for findings suggestive of an inflammatory or infectious process including mucosal hyperemia, edema, polyps, or excessive mucin. Treatment with topical steroid medications is considered a first line treatment in patients with nasal obstruction with underlying mucosal disease, and similar to nonpreservation rhinoplasty, patients should be counseled on the potential need to continue medical management postoperatively.

Conventional hump resection procedures can result in disruption of nasal mucosa given their excisional nature. This disruption may contribute to vasomotor disturbances given the sensitivity of the nasal mucosa.[12] Because DP procedures do not violate the nasal roof and the underlying lining, there is less risk of this "open roof" syndrome.[12] By maintaining the natural protective capacity of the nasal mucosa, there is theoretically less reactivity and fewer inflammatory sequela (eg, sensitivity to temperature changes, watery rhinorrhea) from rhinoplasty with DP procedures. A comparative study between conventional and

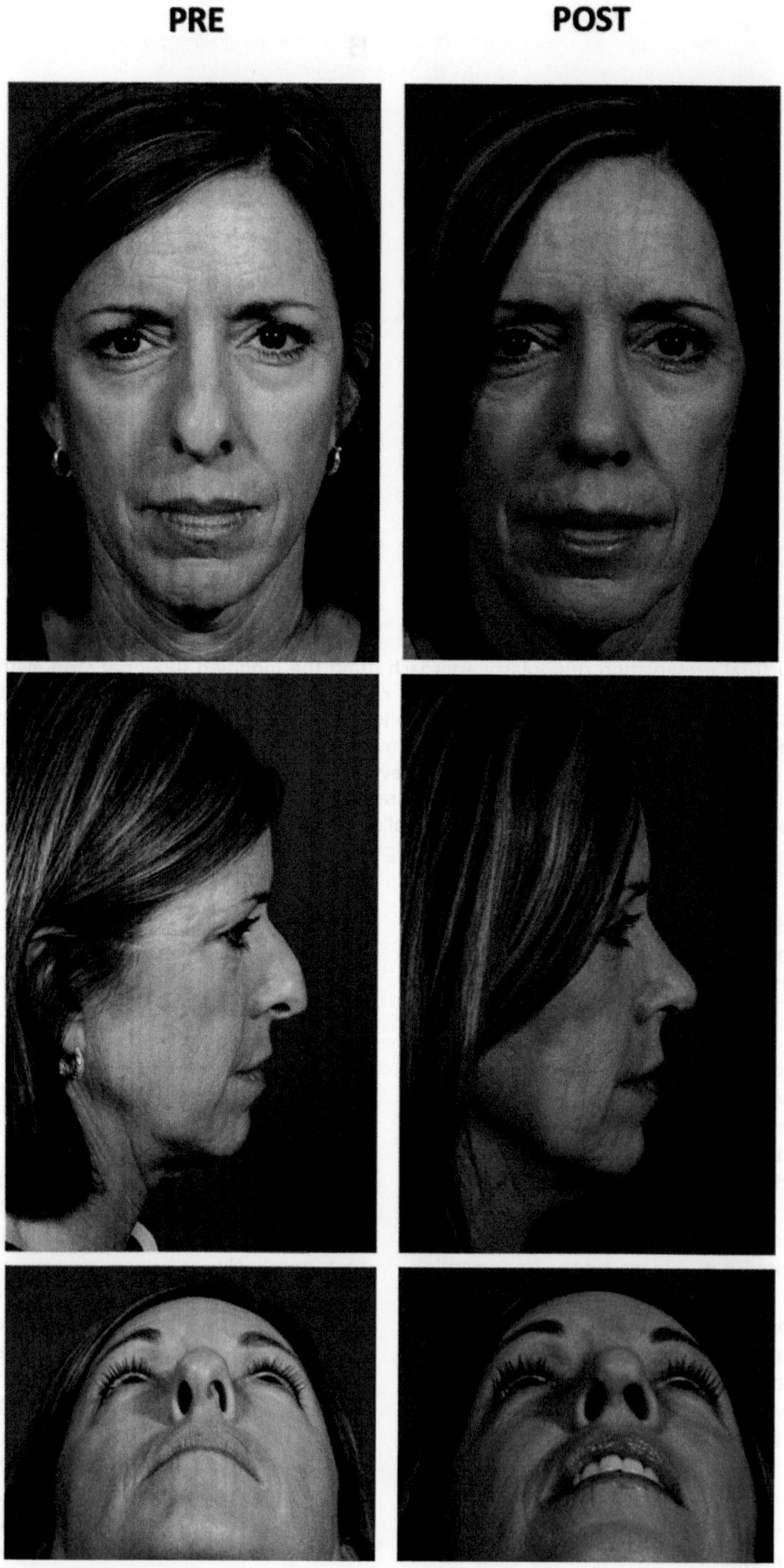

Fig. 3. Representative photographs of a patient undergoing a LD procedure with a modified subdorsal strip method. This patient also underwent an ASR. Improvements in external nasal contour with dorsal reduction and improvement in caudal septal position is noted when comparing preoperative (*left*) and 6-month postoperative (*right*) images.

dorsal preservation procedures in this regard is needed to further evaluate the changes to nasal mucosa between these methods.

NASAL LIGAMENTS

The complex fibrous attachments of the nose are important in providing structural support to the nose. Ligaments between the nasal cartilages have continuity with the overlying superficial musculo-aponeurotic system, nasal soft tissue, or maxillary bone and thereby provide suspensory support to the nasal framework.[40] These structures includes the scroll ligament and the vertical pyriform attachment, which play an important role in ensuring the upper lateral cartilages do not collapse and cause internal nasal valve narrowing. Release of these ligaments, therefore, may result in disruption of nasal support although this has not been previously studied.

Given this theoretic risk of nasal obstruction, many DP surgeons describe an endonasal (closed) technique with limited soft tissue dissection, although several use an external approach.[4,13,14,41] In the external approach, given release of nasal ligaments and soft tissue attachments, care to prevent overmobilization of bone should be emphasized. At present, in DP surgery, there is no consensus about the best approach as it relates to structural support, functional outcomes, and nasal aesthetics.[13]

PATIENT-REPORTED OUTCOMES

Despite the theoretic benefits of DP surgery and the single cadaveric study on internal nasal valve dimensions, robust outcome studies that (1) elucidate the functional implications of DP surgery and (2) compare breathing outcomes between conventional and preservation hump reduction techniques are lacking.

Several authors have suggested excellent functional results with DP. Using the subdorsal resection technique, Saban and coworkers (n = 320), Gola (n = 1000), and Tuncel and Aydogdu (n = 520) comment on great functional and aesthetic success.[4,12,42] Unfortunately, this assessment is largely based on physician subjective assessment. Saban and colleagues administered the Nasal Obstruction Symptom Evaluation (NOSE) questionnaire to 30 of the 320 patients in their study who underwent the subdorsal resection technique with endoscopic visualization and either the PD or LD procedure. Twenty-seven patients (90%) reported improvements in nasal obstruction; the remaining 3 patients described no change (but no worsening) in symptoms. Santos and colleagues, in a cohort of 100 patients who underwent a cartilaginous preservation surgery (spare roof technique), found there was an improvement in functional visual analog scale scores at 12 months postoperatively on the right side (5.13–8.62; $P<.001$) and left side (4.49–8.72; $P<.001$).[26] As mentioned elsewhere in this article, this technique does not preserve the bony dorsum and is thus differentiated from other DP surgery. Nonetheless, this work suggests that preservation and descent of the midvault may result in a widening of the interval nasal valve with subsequent functional improvement in the nasal airway.

Of 22 patients at our institution who underwent the modified subdorsal strip method, 10 had functional breathing complaints with documented anatomic obstruction noted on preoperative examination. These patients, in addition to preservation dorsal hump surgery, underwent functional surgery (9 underwent turbinate reduction, 9 underwent septoplasty, and 2 underwent placement of lateral crural strut grafts). The standardized cosmesis and health nasal outcomes survey score (SCHNOS), of which there is an obstructive (SCHNOS-O) and cosmetic (SCHNOS-C) domain, was administered to these patients. The mean preoperative SCHNOS-O and -C scores were 66.5 $\pm$ 19.4 and 54.7 $\pm$ 24.9, respectively. These scores improved to 18.0 $\pm$ 14.0 and 11.3 $\pm$ 15.5, respectively ($P<.001$). As such, when functional surgery is combined with DP hump reduction, there is a clear benefit in both nasal functionality and aesthetics. Notably, 3 patients within this group underwent an ASR for significant caudal septal deviation, as is possible with the modified subdorsal resection technique. In these patients, the mean SCHNOS-O scores improved from 73.3 $\pm$ 12.6 to 13.3 $\pm$ 5.8 ($P = .007$).

In patients who did not undergo functional surgery (n = 12), the mean SCHNOS-C scores significantly improved (68.3–3.3; $P<.001$), although there was no significant change in the SCHNOS-O scores (20.8–24.9; $P = .314$). When considering the entire cohort (n = 22), 8 patients underwent a PD procedure and 14 underwent an LD procedure. In patients who underwent the PD procedure, the mean SCHNOS-O score improved from 41.3 $\pm$ 32.6 to 16.3 $\pm$ 13.8 ($P = .06$). Patients who underwent an LD procedure had an improvement from 48.8 $\pm$ 28.3 to 24.6 $\pm$ 17.1 ($P = .05$). No patient in the cohort experienced any lateral wall insufficiency or valve collapse postoperatively. As such, from this limited data, DP does not seem to worsen nasal obstruction. How this result compares to conventional dorsal hump reduction strategies is unclear and remains an area of ongoing research at our center.

SUMMARY

In DP surgery, the nasal vault is treated en bloc without disarticulation of the upper lateral cartilages from the septum with resulting functional implications. Importantly, the internal nasal valve—the narrowest aspect of the nasal passage—is not disrupted and midvault reconstruction is not required. In addition, there is limited damage to nasal mucosa and nasal ligaments, which may limit nasal sidewall collapse and prevent vasomotor changes that may be seen with conventional hump take down techniques. In DP, the bony pyramid can be managed using 1 of 2 techniques: either the LD or PD techniques. The latter may be inferior with regards to narrowing of the nasal passageway. The techniques used to treat the septum in DP surgery differ in location of septal cartilage resection and thereby impact the nature of functional septoplasty that can be performed for nasal obstruction. Limited patient-reported outcomes demonstrate that DP techniques may preserve the nasal airway. However, more robust studies are needed to elucidate the functional implications of DP surgery and compare breathing outcomes between conventional and preservation hump reduction techniques.

CLINICS CARE POINTS

- In dorsal preservation surgery, the internal nasal valve is not compromised and midvault reconstruction is therefore not required.
- The let-down dorsal preservation procedure is radiologically superior to the push-down procedure in preserving the internal nasal valve dimensions, although the clinical implications of this are unclear.
- The techniques used to manage the septum in dorsal preservation surgery differ in location of septal cartilage resection and thereby impact the nature of functional septoplasty that can be performed for nasal obstruction.

REFERENCES

1. Joseph J. The classic reprint: nasal reductions. Plast Reconstr Surg 1971;47(1):79–83.
2. Azizzadeh B, Reilly M. Dorsal Hump Reduction and Osteotomies. Clin Plast Surg 2016;43(1):47–58.
3. Daniel RK. The preservation rhinoplasty: a new rhinoplasty revolution. Aesthet Surg J 2018;38(2): 228–9.
4. Saban Y, Daniel RK, Polselli R, et al. Dorsal preservation: the push down technique reassessed. Aesthet Surg J 2018;38(2):117–31.
5. Patel PN, Abdelwahab M, Most SP. A review and modification of dorsal preservation rhinoplasty techniques. Facial Plast Surg Aesthet Med 2020; 22(2):71–9.
6. Barelli PA. Long term evaluation of "push down" procedures. Rhinology 1975;13(1):25–32.
7. Pinto RM. On the "let-down" procedure in septorhinoplasty. Rhinology 1997;35(4):178–80.
8. Rohrich RJ, Muzaffar AR, Janis JE. Component dorsal hump reduction: the importance of maintaining dorsal aesthetic lines in rhinoplasty. Plast Reconstr Surg 2004;114(5):1298–308 [discussion: 1309–2].
9. Ishida J, Ishida LC, Ishida LH, et al. Treatment of the nasal hump with preservation of the cartilaginous framework. Plast Reconstr Surg 1999;103(6): 1729–33 [discussion: 1734–5].
10. Çakir B, Saban Y, Daniel RK, et al. Preservation rhinoplasty book. Istanbul (Turkey): Septum Publishing; 2018.
11. Tuncel U, Aydogdu O. The probable reasons of dorsal hump problems following let-down/push-down rhinoplasty and solution proposals. Plast Reconstr Surg 2019;144(3):378e–85e.
12. Gola R. Functional and esthetic rhinoplasty. Aesthetic Plast Surg 2003;27(5):390–6.
13. Montes-Bracchini JJ. Nasal Profile Hump Reduction Using the Let-Down Technique. Facial Plast Surg 2019;35(5):486–91.
14. Kosins AM, Daniel RK. Decision making in preservation rhinoplasty: a 100 case series with one-year follow-up. Aesthet Surg J 2020;40(1):34–48.
15. Abdelwahab MA, Neves CA, Patel PN, et al. Impact of dorsal preservation rhinoplasty versus dorsal hump resection on the internal nasal valve: a quantitative radiological study. Aesthetic Plast Surg 2020; 40(1):34–48.
16. Fettman N, Sanford T, Sindwani R. Surgical management of the deviated septum: techniques in septoplasty. Otolaryngol Clin North Am 2009;42(2): 241–52, viii.
17. Abdelwahab M, Yoon A, Okland T, et al. Impact of distraction osteogenesis maxillary expansion on the internal nasal valve in obstructive sleep apnea. Otolaryngol Head Neck Surg 2019;161(2):362–7.
18. Schlosser RJ, Park SS. Functional nasal surgery. Otolaryngol Clin North Am 1999;32(1):37–51.
19. Sheen JH. Spreader graft: a method of reconstructing the roof of the middle nasal vault following rhinoplasty. Plast Reconstr Surg 1984;73(2):230–9.
20. Grymer LF. Reduction rhinoplasty and nasal patency: change in the cross-sectional area of the nose evaluated by acoustic rhinometry. Laryngoscope 1995;105(4 Pt 1):429–31.
21. Rudy S, Moubayed SP, Most SP. Midvault reconstruction in primary rhinoplasty. Facial Plast Surg 2017;33(2):133–8.
22. Jobe R. En bloc nasal shift rhinoplasty–an approach to the small crooked nose. Ann Plast Surg 1981;7(2): 120–5.

23. Huizing EH. Push-down of the external nasal pyramid by resection of wedges. Rhinology 1975;13(4):185–90.
24. Lopez Úlloa F. Let down technique. 2011. Available at: https://www.rhinoplastyarchive.com/articles/let-down-technique. Accessed December 12, 2019.
25. Lothrop O. An operation for correcting the aquiline nasal deformity; the use of new instrument; report of a case. Boston Med Surg J 1914;170:835–7.
26. Santos M, Rego AR, Coutinho M, et al. Spare roof technique in reduction rhinoplasty: Prospective study of the first one hundred patients. Laryngoscope 2019;129(12):2702–6.
27. Goodale JL. A new method for the operative correction of exaggerated roman nose. Boston Med Surg J 1899;140:112.
28. Goodale JL. The correction of old lateral displacements of the nasal bones. Boston Med Surg J 1901;145:538–9.
29. Cottle MH, Loring RM. Corrective surgery of the external nasal pyramid and the nasal septum for restoration of normal physiology. Ill Med J 1946;90:119–35.
30. Most SP, Rudy SF. Septoplasty: basic and advanced techniques. Facial Plast Surg Clin North Am 2017;25(2):161–9.
31. Paradis J, Rotenberg BW. Open versus endoscopic septoplasty: a single-blinded, randomized, controlled trial. J Otolaryngol Head Neck Surg 2011;40(Suppl 1):S28–33.
32. Becker DG. Septoplasty and turbinate surgery. Aesthet Surg J 2003;23(5):393–403.
33. Haack J, Papel ID. Caudal septal deviation. Otolaryngol Clin North Am 2009;42(3):427–36.
34. Most SP. Anterior septal reconstruction: outcomes after a modified extracorporeal septoplasty technique. Arch Facial Plast Surg 2006;8(3):202–7.
35. Surowitz J, Lee MK, Most SP. Anterior septal reconstruction for treatment of severe caudal septal deviation: clinical severity and outcomes. Otolaryngol Head Neck Surg 2015;153(1):27–33.
36. Toriumi DM. Subtotal reconstruction of the nasal septum: a preliminary report. Laryngoscope 1994;104(7):906–13.
37. Toriumi DM. Subtotal septal reconstruction: an update. Facial Plast Surg 2013;29(6):492–501.
38. Larrabee YC, Kacker A. Which inferior turbinate reduction technique best decreases nasal obstruction? Laryngoscope 2014;124(4):814–5.
39. Ghanaatpisheh M, Sajjadian A, Daniel RK. Superior rhinoplasty outcomes with precise nasal osteotomy: an individualized approach for maintaining function and achieving aesthetic goals. Aesthet Surg J 2015;35(1):28–39.
40. Daniel RK, Palhazi P. The nasal ligaments and tip support in rhinoplasty: an anatomical study. Aesthet Surg J 2018;38(4):357–68.
41. Gola R, Nerini A, Laurent-Fyon C, et al. [Conservative rhinoplasty of the nasal canopy]. Ann Chir Plast Esthet 1989;34(6):465–75.
42. Tuncel U, Aydogdu O. The probable reasons for dorsal hump problems following let-down/push-down rhinoplasty and solution proposals. Plast Reconstr Surg 2019;144(3):378e–85e.

Preservation Rhinoplasty and the Crooked Nose

Charles East, MD, FRCS

KEYWORDS

• Rhinoplasty • Preservation rhinoplasty • Crooked nose • Septoplasty

KEY POINTS

- Crooked noses are among the most difficult cases in rhinoplasty.
- A partially structural approach may be required while adhering to preservation techniques.
- Careful examination of facial bony asymmetry is paramount.

INTRODUCTION

The principles of preservation rhinoplasty are to respect conserve or restore the soft tissue envelope ligaments, minimize the resection of cartilage through reorientation and to keep the dorsal continuity of the patient's own bridge. The origins of the operation date back to the beginning of the 20th century.[1] Although initially described as an endonasal procedure, preservation rhinoplasty can be performed via open or closed approaches.

Crooked or deviated noses pose a specific challenge, as many of the elements in a deviated nose are not symmetric and therefore not ideal for preservation techniques.[2–4] Indeed, deviated noses are often where there is a hybridization between preservation and structural rhinoplasty.

The first question to ask is whether the deviation is part of a facial asymmetry—that is, the underlying foundation of the nose (maxilla) is different between left and right sides either in left to right vertical height or anterior posterior discrepancy. This is usually obvious by looking at the orbit or brow position, the insertion of the alar base of the cheek, the cant of the smile, and the dentition if the patient has not undergone orthodontic treatment. It is easy to assess bony asymmetries by using a head down frontal photograph or by walking round behind the patient to examine the nose from above. This ascertains whether the deviation involves predominantly the bony pyramid, the cartilaginous part of the nose, or the whole nasal structure. It also permits assessment of asymmetries in the nasal sidewalls and the tip. The axis of a nose can be straight but sidewall asymmetry can create the appearance of deviation.[4,5]

Trauma in childhood often results in a similar growth-related disorder to the developmentally deviated nose without a history of injury, except here there will be evidence of the previous injury with angulations in the cartilaginous and bony dorsum. The septum has a major role to play in deviated or crooked noses particularly as it may contribute to a dysfunctional airway due to compromise of the nasal valve—anywhere from the front of the nostril to behind the head of the inferior turbinate. The secondary changes in the turbinate size or shape usually demand that lateral nasal wall surgery will be combined with rhinoplasty or endoscopic sinus surgery.

This makes an external and internal and functional assessment so important in deciding the appropriate procedure. Careful palpation of the nasal pyramid and CT scanning is highly recommended in evaluating the underlying architecture nose and septum plus examination of the nose by endoscopy (**Fig. 1**).

CROOKED OR DEVIATED NOSES

The working definition for deviation can be any deviation of the nasal form from a vertical line dropped from the midpoint of the intercanthal distance.[2] This of course is an approximation as in facial asymmetry the midline between the

UCL, Rhinoplasty London, London SW1W 8TW, UK
E-mail address: eastca@gmail.com

Facial Plast Surg Clin N Am 29 (2021) 123–130
https://doi.org/10.1016/j.fsc.2020.09.007

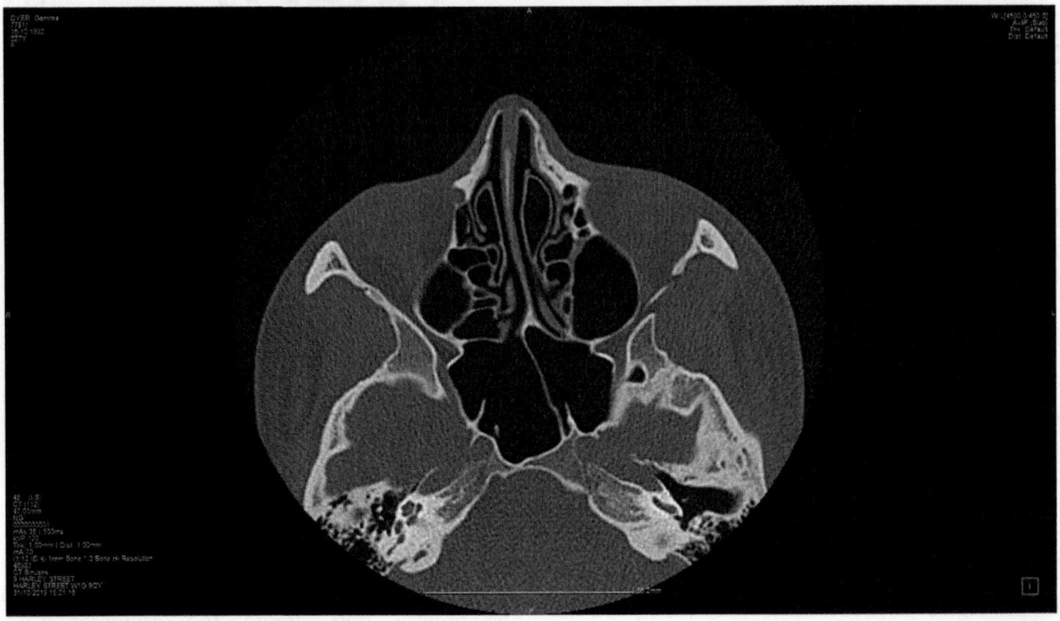

Fig. 1. Axial CT of nasal pyramid with deviation, different bone thickness, septal deviation, and pneumatized expansion of the left middle turbinate.

eyes, the philtrum the dental midlines and the chin point may not lie on the same vertical axis. However, we assume that the nose is the central feature about which we evaluate the whole face; however, this seems to vary between Western and Asian cultures. For facial learning and recognition, westerners focus more on the eyes and mouth in a triangular pattern, whereas Eastern Asians rely more on the central face, mainly the nose. So the perception of facial deformity and tolerance of deformity particularly with respect to the nose may differ between different cultures.[6]

In Western noses which in general are slimmer with a higher dorsum and have more projection, deviation of the nose creates very different profiles particularly in the three-quarter view often leading to the adoption of 'head tilt'—an adaptive mechanism whereby an individual often subconsciously presents the perceived least deformed side in pictures or face-to-face meetings.

These variations in perception may need to be accounted for in a patient's acceptance of improvement over perfection—something that is very difficult to achieve in deviated noses, that is, an improvement is possible, symmetry is not, especially from all the different angles. A straighter nose is possible on an asymmetric face.

In the history of preservation rhinoplasty, one of the reasons dorsal preservation may not have been adopted for deviated or crooked noses was the inability to correct a deformed or twisted bridge and for the need to correct a complex septal deformity. There may be several reasons why preservation techniques are now being reapplied to deviated noses. The first is the ability to accurately image by CT or cone-beam CT, the second is the ability to reshape and move nasal bones using the piezoelectric technology, and the third is a reappraisal of the management of the nasal septum in deviated noses, moving away finally from the 'L strut'. Fundamentally therefore, the ability to change the foundation of the nose (maxilla) or the roof (dorsal profile) safely and predictably means the preservation techniques can be applied to noses other than those that have existing pleasing dorsal aesthetic lines.

The basis of a straight nose is to have a central septum fixed to a midline nasal spine and equal sidewall slopes in terms of angulation, if not length. Creating more symmetric dorsal aesthetic lines but perhaps not symmetric lateral aesthetic lines is probably a realistic goal in correcting nasal deviations by preservation. Additional augmentation of one side of the maxilla is possible with diced cartilage or fat transfer.

THE SKIN ENVELOPE

Developmentally deviated noses invariably have differences in the size of the soft tissue envelope—not only skin but also the muscles and ligaments. The soft tissue envelope has an ability to adapt or contract there is often considerable difference in the healing response from a deception in the subperichondrial/periosteal plane compared with the sub-SMAS. Although it may be possible to preserve many of the ligaments in deviated noses, some may have to be modified. In particular, the position of insertion of the vertical scroll ligament on the short side of the deviated nose will be different with the repositioned nasal pyramid. Release of certain ligaments, for example, the pyriform ligament and adjacent upper lateral/nasal junction may be necessary to create length on the short side of the nose. When an overprojected deviated nose is reduced, however, there will be a relative excess of the envelope. If there is little need to adjust the profile, a straight nose that has axis deviation to one side may not need a soft tissue dissection over the upper laterals or nasal bones and shifting the pyramid to one side can readily correct minor axis deviations (**Fig. 2**).

In general, it is the author's preference to undertake a subperichondrial/periosteal dissection especially in the middle and upper third of the nose. Wide dissection down to the face of the maxilla is required for piezo sculpting. A limited dissection or sometimes no soft tissue elevation is required for simple rotation of the pyramid through a closed approach.

The Dorsum: Bony Pyramid/Bone Cap Cartilage Complex

CT scanning can be very helpful in determining, first, the slope angle of each nasal sidewall and second, the shape of the sidewall being straight convex or concave.

Straight bones that lean to one side lend themselves ideally to a preservation technique,

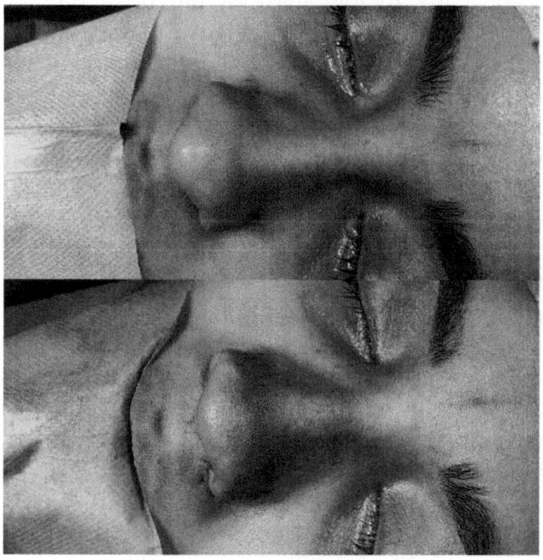

Fig. 2. Straightening an axis deviation without dorsal soft tissue elevation.

whereby the osteotomy on the more oblique bone is combined with an ostectomy in the nasomaxillary groove (**Fig. 3**A). A sagittal lateral osteotomy having removed Webster's triangle with elevation of the internal periosteum will create the space allowing the bony sidewall to slide down on the inner aspect of the piriform aperture. On the opposite more vertical nasal bone, a transverse cut is made without internal mucoperichondrial elevation allowing this side to be a hinge, as the oblique side impacts downward on the inner aspect of the piriform aperture. The transverse osteotomy between the lateral and the radix cuts may be performed percutaneously with a 2-mm chisel, with a powered instrument or hand saw. The radix cut is usually perpendicular to the nasal bone connecting the transverse cuts (**Fig. 3**B, C). An oblique radix cut may be used to create a rotational hinge of the dorsum, therefore preventing posteriorly displacement of the radix point.

If the dorsal aesthetic lines are already slim, this is a very effective way of treating a nasal dorsum that has purely axis deviation, combined with a reposition of the nasal septum to the midline affixing it to the spine with a secure suture through a drill hole (**Figs. 4 and 5**).

With increasing degrees of axis displacement, not only is there a discrepancy in the anterior/posteriorly length of the nasal bones but also in the length vertically of each nasal sidewall.

Without compensating for this, there is a limit to how far the whole dorsal unit can just be aligned by osteotomies. More severe asymmetries occurring in the middle third cartilaginous portion additional maneuvers may be necessary to lengthen one side compared with the other.

Partial release of the upper lateral/bony junction known as the lateral K area can gain the required length to achieve symmetry. The pyriform ligament is sectioned and released across the mucosal space of the nose. Sharp dissection of the upper lateral, nasal bone overlap parallel to the upper lateral cartilage and extending up to within 5 mm of the dorsum will allow the vertically short side to elongate minimizing the risk of redeviation. This will almost always be necessary in concert with repositioning of the quadrangular cartilage of the septum (**Fig. 6** A,B).

RHINOSCULPTING

Modifying the shape of asymmetric nasal bones has a limited value in achieving a straighter looking nose and depends on the thickness and shape of the bone. CT scanning is an important investigation in ascertaining the limits of rhinosculpting. Thicker convex bones can be thinned but not to

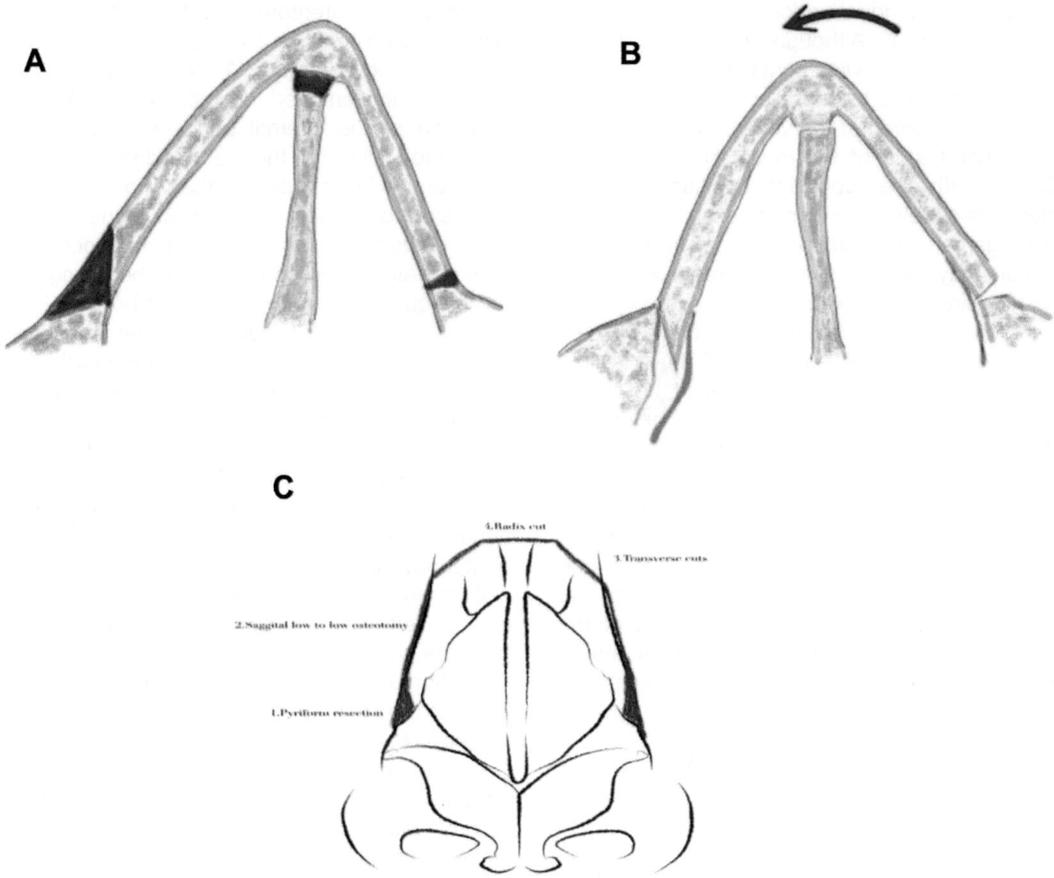

Fig. 3. Schematic for preservation osteotomies in a deviated nose.

the point where there is a risk of fracture. An alternative way to change the convexity of a nasal bony sidewall is to perform a series of criss-cross cuts using the fine piezo saw but not damaging the deep mucoperiosteum. This is analogous to a series of tiles on a flexible backing and will allow subtle convexity is to be flattened without performing longitudinal or transverse osteotomies using osteotomes. In the same degree, modification of the bony nasal can be performed by local rasping or contouring with powered instruments and this may be all that is necessary in a post-traumatic nose correction that involves the rhinion.

THE CARTILAGINOUS VAULT

Distortions in the cartilaginous vault are difficult to correct in dorsal preservation—marked twists in this area invariably need release of the upper laterals from the septum possibly with spreader graft or flap reconstruction.

Where the upper laterals are of a similar length but displaced along with the dorsal more caudal septum, the middle third of the nose can be controlled by a complete release of the septum via a low strip section from the vomer and release from the perpendicular plate of the ethmoid together with if necessary resection of a triangular piece of perpendicular plate under the nasal bones. This allows the septum and the cartilaginous vault as one unit to be rotated back to the midline. This may also be facilitated by removal of the bony cap, still preserving the whole cartilaginous dorsum intact (see **Fig. 5**).

A variation of preservation rhinoplasty called 'spare roof technique' allows the dorsal cartilage vault separation from the septum after removal of the bone cap.[7] By releasing the cartilaginous vault completely including a lateral K area dissection, the bony sidewalls can be treated by paramedian and lateral osteotomies to narrow the bony base. The cartilage roof is either pushed down or centralized and then reattached to an

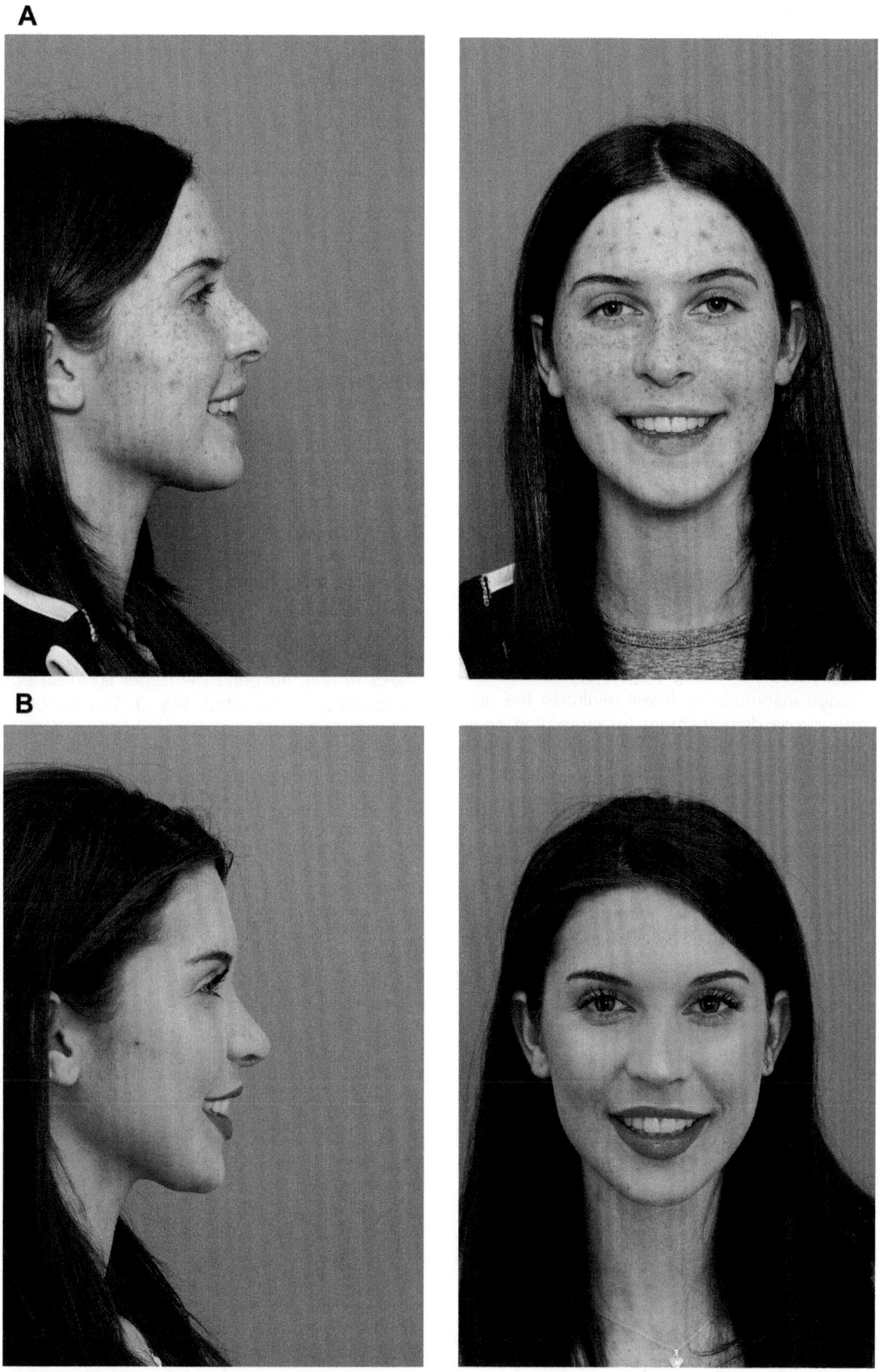

Fig. 4. (*A, B*) Low strip, dorsal preservation septorhinoplasty.

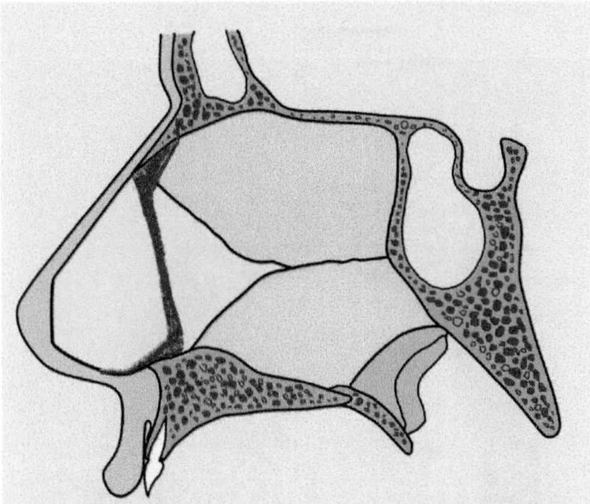

Fig. 5. The septal cuts for a low strip preservation rhinoplasty with deviation. The vertical cut is made at the maximum convexity of the rhinion and the caudal septum advanced and sutured to the spine moving the whole axis to the midline.

independently repaired septum by suturing. This almost certainly requires an open approach, as there is frequently a widening effect in the middle third which will need suture control ideally with a criss-cross technique to achieve the correct contour. It must be inserted behind the W point to avoid valvular narrowing (**Fig. 7**). This has an advantage insomuch as it will minimize the risk of further axis displacement by overriding segments of the neodorsum on an underlying unfavorable high septal deformity and overcomes the limitations of high strip excision in preservation rhinoplasty where extensive septal surgery is required—an extracorporeal septal reconstruction is possible before replanting and fixation at the nasal spine and to the upper lateral 'roof' (**Fig. 8** reproduced by permission M GF).

SOFT TISSUE LIGAMENT REPAIR

The reliance on the support of the soft tissue ligaments, for example, scroll ligament the deep and superficial medial SMAS after rhinoplasty for a deviated nose is still unclear.[8] It is the authors' experience that in correcting some deviated noses, it has been preferable to excise the sesamoid cartilages in the scroll and not reattach the ligament particularly on the shorter side. First, the discrepancy in the skin envelope may recreate a deformity and second, the scroll cartilages may displace cranially producing an unfavorable supratip bulge which can need to be excised endonasally in a minor revision procedure. Where a caudal septal reconstruction with an extension graft or strut is used to support the nasal tip, there is little point in re-establishing the deep medial SMAS. However, refixation of the dorsal perichondrium/periosteal flap by fixation to the anterior septal angle and repair of the superficial medial SMAS to help suspend the upper lip in an open approach are advocated. **Fig. 9**. The periosteal/perichondrial flap tensioning is analogous to plicating or tightening the SMAS in a facelift and has a considerable effect in helping the soft tissue envelope redrape as well as closing dead spaces.

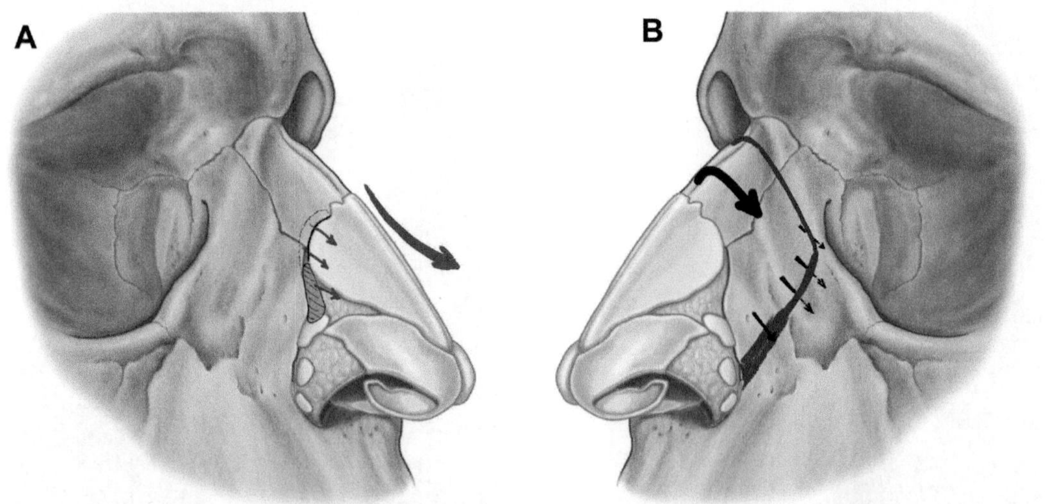

Fig. 6. (*A*) Section of the pyriform ligament (cross hatched) and separation of the lateral keystone will allow a rotational lengthening of a short middle third. (*B*) Rotation of the whole dorsum impacting the longer wall inside the pyriform aperture.

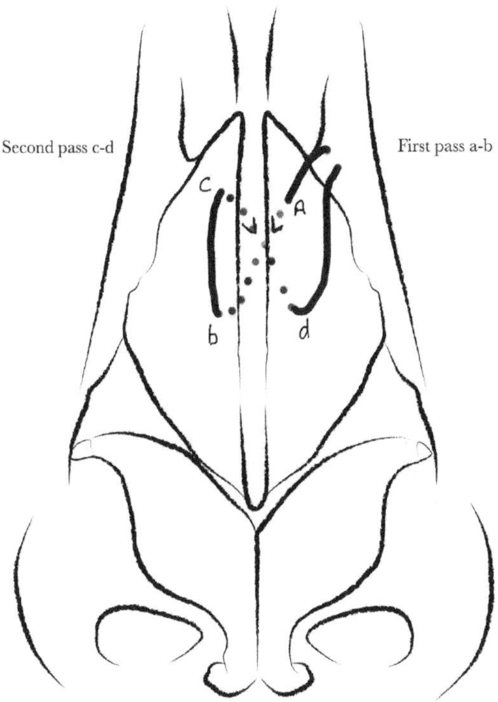

Fig. 7. Criss-cross suture fixation.

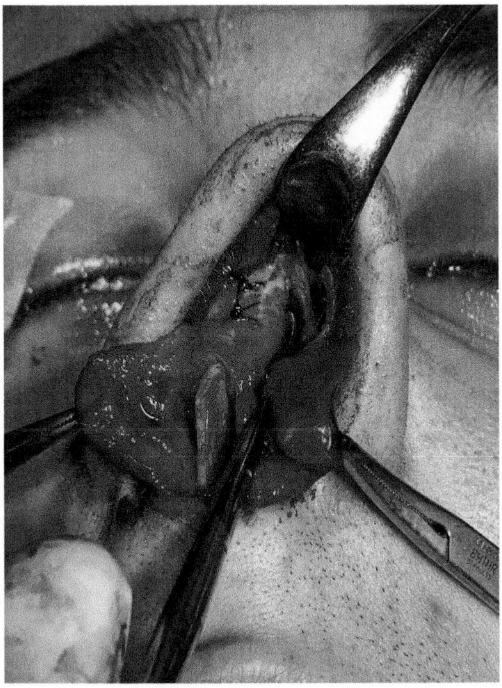

Fig. 8. Fixation of the cartilage vault to the lowered septum. Note the lateral K release to allow flattening of the rhinion. The bone cap has been removed creating a near complete cartilaginous dorsum.

THE NASAL TIP

Developmentally deviated noses will invariably have a degree of asymmetry in the nasal base in a vertical or an anteroposterior plane. There may be pre-existing nostril asymmetry and a need for differential alar base reduction. In principle, the more vertical side of the nasal tip will need to be lengthened to allow the dome to be approximated in the midline with its opposite number. A form of lateral crural steal on one side or release at the junction of the A—A1 cartilage supported with a lateral crural strut graft or rim graft may be required. The use of a lateral crural strut together with sectioning of the levator labii alaeque nasi muscle can lower high insertion of the alar on to the cheek skin. In all these instances, there is a departure from pure preservation rhinoplasty and in general a form of hybrid operation is invariably performed but with the principles of suturing and reorientation with minimum cartilage resection.

The use of a septal extension graft attached to the midline septum is an excellent anchor point for creating tip symmetry, and although there is a tendency to stiffness in the nasal tip, this is preferable to recurrence of deviation. Release of the nasal tip from the muscles around the piriform aperture may be required together with augmentation of the premaxilla under the alar using free segments of cartilage or diced cartilage injected via an incision in the floor of the nasal vestibule in a similar fashion to augmenting a depressed alar sidewall in a cleft nose.

Otherwise the principles of preservation by minimum cephalic resection, lateral crural underlay techniques, dome suturing and lateral crural flare sutures are used to build a symmetric tip on a stable midline medial crural column.

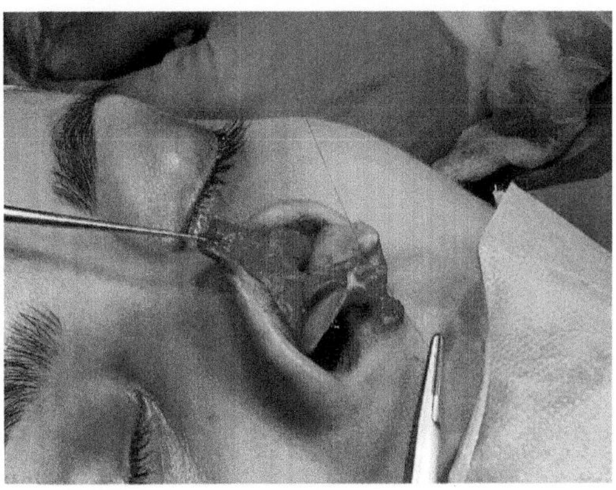

Fig. 9. Retensioning the deep soft tissues to close a dead space.

SUMMARY

Although it is clear that the most deviated or twisted noses will require a reconstructive approach to septorhinoplasty, the principle of deep dissection in a subperichondrial periosteal plane in the upper two-thirds and the realigning of a mild axis deviated nose via transverse lateral and radix osteotomies are all achievable goals following the goals in preservation techniques.[9] Therefore, apart from simple axis deviation of the nose with good aesthetic lines, corrections of deviated noses tend to need a hybrid approach often with minor grafting.

CLINIC CARE POINTS

- Ostectomy and saggital osteotomies allow impaction techniques in preservation rhinoplasty.
- Lateral K release permits lengthening of a short midvault and permits flexion of the central K area.
- Fixation of the quadrangular cartilage on the centralised nasal spine is key to stability.

DISCLOSURES

None.

REFERENCES

1. Goodale JL. The correction of old lateral displacements of the nasal bones. Boston Med Surg J 1901;20:538–9.
2. Ellis D, Gilbert R. Analysis and correction of the crooked nose. J Otolaryngol 1991;20(1):14–8.
3. Preservation Rhinoplasty, 2019 Saban Y, Cackir B,Daniel R, Palhazi P. ISBN 978-605-5322-49-6.
4. Kosins A, Daniel RK, Nguyen DP. Rhinoplasty: The asymmetric deviated nose-an overview. Facial Plast Surg 2016;32(4):361–73.
5. Daniel R, Palhazi P. Rhinoplasty. An anatomical and clinical Atlas. Springer; 2018.
6. Blais C, Jack R, Christoph S, et al. Culture shapes how we look at faces. PLoS Journal, San Francisco 2008;3(8):e3022.
7. Ferreira MG, Monteiro D, Reis C, et al. spare roof technique: middle third new technique. Facial Plast Surg 2016;32(1):111–6.
8. Palhazi P, Daniel R, Kosins A. The osseocartilagenous vault: anatomy and surgical observations. Aesthet Surg J 2015;35(3):242–51.
9. Cakir B, Ali Riza O, Teoman D, et al. A complete subperichondrial dissection technique for rhinoplasty with management of the nasal ligaments. Aesthet Surg J 2012;32(5):564–74.

Modified Skoog Method for Hump Reduction

Jennifer C. Fuller, MD[a], Peter A. Hilger, MD[b,*]

KEYWORDS

• Rhinoplasty • Skoog • Dorsum • Dorsal hump

KEY POINTS

- The evolution of dorsal hump reduction has been toward that of preservation and use of grafts that resist the contractive forces of healing.
- The modified Skoog technique uses a modified composite dorsal segment as an onlay spreader graft to maximize aesthetic and functional outcomes.
- The modified Skoog technique is ideal for patients with short nasal bones, a predominantly cartilaginous dorsal hump, normal to narrow nasal width, and thin skin.

INTRODUCTION

Nasal hump reduction is a key component of rhinoplasty. Western ideals of nasal aesthetics emphasize a straight dorsal profile, thin nasal dorsum, and smooth dorsal lines.

In the past decades, aesthetic surgery has seen great emphasis, by surgeons and patients alike, on minimally invasive procedures that use less tissue resection, anatomic preservation, and tissue repositioning to create a more natural, flattering change with less risk of revision surgery.

There has been a trend toward preservation, reshaping, and realignment rather than reduction and removal.[1] Rather than mere reduction, the importance of adding structural grafts to create definition and resist the contractive forces of healing to preserve normal nasal function while also controlling aesthetic outcomes has gained esteem. In the area of rhinoplasty, this technique has been referred to as preservation rhinoplasty.[1] We embrace these concepts whenever possible and the approach to nasal hump reduction has followed suit. Herein, we discuss the evolution of dorsal modification and focus on a preservation technique, the modified Skoog method.

THE EVOLUTION OF NASAL HUMP REDUCTION

Composite Resection

The classic technique for nasal hump reduction was first introduced by Joseph in 1931.[2] This procedure involves an en bloc resection of the dorsal hump. A scalpel is used to cut through the cartilaginous dorsal septum and upper lateral cartilages, and an osteotome is used to resect the bony dorsum. The resected hump is discarded and lateral osteotomies are used to medialize the bony side walls and close the open roof deformity. Although effective for hump reduction, this method can be wrought with adverse sequelae including uneven resection of the dorsum, inadvertent over-resection, destabilization of the keystone area, creation of dorsal irregularities, excessive dorsal narrowing, and midvault collapse, resulting in both an unnatural appearance and poor nasal function.

Push-Down Technique

In response, Cottle[3] introduced his push down technique in 1954, aimed at reducing the dorsal profile while preserving the nasal dorsum and

[a] Department of Otolaryngology- Head and Neck Surgery, Division of Facial Plastic and Reconstructive Surgery, Loma Linda University, 11234 Anderson Street, Room 2586A, Loma Linda, CA 92354, USA; [b] Department of Otolaryngology-Head and Neck Surgery, Division of Facial and Plastic and Reconstructive Surgery, University of Minnesota, 7373 France Avenue South, Suite 410, Edina, MN 55435, USA
* Corresponding author.
E-mail address: hilge006@umn.edu

Facial Plast Surg Clin N Am 29 (2021) 131–139
https://doi.org/10.1016/j.fsc.2020.09.008

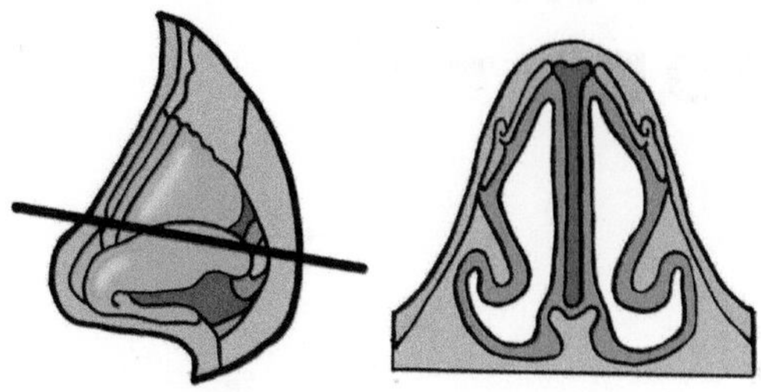

Fig. 1. Internal nasal valve. The internal nasal valve in cross-section (*right*) is bound by the septum, upper lateral cartilages, head of the inferior turbinate, and nasal floor.

midvault. In this technique, lateral osteotomies are performed and an inferior strip of the septum is removed, allowing for mobilization of the entire bony and cartilaginous nasal pyramid. The nasal pyramid is then pushed down into the piriform aperture, reducing the dorsal profile. Although this technique did not disturb the native dorsum or midvault, the amount of reduction was limited and it did not gain widespread popularity in the United States.

The Skoog Technique

In 1966, Skoog[4] introduced an alternative method for dorsal hump reduction that similarly aimed to preserve the nasal dorsum and midvault. In this method, an en bloc resection of the cartilaginous and bony dorsum is performed in the same manner as that described by Joseph. The mucosa is then removed from the undersurface of the resected composite dorsum. The lateral walls of the hump are shaped, leaving the dorsum with the desired width. The bony and cartilaginous septum are then removed from the undersurface with a Ronguer, allowing the angle between the bone and cartilage to flatten. The remaining flattened dorsum is then replaced over the dorsum as a free graft. Although this technique minimized dorsal irregularities, the upper lateral cartilages were not resuspended, and nasal function continued to suffer.

Understanding the Internal Nasal Valve

Although first described by Mink[5] in 1903, the importance of maintaining the internal nasal valves for proper nasal function was not fully understood until more recently. This new appreciation further impacted the evolution of dorsal hump reduction and created a greater emphasis on preserving the middle vault to achieve not only excellent aesthetic results but functional outcomes as well.

The internal nasal valve, bound by the septum, upper lateral cartilage, head of the inferior turbinate, and nasal floor, is the narrowest portion of the nasal airway (**Fig. 1**). As such, it regulates upper airway resistance and thus nasal airflow. In accordance with Poiseuille's law, resistance is inversely proportional to the radius of cross-sectional area to the fourth power. Thus, small changes in internal nasal valve area can have profound changes on resistance. This was confirmed by Roithmann and colleagues[6] through the use of acoustic rhinometry and rhinomanometry. Furthermore, as the cross-sectional area of the valve decreases, a greater negative pressure is generated within the nasal cavity during inspiration owing to the Bernoulli effect. This pressure in turn can result in a dynamic collapse of the nasal sidewall, depending on the strength of the cartilaginous framework and nasal musculature resisting this pressure. Reduction rhinoplasty was found to be

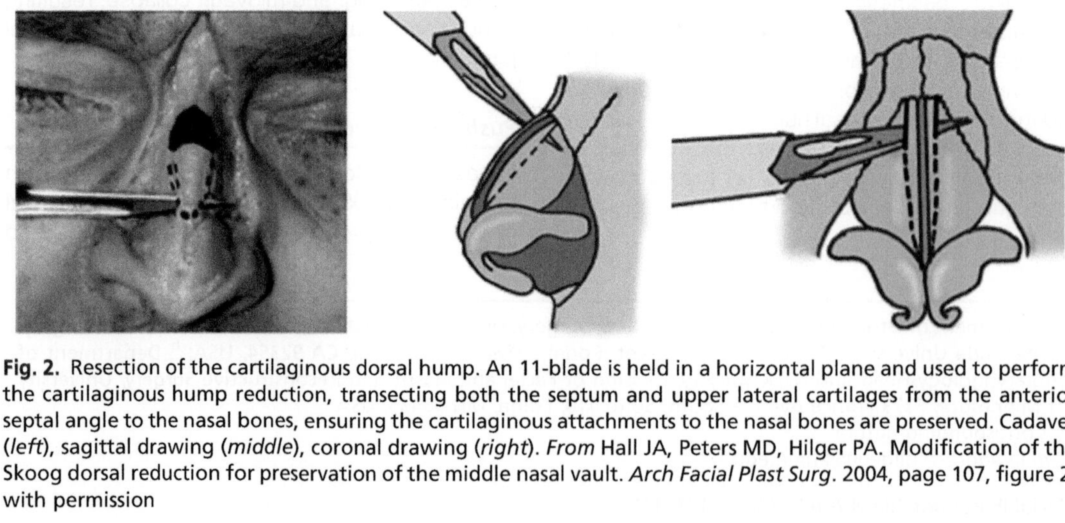

Fig. 2. Resection of the cartilaginous dorsal hump. An 11-blade is held in a horizontal plane and used to perform the cartilaginous hump reduction, transecting both the septum and upper lateral cartilages from the anterior septal angle to the nasal bones, ensuring the cartilaginous attachments to the nasal bones are preserved. Cadaver (*left*), sagittal drawing (*middle*), coronal drawing (*right*). *From* Hall JA, Peters MD, Hilger PA. Modification of the Skoog dorsal reduction for preservation of the middle nasal vault. *Arch Facial Plast Surg*. 2004, page 107, figure 2; with permission

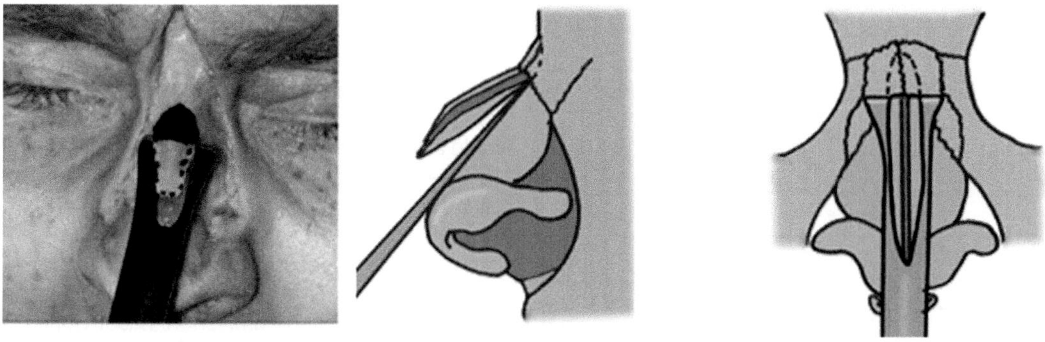

Fig. 3. Resection of the bony dorsal hump. A 10-mm Rubin osteotome is inserted under the cartilaginous segment and the bony dorsum is removed in the desired plane. Cadaver (*left*), sagittal drawing (*middle*), coronal drawing (*right*). *From* Hall JA, Peters MD, Hilger PA. Modification of the Skoog dorsal reduction for preservation of the middle nasal vault. *Arch Facial Plast Surg*. 2004; page 107, figure 3; with permission

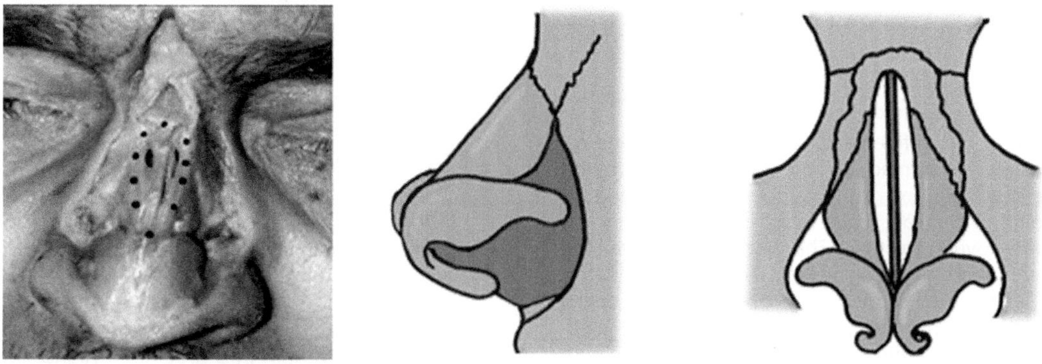

Fig. 4. Nose after removal of composite osseocartilaginous dorsal segment. Cadaver (*left*), sagittal drawing (*middle*), coronal drawing (*right*). *From* Hall JA, Peters MD, Hilger PA. Modification of the Skoog dorsal reduction for preservation of the middle nasal vault. *Arch Facial Plast Surg*. 2004; page 108, figure 4; with permission

the second most common cause of internal nasal valve obstruction, second only to trauma,[7] and a study by Grymer and colleagues demonstrated an average 22% decrease in the cross-sectional area at the internal nasal valve by acoustic rhinometry 6 months after standard reduction rhinoplasty.[8]

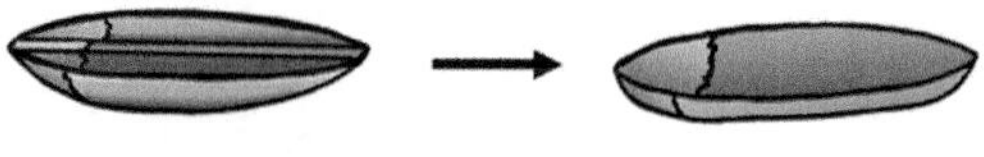

Fig. 5. Modification of the composite osseocartilaginous dorsal segment. The bony and cartilaginous septal remnants are removed from the ventral surface of the dorsal segment. This allows flattening of the segment at the bony–cartilaginous junction and prevents displacement of the dorsal segment off of midline once it is replaced. Premodification (*left*) and postmodification (*right*). *From* Hall JA, Peters MD, Hilger PA. Modification of the Skoog dorsal reduction for preservation of the middle nasal vault. *Arch Facial Plast Surg*. 2004; page 108, figure 5; with permission.

Midvault Grafts

With this new understanding in mind, a number of techniques were introduced to reconstruct the middle vault and internal nasal valves after dorsal hump reduction. In 1984, Sheen[9] introduced spreader grafts to reconstruct the middle vault. Spreader grafts have gained widespread popularity and have been shown to improve nasal airflow.[9–12] In 1999, Alsarraf and Murakami[13] described onlay spreader grafts from septal or conchal cartilage, and more recently, in 2004, the concept of a component dorsal hump resection in which the upper lateral cartilages are released from the septum before hump takedown and then used as autospreader grafts was introduced.[14–17] These advances have greatly advanced the reconstruction of the middle vault and patency of the internal nasal valves, resulting

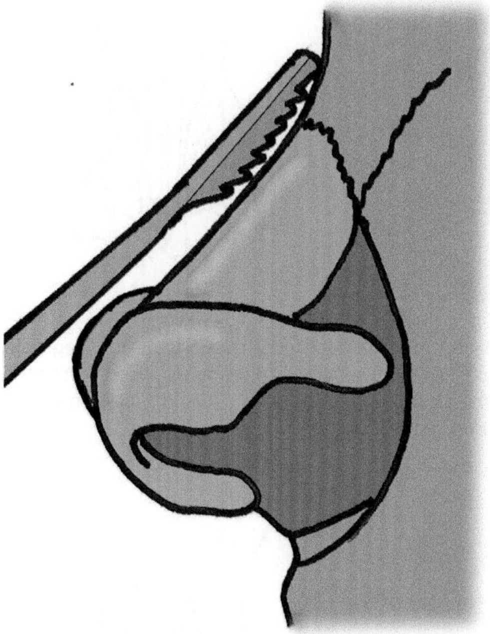

Fig. 6. Dorsal refinement. Further dorsal modifications are performed on the nose gradually with repeated replacement of the dorsal segment and redraping of the soft tissue to assess the changes and prevent over resection. The bony dorsum can be reduced with a rasp as needed. *From* Hall JA, Peters MD, Hilger PA. Modification of the Skoog dorsal reduction for preservation of the middle nasal vault. *Arch Facial Plast Surg*. 2004; page 108, figure 5; with permission.

in improved aesthetic and functional outcomes following dorsal hump reduction; however, they still have the heightened risk of creating dorsal irregularities, particularly in patients with thin skin.

THE MODIFIED SKOOG TECHNIQUE

With both function and aesthetics in mind, the modified Skoog technique was introduced in 2004 as a method of dorsal hump reduction that would allow for the preservation of the middle vault and internal nasal valves while also maintaining a natural, smooth contour of the nasal dorsum, and potentially obviating the need for lateral osteotomies.[18] Ideal candidates for this procedure are patients with an overprojected nasal dorsum, long cartilaginous dorsum, short nasal bones, a normal to narrow bony base, and thin skin.

This technique is performed in the following steps.

1. A standard open septorhinoplasty approach through transcolumellar and marginal incisions is used.
2. The soft tissue envelope is elevated in the standard supraperichondrial, subperiosteal fashion.
3. The anterior septal angle is exposed and bilateral mucoperichondrial flaps are elevated from the septum.
4. The mucosal attachments of the medial aspect of the upper lateral cartilages and nasal bones are released. (Note: this modification was first introduced by Regnault and Alfaro in 1980.[19])
5. Any necessary nasal tip work is performed
6. An 11-blade is held in a horizontal plane and used to perform the cartilaginous hump reduction, transecting both the septum and upper lateral cartilages from the anterior septal angle to the nasal bones, ensuring the cartilaginous attachments to the nasal bones are preserved (**Fig. 2**).

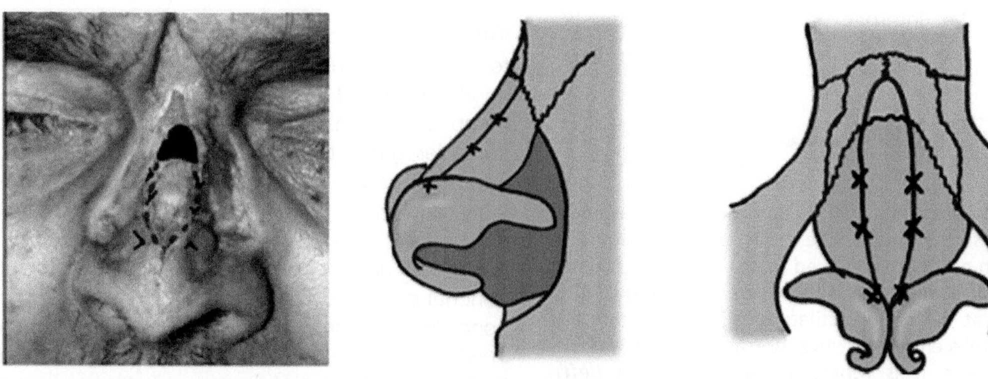

Fig. 7. Replacement and fixation of the composite dorsal segment. Once the desired modifications have been made, the dorsal segment is replaced, and the upper lateral cartilages are resuspended to the graft with 5-0 polydioxanone suture fixation with a minimum of 2 sutures placed on each side. Cadaver (*left*), sagittal drawing (*middle*), coronal drawing (*right*). *From* Hall JA, Peters MD, Hilger PA. Modification of the Skoog dorsal reduction for preservation of the middle nasal vault. *Arch Facial Plast Surg*. 2004; page 108, figure 5; with permission.

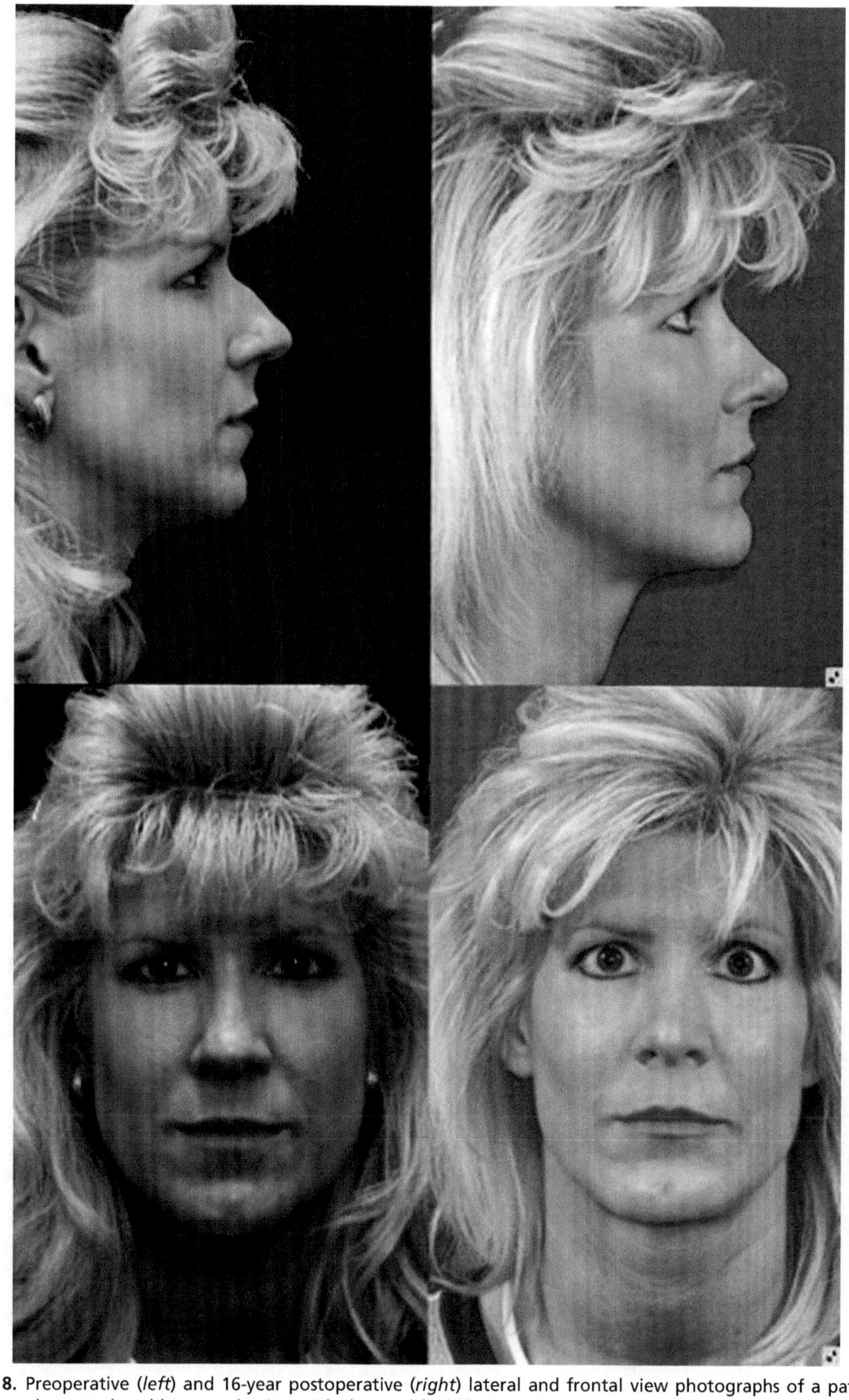

Fig. 8. Preoperative (*left*) and 16-year postoperative (*right*) lateral and frontal view photographs of a patient who underwent dorsal hump reduction with the modified Skoog technique.

7. A 10-mm Rubin osteotome is inserted under the cartilaginous segment and the bony dorsum is removed in the desired plane (**Figs. 3** and **4**).
8. The composite osseocartilaginous dorsal segment is removed and modified on the back table (**Fig. 5**).
   a. The bony and cartilaginous septal remnants are removed from the ventral surface of the dorsal segment. This allows flattening of the segment at the bony–cartilaginous junction and prevents displacement of the dorsal segment off of midline once it is replaced.
9. Further dorsal modifications are performed on the nose gradually with repeated replacement of the dorsal segment and redraping of the soft tissue to assess the changes and prevent over-resection.
   a. The bony dorsum is further reduced with a rasp as needed (**Fig. 6**).

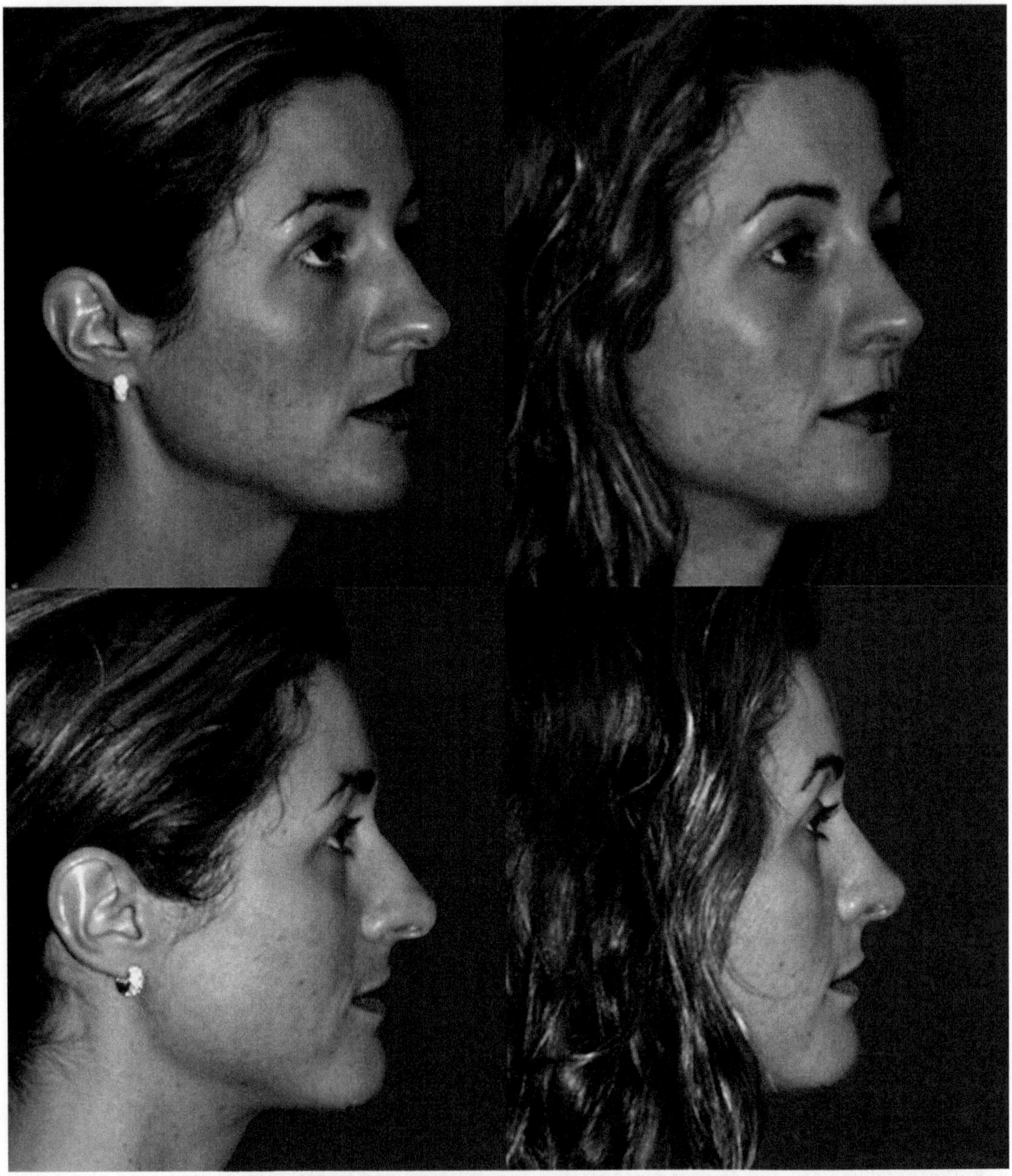

Fig. 9. Preoperative (*left*) and postoperative (*right*) lateral and oblique view photographs of a patient who underwent dorsal hump reduction with the modified Skoog technique.

b. The cartilaginous dorsum and dorsal edges of the upper lateral cartilages are further resected as needed to accommodate replacement of the dorsal segment and achieve the desired hump reduction.

10. Once the desired modifications have been made, the dorsal segment is replaced and the upper lateral cartilages are resuspended to the graft with 5-0 polydioxanone suture fixation with a minimum of 2 sutures placed on each side (**Fig. 7**).

11. The segment is secured caudally to the anterior septal angle or to the cephalic edges of the lower lateral cartilages.

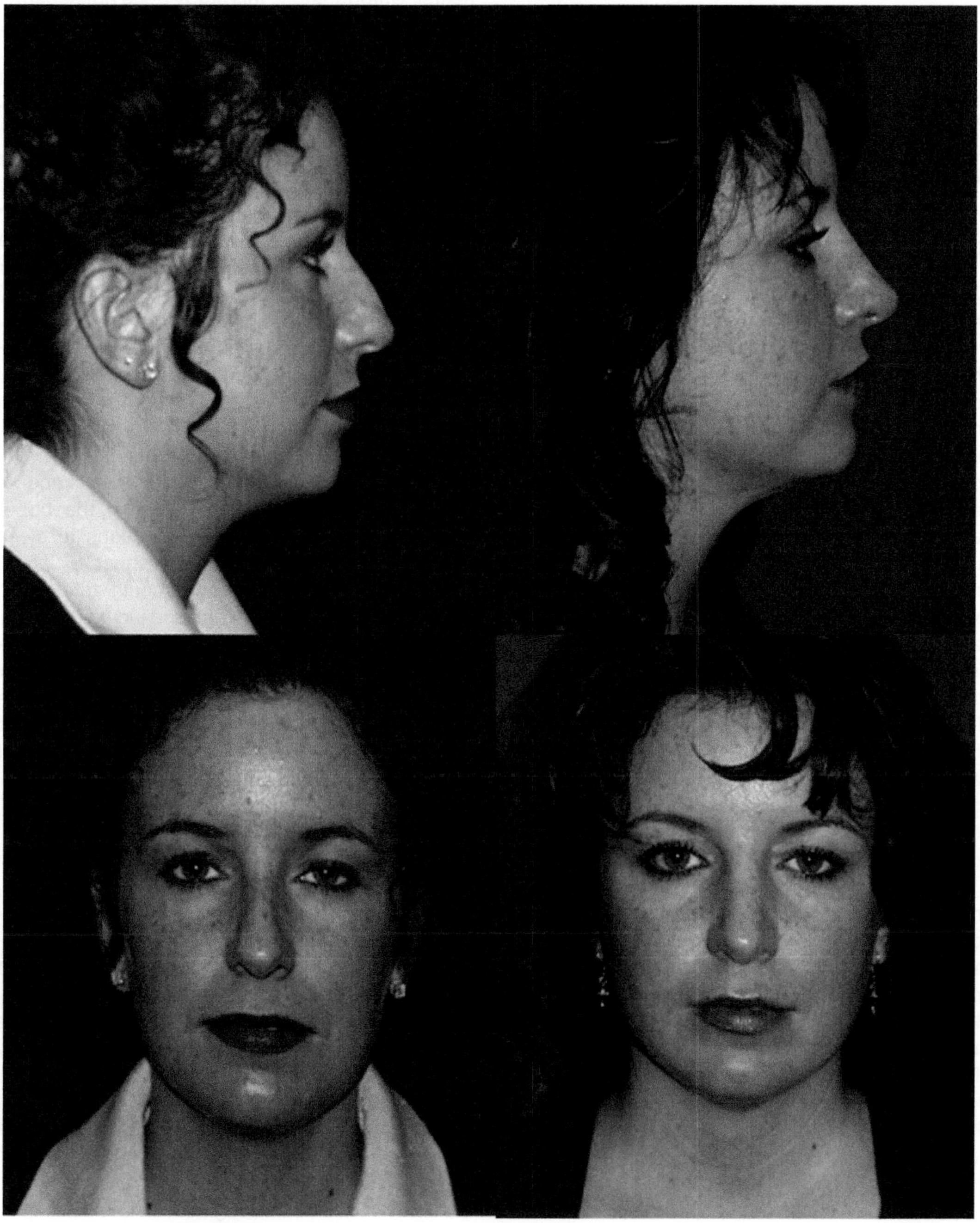

Fig. 10. Preoperative (*left*) and postoperative (*right*) lateral and frontal view photographs of a patient who underwent dorsal hump reduction with the modified Skoog technique.

12. The skin is redraped, the nose is closed, and SteriStrips and a rigid splint are applied and left in place for 1 week.

In this modified Skoog technique, the modified dorsal segment acts as a dorsal onlay spreader, reestablishing the middle vault width and preserving the internal nasal valves. The natural dorsal contour is also preserved. The dorsal segment functions to correct the open roof deformity, thus obviating the need for lateral osteotomies and preventing over narrowing of the nose. In addition, the dorsal segment is one smooth segment, preventing dorsal irregularities that could otherwise be seen in the thin-skinned patient. **Figs. 8–10** demonstrate patients who underwent the modified Skoog technique of dorsal hump reduction.

SUMMARY AND DISCUSSION

Although dorsal hump reduction has long been a primary goal of rhinoplasty, the methods through which it is accomplished have evolved over time. Throughout its history, many techniques have been introduced to address the ever-challenging goal of achieving both aesthetically and functionally superb outcomes. From simple reduction rhinoplasty to the present day understanding of the need to preserve the middle vault and internal nasal valves for improved aesthetic and functional outcomes, the evolution has been toward that of preservation and the addition of structural grafts to resist the contractive forces of healing. Unfortunately, the addition of various grafts may lead to visible dorsal irregularities, particularly in patients with thin skin. The modified Skoog technique aims to accomplish dorsal hump reduction while preserving the middle vault, maintaining internal nasal valve patency, and creating smooth dorsal lines, all while minimizing the risk of generating dorsal irregularities and an overly narrowed dorsum.

Hall and colleagues[18] studied 22 patients who underwent a modified Skoog dorsal hump reduction and had at least 9 months of follow-up. In this cohort, there was 1 complication, a visible ridge at the lateral aspect of the dorsal segment at the junction with the upper lateral cartilage that required an endonasal revision with shaving of the ridge through an intercartilaginous incision. No patients experienced nasal obstruction and all patients had adequate reduction without malpositioning or resorption of the dorsal segment, and all had normal nasal width and natural appearing dorsal aesthetic lines. The lack of resorption found is consistent with a study by Lejour and colleagues[20] that looked at resorption of the reinserted dorsal segment in patients who underwent a standard Skoog dorsal hump reduction. The study found no evidence of dorsal segment resorption in any of the included 29 patients by radiographic evaluation.[20]

In 2011, Niechajev and colleagues[21] presented a study of 44 patients who underwent either a Skoog or modified Skoog nasal hump reduction via a predominantly endonasal approach (40 patients). Unfortunately, this study does not separate outcomes based on technique used. However, the study found overall favorable results with no resorption of the dorsal segment. It did find that very thin, plate-like dorsal segment grafts sometimes resulted in visible edges in patients with thin skin. This necessitated secondary shaving or filing in 4 patients. In response, it was concluded the technique was best used in patients with high dorsal convexities. In addition, this technique was found to be useful in cases of accidental over resection as the dorsum could be more judiciously reduced and replaced.

The modified Skoog technique is ideal for patients with a predominantly cartilaginous dorsal hump, short nasal bones, thin skin, a normal to narrow nasal width, and minimal dorsal deviation. The modified dorsal segment acts as an onlay spreader graft to preserve the middle vault and internal nasal valves by resuspending the upper lateral cartilages to it. It also functions to close the open roof deformity without the need for lateral osteotomies and nasal bone medialization and narrowing. It allows for careful and judicious dorsal hump reduction, decreasing the risk of over resection. Finally, it creates a smooth dorsal contour from the radix to the anterior septal angle. The modified Skoog technique is an excellent method of nasal hump reduction in select patients that maximizes aesthetic and functional outcomes.

CLINICAL CARE POINTS

- Dorsal contour correction is a common objective in rhinoplasty. Preservation or enhancement of the internal nasal valve is important in nasal physiology.
- Creating a smooth dorsal line with adequate midvault width is a challenge in rhinoplasty particularly for the patient with thin skin, a narrow vault or narrow bony base. Traditional spreader grafts or onlay spreader grafts have been utilized to address these challenges.
- The modified Skoog technique achieves several objectives: preservation of midvault width, and airway, and preservation of the

natural interface between the nasal frame and soft tissue envelope.

- This technique achieves many of the goals of the revitalized "preservation rhinoplasty" concept but utilizes many of the technical steps in rhinoplasty with which most surgeons are familiar as compared to developing competence in the let down or push down techniques.

DISCLOSURE

The authors have nothing to disclose.

REFERENCES

1. Patel PN, Abdelwahab M, Most SP. A review and modification of dorsal preservation rhinoplasty techniques. Facial Plast Surg Aesthet Med 2020. https://doi.org/10.1089/fpsam.2020.0017.
2. Joseph J. Nasenplastik und sonstige Gesichtsplastik, nebst einem Anhang über Mammaplastik und einige weitere Operationen aus dem Gebiete der ausseren Körperplastik. By Prof. Dr. J. Joseph (Berlin). Imperial 8vo. Pp. 843 + xxxi, with 1718 illustrations, many in colo. Br J Surg 1931. https://doi.org/10.1002/bjs.1800197416.
3. Cottle MH. Nasal roof repair and hump removal. AMA Arch Otolaryngol 1954. https://doi.org/10.1001/archotol.1954.00720010420002.
4. Skoog T. A method of hump reduction in rhinoplasty: a technique for preservation of the nasal roof. Arch Otolaryngol 1966. https://doi.org/10.1001/archotol.1966.00760020285020.
5. Mink J. Le nez comme voie respiratory. Belgium: Press Otolaryngol; 1903. p. 481–96.
6. Roithmann R, Cole P, Chapnik J, et al. Acoustic rhinometry, rhinomanometry, and the sensation of nasal patency: a correlative study. J Otolaryngol 1994; 23(6):454–8.
7. Kasperbauer JL, Kern EB. Nasal valve physiology. Implications in nasal surgery. Otolaryngol Clin North Am 1987;20(4):699–719.
8. Grymer LF. Reduction rhinoplasty and nasal patency: change in the cross-sectional area of the nose evaluated by acoustic rhinometry. Laryngoscope 1995. https://doi.org/10.1288/00005537-199504000-00017.
9. Sheen JH. Spreader graft: a method of reconstructing the roof of the middle nasal vault following rhinoplasty. Plast Reconstr Surg 1984. https://doi.org/10.1097/00006534-198402000-00013.
10. Fuller JC, Gadkaree SK, Levesque PA, et al. Peak nasal inspiratory flow is a useful measure of nasal airflow in functional septorhinoplasty. Laryngoscope 2019. https://doi.org/10.1002/lary.27566.
11. Fuller JC, Levesque PA, Lindsay RW. Analysis of patient-perceived nasal appearance evaluations following functional septorhinoplasty with spreader graft placement. JAMA Facial Plast Surg 2019. https://doi.org/10.1001/jamafacial.2018.2118.
12. Constantinides MS, Adamson PA, Cole P. The long-term effects of open cosmetic septorhinoplasty on nasal air flow. Arch Otolaryngol Head Neck Surg 1996. https://doi.org/10.1001/archotol.1996.01890130035005.
13. Alsarraf R, Murakami C. The saddle nose deformity. Facial Plast Surg Clin North Am 1999;7:303–10.
14. Barrett DM, Casanueva F, Wang T. Understanding approaches to the dorsal hump. Facial Plast Surg 2017. https://doi.org/10.1055/s-0037-1598033.
15. Rohrich RJ, Muzaffar AR, Janis JE. Component dorsal hump reduction: the importance of maintaining dorsal aesthetic lines in rhinoplasty. Plast Reconstr Surg 2004. https://doi.org/10.1097/01.PRS.0000135861.45986.CF.
16. Gruber RP, Park E, Newman J, et al. The spreader flap in primary rhinoplasty. Plast Reconstr Surg 2007. https://doi.org/10.1097/01.prs.0000259198.42852.d4.
17. Yoo S, Most SP. Nasal airway preservation using the autospreader technique: analysis of outcomes using a disease-Specific quality-of-life instrument. Arch Facial Plast Surg 2011. https://doi.org/10.1001/archfacial.2011.7.
18. Hall JA, Peters MD, Hilger PA. Modification of the Skoog dorsal reduction for preservation of the middle nasal vault. Arch Facial Plast Surg 2004. https://doi.org/10.1001/archfaci.6.2.105.
19. Regnault P, Alfaro A. The Skoog rhinoplasty: a modified technique. Plast Reconstr Surg 1980. https://doi.org/10.1097/00006534-198010000-00013.
20. Lejour M, Duchateau J, Potaznik A. Routine reinsertion of the hump in rhinoplasty. Scand J Plast Reconstr Surg Hand Surg 1986. https://doi.org/10.3109/02844318609006293.
21. Niechajev I. Skoog rhinoplasty revisited. Aesthetic Plast Surg 2011. https://doi.org/10.1007/s00266-011-9692-1.

Dorsal Preservation Rhinoplasty

Measures to Prevent Suboptimal Outcomes

Dean M. Toriumi, MD[a,*], Milos Kovacevic, MD[b]

KEYWORDS

• Preservation rhinoplasty • Dorsal preservation • Rhinoplasty

KEY POINTS

- Preservation rhinoplasty is making a resurgence as a reliable method of performing primary rhinoplasty.
- Various septal approaches exist.
- Patient selection and careful execution are paramount.

INTRODUCTION

Preservation rhinoplasty has reemerged as a popular option for managing the dorsum and is changing the manner in which rhinoplasty is performed. It is apparent that the trend is toward preservation of structure to provide a natural and long-lasting outcome.[1–3] There are many components of preservation rhinoplasty, including dorsal preservation and subperichondrial dissection with preservation of the ligaments in the nose. The primary concept of dorsal preservation is to avoid creating the open-roof deformity that is seen with classic hump reduction and to preserve favorable dorsal contours.[1,2] By using the push-down or let-down technique, there is no need to reconstruct the middle nasal vault with spreader grafts or spreader flaps and potentially create irregularity with dorsal hump reduction. Clinicians who argue in favor of dorsal preservation point to the complications, extra time, or additional effort required to reconstruct or the additional cartilage needed to reconstruct the middle vault. These points are all valid but the significance of these issues varies from surgeon to surgeon. Less experienced surgeons may have difficulty taking down a dorsal hump with a Rubin osteotome. In addition, the same less experienced surgeons may have difficulty reconstructing the middle nasal vault with spreader grafts. In contrast, experienced surgeons are very comfortable taking down a dorsal hump with a rasp or osteotome or reconstructing the middle nasal vault with spreader grafts or spreader flaps. The less experienced surgeons who perform the push-down or let-down can have complications such as saddle nose, asymmetries of the bony pyramid, cerebrospinal fluid (CSF) leak, radix step-off, or hump recurrence. Dorsal preservation is not free of potential complications. This article discusses measures that can be taken to try to avoid some of the potential complications associated with dorsal preservation techniques.

PREOPERATIVE ANALYSIS

Analysis of whether dorsal hump reduction is even necessary is the first step in treating the profile. If the patient has a low radix and underprojected nasal tip (pseudohump), it is more beneficial to raise the radix, increase tip projection, and limit the amount of dorsal hump reduction (**Fig. 1**). This approach is particularly helpful in patients who have thicker skin or are wide on frontal view. By leaving the nose more projected with a higher dorsum, the nose will look narrower on frontal view.[4] If this approach is taken, the surgeon

[a] Department of Otolaryngology–Head and Neck Surgery, Rush University Medical School, 60 East Delaware Pl, Suite 1425, Chicago, Illinois 60611, USA; [b] Private Practice, Gerhofstrasse 2, 20354 Hamburg, Germany
* Corresponding author.
E-mail address: deantoriumi@toriumimd.com

Facial Plast Surg Clin N Am 29 (2021) 141–153
https://doi.org/10.1016/j.fsc.2020.09.009
1064-7406/21/

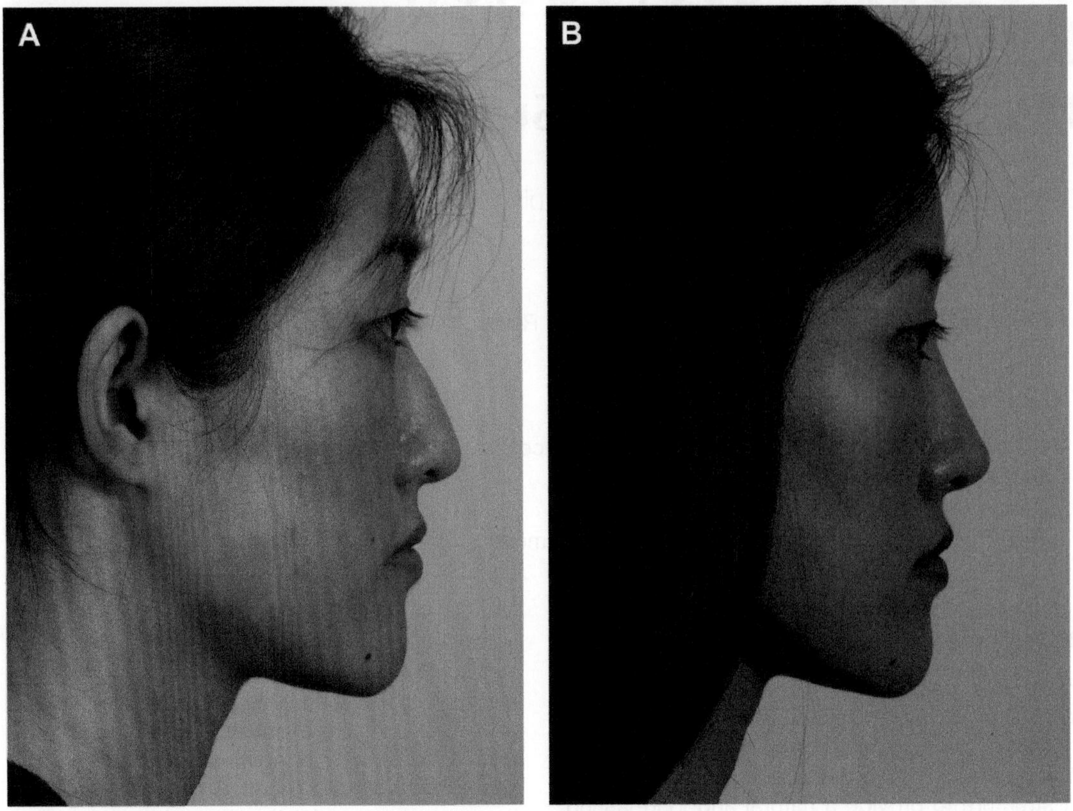

Fig. 1. Asian patient with dorsal convexity, low radix, and underprojected nasal tip. Rather than perform a dorsal hump reduction in this patient, her radix was elevated and her tip projection was increased. This technique allows better narrowing on frontal view and provides a more elegant nasal contour. (*A*) Preoperative lateral view. (*B*) One-year postoperative lateral view.

must be able to reliably increase tip projection. In order to increase projection, it may be necessary to stabilize the nasal base with a caudal septal extension graft.[4] This approach can be helpful in ethic patients who tend to lack good tip support (see **Fig. 1**). In many of these patients, the authors limit hump reduction to the bony cap. This anatomic structure has been described by Daniel and Palhazi.[5] By simply removing the bony cap, there is no need to perform a reconstruction of the bony or cartilaginous middle nasal vault. In some cases, when the bony cap is removed, the horns of the upper lateral cartilages can pop up, leaving a dorsal convexity requiring some minor reduction. In many ethnic patients, the surgery is augmenting the dorsum and not reducing it. By augmenting the dorsum, the upper two-thirds of the nose can be made narrower without manipulating the bony vault with osteotomies.

PATIENT SELECTION

If profile alignment requires reduction of the height of the dorsum, the surgeon can consider dorsal preservation. Ideal patients have a normal radix and smaller, cartilaginous, or V-shaped hump. A V-shaped hump has only 1 curvature, which can be more readily flattened, whereas an S-shaped hump has 2 curvature points and is more difficult to flatten. Patients with a narrow bony and cartilaginous dorsum that is straight and favorable in appearance on frontal view also have favorable characteristics. If the patient can benefit from slight widening of the middle nasal vault or preservation of the existing dorsal aesthetic lines, the authors strongly consider a push-down or let-down technique. Other important parameters include shorter nasal bones, and a primarily cartilaginous dorsal hump. In such patients, we consider removing a subdorsal strip of cartilage to allow the cartilaginous hump to be pushed down and sutured into proper position. We may perform a bony cap removal or some rasping to contour the bone with release of the upper lateral cartilages from the lateral keystone as described by Jankowski and Ferreira.[6,7] This technique avoids the need for a bony push-down, limiting the push-down to the cartilaginous vault and eliminating the need for more extensive osteotomies. Care must be taken to prevent visibility after the bone is removed and recognize if the cartilaginous vault pops up or deforms.

POTENTIAL SEQUELAE

One of the most common complications of the dorsal preservation technique is the radix step, which occurs if a larger strip of bone and cartilage is resected below the radix and the cut below the dorsum is very deep into the ethmoid (**Fig. 2**A). In this case, the entire pyramid can drop excessively, creating a visible step that cannot be hidden by the thicker skin over the radix. This situation occurs if the surgeon tries to use dorsal preservation techniques on noses with a very depressed kyphotic hump, without considering the option of longitudinal stretching of the pyramid. One method to minimize the step-off is to make an oblique transverse osteotomy that allows the bone to slide instead of drop vertically.

When performing a push-down, there are several potential complications that must be considered. One of the most consequential, but rare, complications is a CSF leak. CSF leak can occur when excessive force is applied to the ethmoid bone, which then can disrupt or fracture the cribriform plate, resulting in a skull base defect that can leak CSF.[8] This complication must be avoided at all cost because the consequences, such as intracranial spread of infection, can be life threatening. Surgical repair can be difficult and fraught with its own complications. The problem lies in the transfer of energy to the ethmoid plate and skull base. When performing a push-down or let-down, a subdorsal strip is removed that may extend into the ethmoid bone, creating a subdorsal space (see **Fig. 2**A). It is recommended that a subdorsal stump be left attached to the undersurface of the cartilaginous dorsum for stability purposes (see **Fig. 2**A). The subdorsal stump should be approximately 2 mm to 3 mm in vertical height. If necessary, some vertical cuts are made in the subdorsal stump to allow flexion of the dorsum and allow straightening when the push-down is completed (**Fig. 2**B). In most methods of the push-down, the subdorsal stump is rectangular (see **Fig. 2**). The problem occurs when the cuts are made in the bony dorsum and the nasal bones are pushed down excessively. With the complete release of the bony vault through the lateral and transverse osteotomies, impaction onto the underlying ethmoid bone can result in excessive force on the skull base or if the osteotomy below the dorsum is executed with too much force and the fracture extends superiorly (**Fig. 3**).

ADJUSTMENTS TO MINIMIZE SUBOPTIMAL OUTCOMES

Kovacevic[9] describes a modification of the subdorsal strip and bone cuts to help minimize force on the ethmoid/skull base complex and limit the radix step. His modification involves making a triangular instead of a rectangular subdorsal stump (**Fig. 4**). In this modification, the first step is to perform the left-sided lateral osteotomy. A subperiosteal tunnel is created around the proposed osteotomy site to allow proper mobilization of the nasal bone. In the absence of piezo, a 3-mm straight osteotome can be used to complete the lateral osteotomy. In some cases, a 3-mm bony wedge resection is performed at the site of the lateral osteotomy to allow the bony pyramid to slide down without any resistance (**Fig. 5**). In many patients with smaller dorsal humps, the bony vault moves readily without the 3-mm wedge excision. Then a convex radix saw (Marina

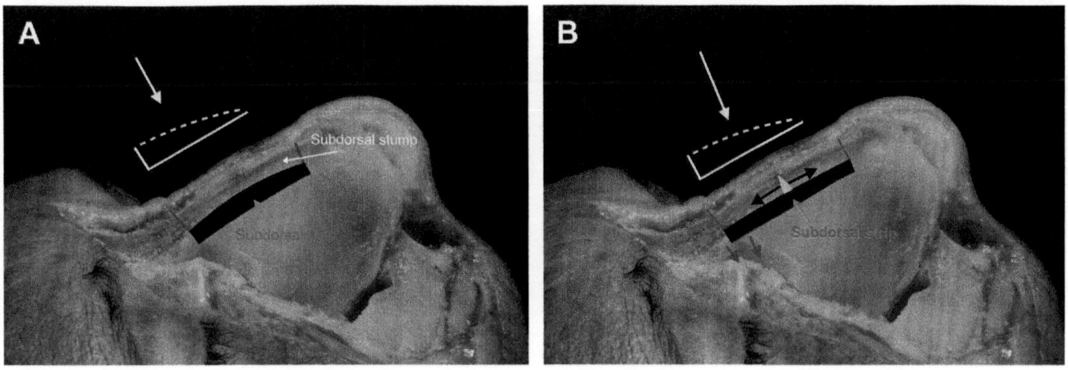

Fig. 2. (*A*) Push-down technique showing subdorsal stump and rectangular subdorsal strip. (*B*) Vertical cut through the subdorsal stump (*pink*) to allow flexion of the dorsal hump. The red arrows show downward movement of upper dorsum and potential pressure on the ethmoid bone.

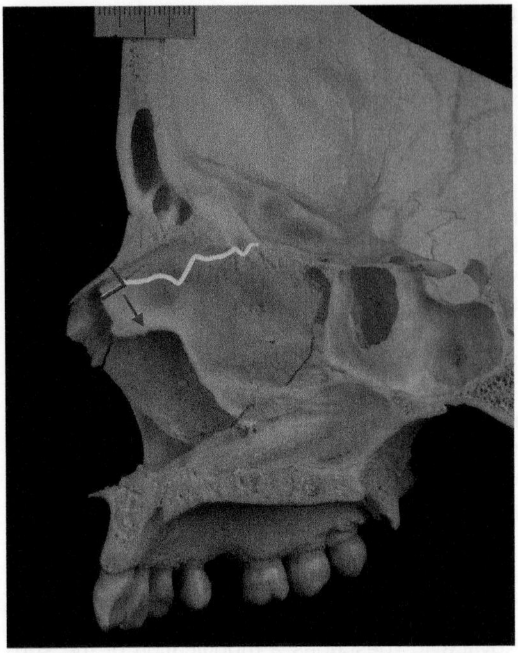

Fig. 3. Pink line shows potential site where fracture could extend to the skull base if excessive force is applied to the ethmoid plate (*arrow*) when the bony dorsum is pushed down. Note extension to skull base in pink.

Medical, Davie, FL) is used to complete the transverse and radix osteotomies (see **Fig. 5**). The transverse osteotomy can also be made using a 2-mm transcutaneous bone cut. This bone cut is made just above the dorsal convexity and extends through the bone and then about 4 mm into the ethmoid bone. If made obliquely, the bone tends to hinge or slide, decreasing the chance of a step-off. The bone cut is extended to the left lateral osteotomy. This cut can be accomplished without dissecting the entire bony dorsum down to the lateral osteotomy. If using piezo, the entire bony dorsum is exposed and the bone cuts are connected under direct visualization. The bone cuts can be made using conventional osteotomes; however, the convex radix saw is helpful to make the transverse and radix osteotomies. The reason for not completing the right lateral osteotomy is to preserve the position of the bony vault until the septal work is completed and to avoid any septal disruption close to the skull base. In addition, extending the radix osteotomy 4 mm into the ethmoid avoids transfer of energy to the subdorsal osteotomy cranially.

Then the septal work is completed. The first step is make the septal incision cut 3.5 mm to 4 mm cephalad to the W area (where the upper lateral cartilages meet the dorsal septum) and about 2.5 to 3 mm deep to the roof of the middle vault. This cartilaginous cut extends to the height of the dorsal hump and close to where the cartilaginous septum meets the ethmoid plate creating a subdorsal triangle (**Fig. 6**). This cut creates a triangular cartilage stump under the roof of the middle vault. The next step is to score the bone directly under the bony hump inferior to the transverse bone cut. This step can be accomplished with a sharp osteotome or knife blade. Then a 3-mm osteotome is used to carefully cut the ethmoid bone directly under the hump and extending to the transverse osteotomy. This step can be completed with gentle force applied through the osteotome. Because the transverse bone cut extends 4 mm through the ethmoid bone, the cut made directly under the bony dorsum is isolated from the cranial segment of ethmoid bone and there is no transfer of force to the skull base (see **Fig. 6**). This bone cut can be made easily and can be visualized with an endoscope, or the mucosa can be dissected from the undersurface of the hump and the subdorsal osteotomy can be performed under direct

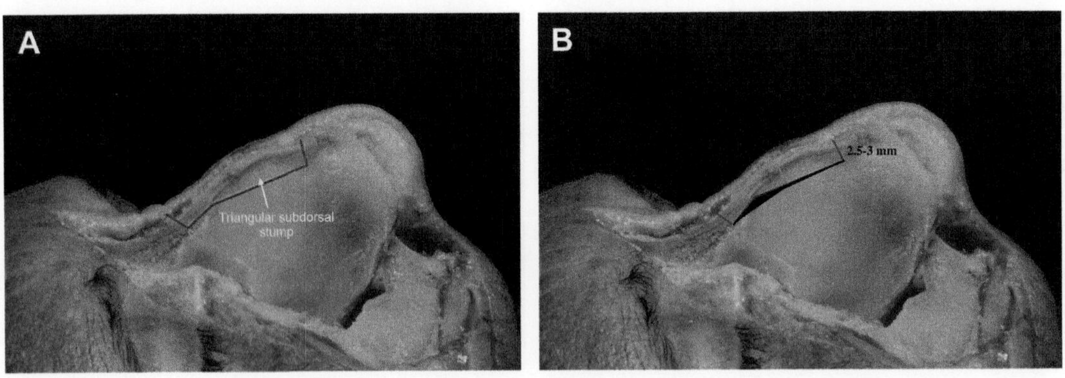

Fig. 4. Kovacevic modification of push-down showing triangular subdorsal stump. (*A*) Septal cartilage and bone cuts. (*B*) Incremental triangular subdorsal strip excision with triangular subdorsal stump. A 2.5-mm to 3-mm subdorsal stump is left near W area and vertical incision (*pink*) to allow flexion of the dorsal convexity.

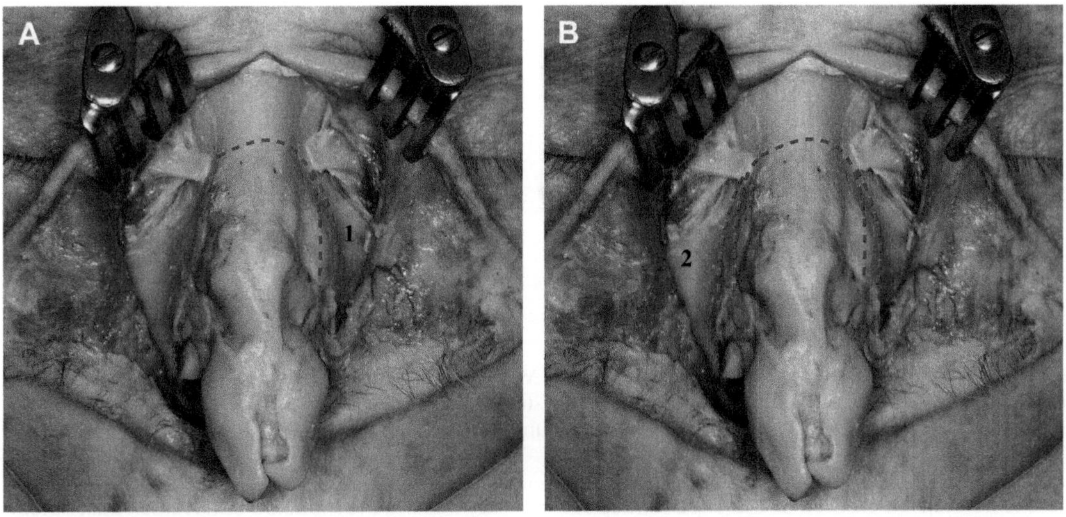

Fig. 5. Bony osteotomies. (*A*) Left lateral osteotomy and transverse/radix osteotomy completed before septal work. (*B*) After septal work completed, the right lateral osteotomy is completed. Also shows bone resection of let-down if executed.

visualization. It may also be possible to gently lift the bony dorsum to gain direct visualization. Once the subdorsal cuts are completed, a small strip (1–2 mm) of ethmoid bone can be resected to provide room for the bony dorsum to be pushed down. A bone scissor, narrow rongeur, or piezo rasp can be used, but this should not be done blindly. Avoid taking out too much bone to avoid excessive lowering of the bony dorsum and creating a radix step.

Another problem that can create deformity is when the subdorsal bony stump lodges on 1 side of the remnant bony septum, resulting in shifting of the bony vault to 1 side. By making the bone cut directly under the bony hump, there is no bony stump that can lodge on 1 side of the remnant ethmoid bone (**Fig. 7**A). In some patients with a deviated ethmoid bone/deviated bony dorsum, it may be helpful to keep a 2-mm to 3-mm bony stump to allow the bony dorsum to lodge on the side opposite the deviation to help straighten the nose (**Fig. 7**B). It is important to preserve a 2.5-mm cartilaginous subdorsal stump caudally close to the W area in the cartilaginous portion of the dorsal hump. If the cuts are made directly under the cartilaginous dorsum, scar contracture can deform the middle vault over time. This point is particularly important in patients with thinner skin.

Once the septal work is completed, the right lateral osteotomy can be performed and a bone wedge can be removed. Then the right lateral osteotomy is connected to the transverse and radix osteotomies, using a radix saw or the piezo. Now that all of the bone cuts are completed, the bony vault in continuity with the cartilaginous vault can be pushed down to reduce the dorsal hump. It may be necessary to make vertical cuts in the cartilaginous subdorsal stump to allow flexing of the dorsal convexity and flattening of the hump. The nasal bones can move medial to or inside the ascending process of the maxilla to allow the dorsum to reduce. The bony vault is essentially hinged at the cranial extent of the hump where the transverse osteotomy was made and the bony dorsum can pivot around this point (**Fig. 8**). The pivot point is located close to the radix. The hinge is created because of the orientation of the subdorsal triangle and the oblique transverse osteotomy. Because the hinge is located cranially,

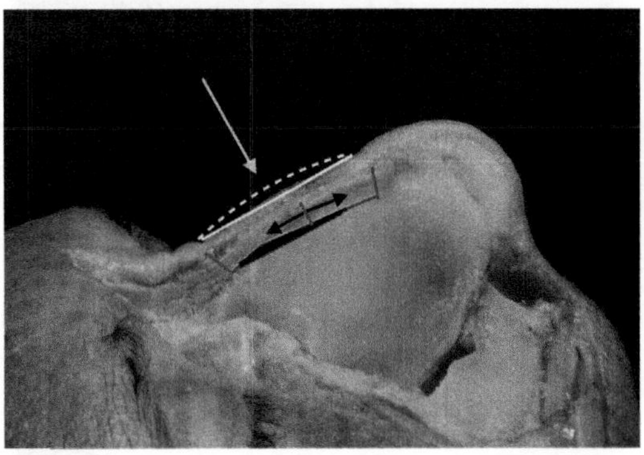

Fig. 6. Modified push-down showing subdorsal excision to accommodate inferior movement of the nasal dorsum with greatest movement at point of maximal dorsal convexity.

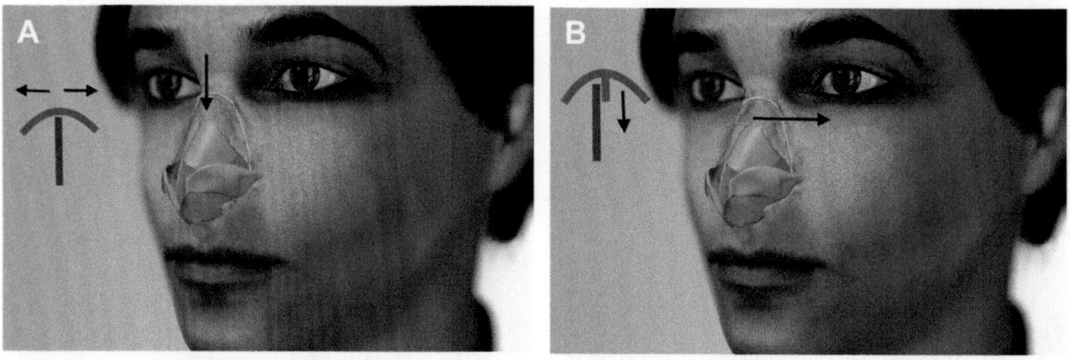

Fig. 7. Ethmoid bone alignment under bony hump. (*A*) With straight bony dorsum, ethmoid cut made directly below the bony hump to allow alignment in the midline. (*B*) With deviated ethmoid bone/deviated bony dorsum, a subdorsal bony stump is left to allow situating the stump on opposite side of the ethmoid bone deviation.

there is no step-off created at the superior aspect of the hump reduction. A large bony step-off can be problematic with the dorsal preservation techniques because the bony dorsum can move inferiorly and create an infantile-appearing dorsum. If a larger dorsal convexity is treated, there is the possibility that a step-off will form. If a radix step-off does form, a rasp or piezo can be used to smooth out the defect.

The final step is to suture fixate the lowered dorsum into proper position. The authors prefer to place 2 to 3 PDS sutures to fixate. The sutures are placed from the dorsal septal segment of the L strut to the upper lateral cartilages. The sutures can be placed in many different ways but should not be tied too tightly to avoid distorting the middle vault. A suture can be placed through the bony vault as well to fixate. Some surgeons place a lateral suture from the bony sidewalls to the ascending process of the maxilla.[3,10]

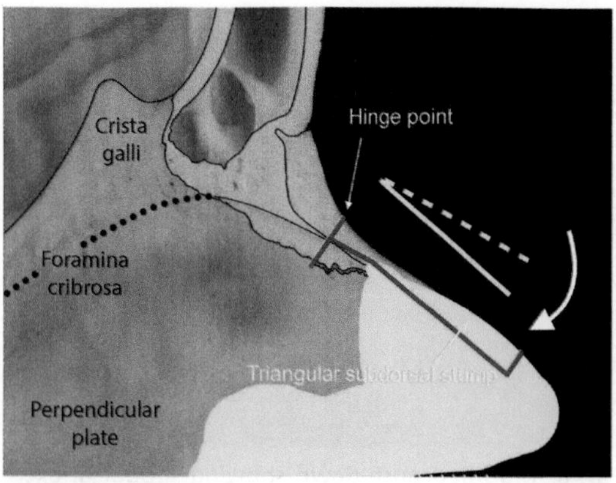

Fig. 8. Modified push-down showing triangular subdorsal stump and cranially positioned hinge point with minimal step-off.

By making the modified transverse/radix osteotomy (4 mm into the ethmoid), a safety zone is created to isolate the bony pyramid and the ethmoid bone that is still attached to the skull base. With this safety zone, there is a buffer that acts to protect the ethmoid bone as it meets the skull base to mitigate the possibility of CSF leak. This cautious approach to dorsal preservation is helpful to prevent unnecessary complications. These precautions are particularly important for surgeons that are starting to perform dorsal preservation and do not have access to piezo. The maneuvers are far from conventional and extend beyond the boundaries of conventional osteotomies.

Kovacevic[9] prefers the let-down, removing a strip of bone along the ascending process of the maxilla. He believes this decreases the likelihood of recurrence of the dorsal hump because a lateral bony space is created to allow the bony vault to shift into proper position. The let-down requires more involved bone cuts and is much easier to perform with wider dissection and use of piezo.

MODIFICATION TO THE CLASSIC COTTLE TECHNIQUE

The classic Cottle technique incorporates a reverse Z cut made through the whole vertical axis of cartilaginous septum.[11] In patients with a larger dorsal hump, a longitudinal stretching of the dorsum can be helpful, which is the inherent component of the classic Cottle technique. In this technique, a reverse Z cut is completed through the vertical axis of the cartilaginous septum. Then a cartilage/bone strip is removed just below the dorsum and an inferior partial-length strip of septum is removed to lower the dorsum (**Fig. 9**). The septum is then pulled/rotated forward and fixed with one 5-0 PDS suture to the

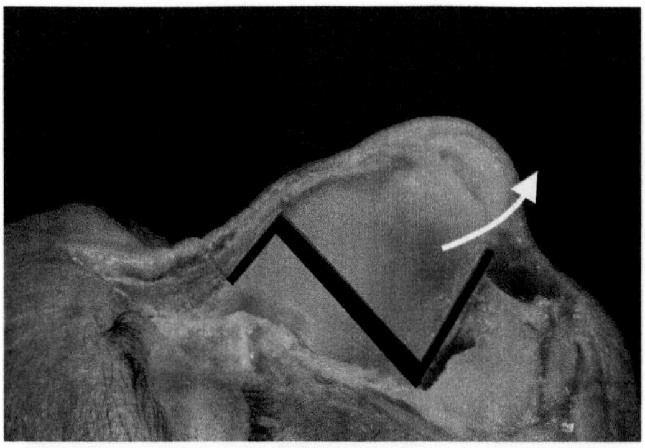

Fig. 9. The classic Cottle technique incorporating a reverse Z cut made through the whole vertical axis of cartilaginous septum. White arrow shows rotation of the cartilage segment.

nasal spine (see **Fig. 9**). Several problems can occur with this technique. A saddle-nose deformity can occur if the fixation to the anterior nasal spine fails. In addition, there is a limited amount of septal cartilage grafting material that is available with this technique.

Various modifications of the Cottle method exist. A modification by Kovacevic[9] of the classic Cottle technique that overcomes these issues involves the same reverse Z cut but at a higher, more anterior level. The first part of the Z cut goes vertically from the highest point of the hump and extends to the point in the septum that accommodates the size of the planned hump reduction (**Fig. 10**A), which can be up to 5 mm in height. The next cut connects the W area, creating a triangular subdorsal stump (**Fig. 10**B). The posterior cut connects the transverse osteotomy with the previous vertical cut. Then, a triangular strip of cartilage and bone is removed depending on the desired amount of dorsal reduction (**Fig. 10**C). In addition, the septum is pulled caudally (stretched) in a longitudinal fashion and either sutured end to end with two 5-0 PDS sutures or the segments can be overlapped as much as needed and then sutured (**Fig. 10**D). The overlapping method is a better option if there is a septal deviation because this can act to straighten the dorsal septum and align the nose. From the external skin surface, a needle is placed through the overlapped septum after the desired dorsal height is attained. Two to three 5-0 PDS sutures are placed to fixate the repair in position and to help prevent recurrence of the hump.[10] Release of the lateral keystone area allows flattening of the dorsum. If necessary, the bony cap can be rasped to attain proper dorsal alignment and prevent a residual dorsal convexity.

The advantages of this modification of the classic Cottle technique include having more septal cartilage for potential grafting and also greater stability of the dorsum to help mitigate against saddling of the dorsum (**Fig. 10**E). The side-to-side dorsal overlap also provides increased stability to the reduction and helps to minimize the likelihood of recurrence of the dorsal hump.

Saddling of the nasal dorsum is also a potential complication that can occur after performing the push-down, let-down, or classic Cottle technique. This complication can occur for several reasons. If too large a subdorsal strip is removed, this can result in a saddle-nose deformity. This complication can be prevented by removing only small increments a couple of millimeters at a time. Another possibility is the disruption of the keystone, which is always a possibility whenever manipulating the bony and cartilaginous septum. With the classic Cottle technique, saddling can occur because of the extensive release of the cartilaginous septum from the bony septum and loss of fixation at the anterior nasal spine. The modifications offered in this article can help to mitigate saddling.

WHEN TO CONSIDER CONVENTIONAL METHODS

There are occasions when dorsal preservation is not an option or is less ideal. These occasions include the wide dorsum, S-shaped dorsal hump, low radix, and severely deviated dorsum with underlying septal deformity. In these cases, it may be more appropriate to open the middle vault and perform a conventional dorsal hump reduction. The advantage to opening the bony and cartilaginous vaults is that parameters such as width and contour can be precisely controlled. This method does require more time, effort, and cartilage to complete the reconstructions. In addition, in patients with thin skin, it may be necessary to drape temporalis fascia or costal perichondrium over the dorsum. In patients with damaged, atrophic dorsal nasal skin, surgeons can use temporalis fascia or costal perichondrium infused with microfat or nanofat to camouflage the dorsum and help to recover the skin.[4] Diced fat with platelet-rich plasma is another option for camouflage.[12] There are many different methods of reconstruction to control contour and anatomy, and the intended goals dictate the method used.

One of the primary advantages of performing a reconstruction with spreader grafts and spreader flaps is the ability to stiffen and strengthen the sidewalls of the middle vault. In some patients,

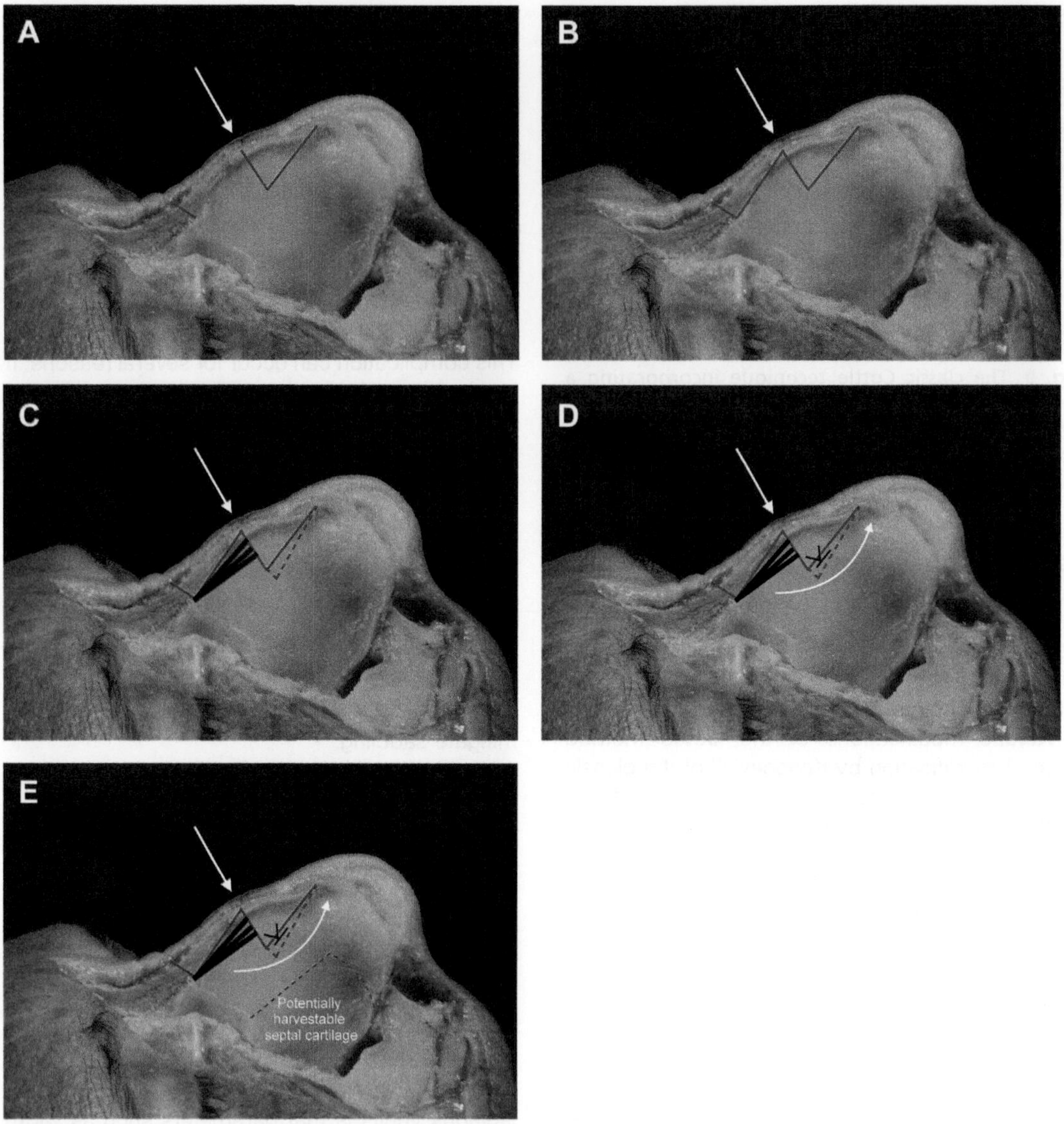

Fig. 10. Modified subdorsal Cottle technique. (*A*) Z cut (up to 5 mm) goes vertically from the highest point of the hump and extends to the point in the septum that accommodates the size of the planned hump reduction. (*B*) Septal cut connecting W area creating a subdorsal triangular stump. (*C*) Triangular strip of cartilage and bone removed depending on the desired amount of dorsal reduction. (*D*) Septum is pulled caudally in a longitudinal fashion and sutured with two 5-0 PDS sutures end to end or overlapped. (*E*) Larger potential area to harvest septal cartilage for grafting purposes.

the upper lateral cartilages are weak and can collapse medially on inspiration. By placing the upper lateral cartilages on tension by inserting spreader grafts and possibly spreader flaps, the sidewalls can be significantly stiffened. This tensioning effect acts to stiffen the sidewall, decrease collapse, and provide an improvement in nasal breathing.[4]

If the upper lateral cartilages are sutured over spreader grafts, the upper laterals can be placed on tension and stiffened, as shown in **Fig. 11**.[4] This effect can provide significant increases in nasal function in zone 1 of the lateral wall.[4,13] The width of the middle nasal vault and the effect on the upper lateral cartilage can be controlled by the thickness of the spreader graft and by how tight the upper lateral cartilages are sutured over the spreader grafts. The bulk under the junction between the dorsal septum and upper lateral cartilage acts to cantilever the upper lateral, stiffen the sidewall, and support the airway. This technique creates a stronger sidewall that helps

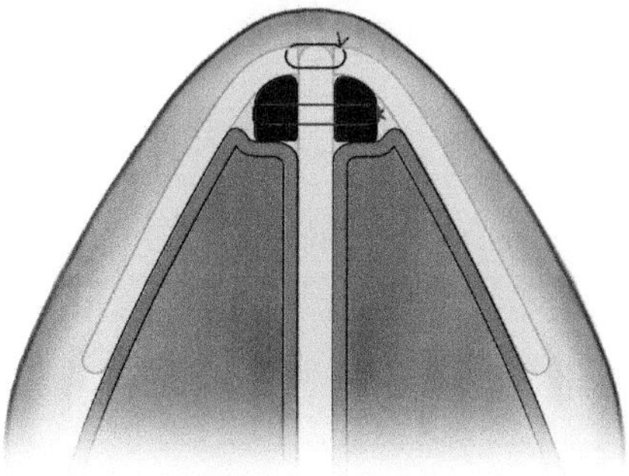

Fig. 11. The upper lateral cartilages can be sutured over the top of spreader grafts that are set back a millimeter or 2 below the leading edge of the dorsal septum to promote outward curvature of the upper lateral cartilages.

prevent medialization on inspiration. With the push-down, the opposite effect may occur, where the upper lateral cartilage is made susceptible to collapse on inspiration because it is less taught. Patients with weaker sidewalls can be identified by watching their sidewalls while they breathe in. If there is weakness, the upper lateral cartilage may move medially on inspiration and the patient may complain of airway obstruction or difficulty breathing through the nose. In patients with stronger upper lateral cartilages, the opposite effect may occur, where the upper laterals can bow outward, creating increased width and potentially improving the airway.

In secondary rhinoplasty, preservation techniques are typically not applicable because most of these patients require some degree of reconstruction of the middle vault and potentially the bony vault as well. If there is collapse or medialization of one of the nasal bones, the nasal bone on the concave side may need to be out-fractured, which is accomplished using the midline vertical osteotomy and then cantilevering the bone out. Lateralization of the nasal bone can also be accomplished by placing a Boise elevator and out-fracturing the nasal bone. A long, thick spreader graft is typically used to hold the nasal bone in a lateralized position. This type of graft typically requires the use of costal cartilage spreader grafts that may be 3 mm thick and more than 40 mm long if they extend beyond the caudal septum. It is usual to place some soft tissue over the extended spreader graft to fill any depressions.

Reconstructing the middle nasal vault in secondary rhinoplasty may require placement of spreader grafts for cosmetic and functional goals. Typically, these grafts are longer and thicker and are usually made of costal cartilage. Excessive widening of the middle vault can be avoided by placing the spreader grafts a millimeter to two below the dorsal margin of the septum and allowing the upper lateral cartilages to arch over the spreader grafts. This arching effect of the upper lateral cartilages creates a narrower-appearing middle vault but provides maximal functional effect by supporting the sidewall.

Some surgeons performing preservation rhinoplasty use tensioning of the lateral crura with articulated rim grafts to manage the nasal tip.[14] Çakir and colleagues[15] use auto rim grafts to support the alar margin. This technique works well in primary rhinoplasty patients. In most secondary rhinoplasty patients, tensioning is not indicated and many of these patients require reconstruction of the tip cartilages. In many secondary rhinoplasty patients, it is necessary to perform lateral crural release, amputation at the level of the medial crura, and placement of lateral crural replacement grafts with lateral crural strut grafts. This approach provides a reliable nasal tip reconstruction that is stable with good control over the lateral wall, nasal valve, alar margin and tip contour.[4] This technique is more complex and requires great attention to detail but is a very effective means of managing the structurally depleted nasal tip.[4]

OVERVIEW

Preservation rhinoplasty techniques are becoming very popular and many surgeons are adopting the methods. As with any technique, there are indications that allow the best outcomes when using these methods. The push-down technique works well in select patients that fit specific criteria: patients with a straight narrow nose, normal radix, and a straight overprojected dorsum; patients with a V-shaped hump; and patients with shorter nasal bones and a hump that is limited to the cartilaginous vault (**Figs. 12** and **13**). In patients with a kyphotic hump, dorsal preservation techniques that create longitudinal stretching of the dorsum are more effective.

It is important for rhinoplasty surgeons to learn how to perform the conventional bony techniques that are necessary in some rhinoplasty patients. Versatile rhinoplasty surgeons are able to manage a multitude of rhinoplasty deformities and problems. If a surgeon is unfamiliar with or is uncomfortable performing osteotomies and hump reduction, this could limit that surgeon's ability to manage the severely deviated nose, wide broad nose, patients with a low radix and S-shaped dorsal hump, and secondary procedures requiring osseous work. By using preservation techniques in appropriate candidates, the likelihood of

A

B

C

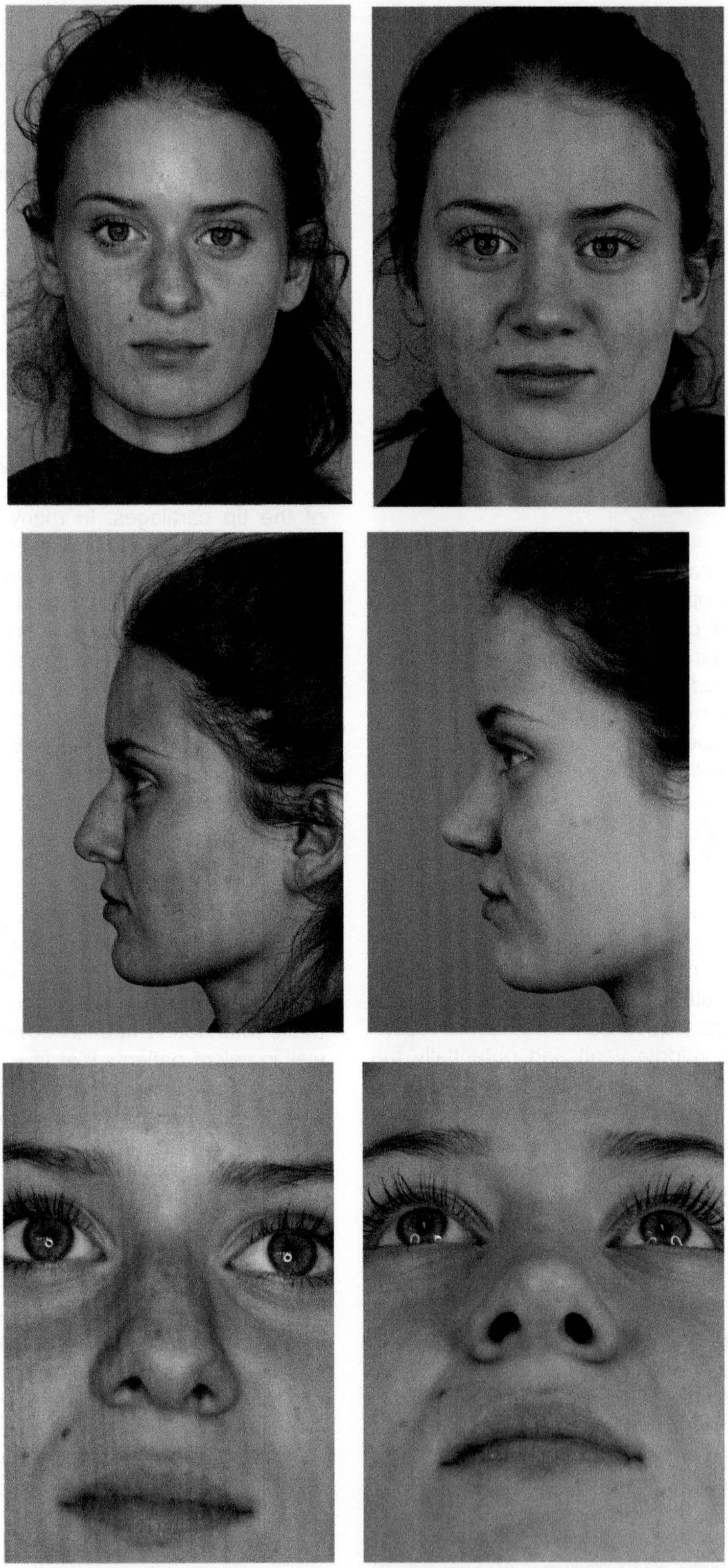

Fig. 12. This patient underwent an open approach with let-down, subdorsal triangular resection with hinge maneuver, bone sculpting with piezo, septal relocation to the right, overlapping septal extension graft on the right side, cephalic trim of LLC, cranial tip suture and articulated rim grafts. (*A*) Preoperative frontal view (*left*). One-year postoperative frontal view (*right*). (*B*) Preoperative lateral view (*left*). Postoperative lateral view (*right*). (*C*) Preoperative base view (*left*). Postoperative base view (*right*).

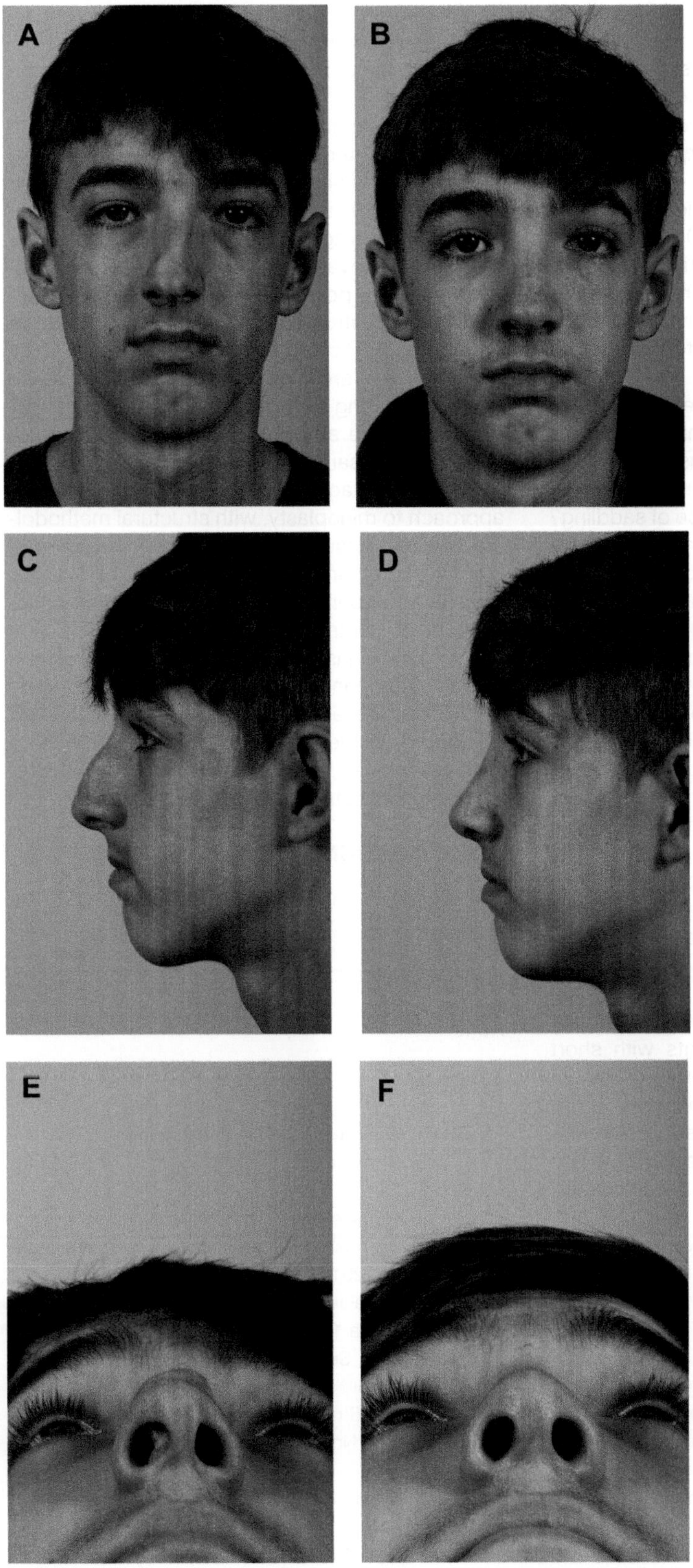

Fig. 13. Patient underwent a let-down, subdorsal Cottle with septal relocation to the left, resection of deviated portion of the caudal septum, caudal septal extension graft and medial crural footplate suture. The tip was treated with lateral crural strut grafts and obliquely oriented dome sutures. A. Preoperative frontal view (left). Four month postoperative frontal view (right). B. Preoperative lateral view (left). Postoperative lateral view (right). C. Preoperative base view (left). Postoperative base view (right).

success will be higher. The natural progression of rhinoplasty surgeons is to take on more complex cases including secondary rhinoplasty as the surgeon's practice matures. This progression requires the surgeons to have a broad armamentarium of surgical techniques available to them.

Even more important is that surgeons must be able to manage their own failures. Once preservation techniques have failed, conventional methods with opening the middle vault and grafting may be necessary to correct the problems at hand. Versatile rhinoplasty surgeons are able to correct any problems they have created.

There remain some unanswered questions. Could the dorsal preservation techniques create instability of the bony or cartilaginous vault? Could trauma to the push-down patient result in more complex injuries or a higher incidence of saddling? Could blunt trauma act to push the nasal structure into the face with loss of projection? Along the same lines, will secondary rhinoplasty performed on a patient who underwent previous preservation techniques present a new set of potential problems, such as loss of dorsal projection, saddling, or irregular bony movement? If septal cartilage is excised for the purpose of cartilage grafting and a subdorsal strip is excised, will this potentially weaken the dorsal strut and make it more susceptible to disruption of the keystone and subsequent dorsal collapse?

Of utmost importance are the long-term consequences of the preservation techniques. How will the push-down technique affect the upper lateral cartilages over time? Will they become less stiff and potentially become more flaccid and deform or medialize over time? This process may be more likely in patients with short nasal bones and long upper lateral cartilages. If the upper lateral cartilages become more flaccid, will they tend to collapse under the forces of negative inspiratory pressure? I am confident that these questions will be answered over time.

With respect to preservation of the Pitanguy ligament and the scroll ligaments, if the nose is lengthened, counterrotated, or has dramatic changes in tip projection, will these ligaments still align properly? For example, if a short nose is lengthened using a caudal septal extension graft, the Pitanguy ligament as it is attached to the skin will be shifted more cranially in relation to the attachments to the cartilages that have been moved caudally. If cephalically positioned lateral crura are repositioned caudally, will the scroll ligament be moved out of alignment as well? In addition, the Pitanguy ligament and the scroll ligaments may have been previously divided in most secondary cases and cannot be realigned.

The use of subperichondrial dissection is also a potential benefit.[16] Our early experience with subperiosteal dissection for open rhinoplasty has not shown long-term benefit. Subperichondrial dissection may change surface tension and could alter cartilage elasticity and strength. The question is how the cartilage will react under potential contractile forces over time. Will there be less contraction or is there potential for deformity over time?

In the end, structure rhinoplasty and preservation rhinoplasty can coexist because the underlying principles are similar: to preserve structure for the best long-term outcome. In the ideal scenario, structure and preservation methods could be used in the same patient where deemed necessary or advantageous. This use of a systematic approach to rhinoplasty, with structural methodology, allows preservation of the good features of the nasal dorsum and middle vault as well as providing the benefits of structural grafting in the nasal tip to control tip position and tip projection and maximize nasal function. Many of the best rhinoplasty surgeons see the benefit of this merging of philosophies and are working to move forward in tandem. In the end, surgeons should all learn both techniques to become well-rounded, versatile rhinoplasty surgeons.

ACKNOWLEDGMENTS

The cadaver images were provided by Peter Palhazi.

DISCLOSURES

None.

REFERENCES

1. Daniel RK. The preservation rhinoplasty: a new rhinoplasty revolution. Aesthet Surg J 2018;38(2):228–9.
2. Saban Y, Daniel RK, Polselli R, et al. Dorsal preservation: the push down technique reassessed. Aesthet Surg J 2018;38(2):117–31.
3. Kosins A, Daniel R. Decision making in preservation rhinoplasty: a 100 case series with one-year follow-up. Aesthet Surg J 2019. https://doi.org/10.1093/asj/sjz107. pii: sjz107.
4. Toriumi DM. Structure rhinoplasty: lessons learned in thirty years. North Salt Lake (UT): DMT publishing; 2019.
5. Daniel RK, Palhazi P. Rhinoplasty: an anatomical and clinical atlas. New York (NY): Springer; 2018.
6. Boulanger N, Baumann C, Beurton R, et al. Septorhinoplasty by disarticulation: early assessment of a

new technique for morphological correction of crooked noses. Rhinology 2013;51(1):77–87.
7. Ferreira MG, Monteiro D, Reis C, et al. Spare roof technique: a middle third new technique. Facial Plast Surg 2016;32:111–6.
8. Youssef A, Ahmed S, Ibrahim AA, et al. Traumatic cerebrospinal fluid leakage following septorhinoplasty. Arch Plast Surg 2018;45(4):379–83.
9. Kovacevic, M. Refinements in Dorsal Preservation, Preservation Rhinoplasty, Third Edition, R. Daniel, P. Palhazi, Y. Saban, B. Cakir. ISBN 978-605-68971-1-1-5, Septum Publisher.
10. Ishida J, Ishida LC, Ishida LH, et al. Treatment of the nasal hump with preservation of the cartilaginous framework. Plast Reconstr Surg 1999;103(6): 1729–33 [discussion: 1734-5].
11. Cottle MH, Loring RM. Corrective surgery of the external nasal pyramid and the nasal septum for restoration of normal physiology. Ill Med J 1946;90: 119–35.
12. Kovacevic M, Riedel F, Goksel A, et al. Options for middle vault and dorsum restoration after hump removal in primary rhinoplasty. Facial Plast Surg 2016;32:374–83.
13. Vaezeafshar R, Moubayed SP, Most SP. Repair of lateral wall insufficiency. JAMA Facial Plast Surg 2018;20(2):111–5.
14. Davis R. Lateral crural tensioning for refinement of the wide and underprojected nasal tip rethinking the lateral crural steal. Facial Plast Surg Clin North Am 2015;23(1):23–53.
15. Çakır B, lu Ö, Ali R, et al. Surface aesthetics in tip rhinoplasty: a step-by-step guide. Aesthet Surg J 2014;34(6):941–55.
16. Cakir B, Oreroğlu AR, Doğan T, et al. A complete subperichondrial dissection technique for rhinoplasty with management of the nasal ligaments. Aesthet Surg J 2012;32(5):564–74.

Printed and bound by CPI Group (UK) Ltd, Croydon, CR0 4YY
08/05/2025
01864692-0010